A COLOR HANDBOOK

OTOLARYNGOLOGY

A COLOR HANDBOOK

OTOLARYNGOLOGY

Edited by

Laura H. Swibel Rosenthal
Loyola University Chicago Stritch School of Medicine
Maywood, Illinois

Monica O. Patadia
Loyola University Chicago Stritch School of Medicine
Maywood, Illinois

James A. Stankiewicz
Loyola University Chicago Stritch School of Medicine
Maywood, Illinois

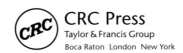

CRC Press
Taylor & Francis Group
Boca Raton London New York

CRC Press is an imprint of the
Taylor & Francis Group, an **informa** business

CRC Press
Taylor & Francis Group
6000 Broken Sound Parkway NW, Suite 300
Boca Raton, FL 33487-2742

© 2017 by Taylor & Francis Group, LLC
CRC Press is an imprint of Taylor & Francis Group, an Informa business

No claim to original U.S. Government works

Printed and bound in India by Replika Press Pvt. Ltd.

Printed on acid-free paper
Version Date: 20160523

International Standard Book Number-13: 978-1-4822-5376-4 (Paperback)

This book contains information obtained from authentic and highly regarded sources. While all reasonable efforts have been made to publish reliable data and information, neither the author[s] nor the publisher can accept any legal responsibility or liability for any errors or omissions that may be made. The publishers wish to make clear that any views or opinions expressed in this book by individual editors, authors or contributors are personal to them and do not necessarily reflect the views/opinions of the publishers. The information or guidance contained in this book is intended for use by medical, scientific or health-care professionals and is provided strictly as a supplement to the medical or other professional's own judgement, their knowledge of the patient's medical history, relevant manufacturer's instructions and the appropriate best practice guidelines. Because of the rapid advances in medical science, any information or advice on dosages, procedures or diagnoses should be independently verified. The reader is strongly urged to consult the relevant national drug formulary and the drug companies' and device or material manufacturers' printed instructions, and their websites, before administering or utilizing any of the drugs, devices or materials mentioned in this book. This book does not indicate whether a particular treatment is appropriate or suitable for a particular individual. Ultimately it is the sole responsibility of the medical professional to make his or her own professional judgements, so as to advise and treat patients appropriately. The authors and publishers have also attempted to trace the copyright holders of all material reproduced in this publication and apologize to copyright holders if permission to publish in this form has not been obtained. If any copyright material has not been acknowledged please write and let us know so we may rectify in any future reprint.

Except as permitted under U.S. Copyright Law, no part of this book may be reprinted, reproduced, transmitted, or utilized in any form by any electronic, mechanical, or other means, now known or hereafter invented, including photocopying, microfilming, and recording, or in any information storage or retrieval system, without written permission from the publishers.

For permission to photocopy or use material electronically from this work, please access www.copyright.com (http://www.copyright.com/) or contact the Copyright Clearance Center, Inc. (CCC), 222 Rosewood Drive, Danvers, MA 01923, 978-750-8400. CCC is a not-for-profit organization that provides licenses and registration for a variety of users. For organizations that have been granted a photocopy license by the CCC, a separate system of payment has been arranged.

Trademark Notice: Product or corporate names may be trademarks or registered trademarks, and are used only for identification and explanation without intent to infringe.

Visit the Taylor & Francis Web site at
http://www.taylorandfrancis.com

and the CRC Press Web site at
http://www.crcpress.com

Contents

Introduction

Laura H. Swibel Rosenthal

A handbook may be used in many ways. It can be particularly useful as a reference tool to learn about a topic of interest. When a handbook contains many images, it can be browsed as a picture book, or it can be read cover to cover like a textbook. A color handbook specifically in otolaryngology can serve in all of these manners. It is expected that most readers will use it in a combination of ways. However, there are many reasons why the subject of otolaryngology makes a very unique type of handbook.

This handbook is partly a reference tool to aid the reader in diagnosis after the examination of a patient, but it can be challenging to encompass the breadth of a surgical field with photos of the disease alone. While photographs from a clinical examination as well as radiographs can partly depict a disease state, to fully encompass the field of otolaryngology, it was important to the editors that surgical management be understood as well. For many chapters, we have therefore attempted to capture this by deviating from a simple format of a photograph associated with a written outline of the disease. Instead, surgical techniques are demonstrated in many sections.

Furthermore, when thinking about the field of head and neck surgery, much of the pathology in the head and neck is buried in bone, beneath the skin or facial bones, deep in the pharynx, or within the complex skull base. Images in this color handbook, therefore, include not only traditional photographs and images from computed tomography or magnetic resonance imaging but also images from rigid or flexible endoscopy, which has become a quintessential tool not only for medical management of otolaryngology but also for teaching. Other miscellaneous tests or diagrams are frequently utilized in the chapters for their unique contributions to diagnosis and management.

While the study of otolaryngology can seem quite narrow to a primary care provider or medical student, for whom the editors hope this book is useful, the field is actually quite broad. The subspecialties, being primarily head and neck surgery, rhinology, skull base surgery, laryngology, neuro-otology, and facial plastic surgery, each lend themselves to a different ratio of focus on diagnosis by physical examination, diagnosis by endoscopy, workup and ancillary studies, medical management, surgical technique, and epidemiology. Some chapters will be more geared toward diagnosis and some will be more oriented toward surgical planning. Inconsistencies in the amount of photographs versus surgical technique between chapters are purposeful and meant to enhance the reader's learning experience.

Otolaryngology is studied by a variety of practitioners. It is the editors' choice to make this text useful not only for experienced otolaryngologists but also for primary care and family practitioners, surgical and nonsurgical residents, medical students, nurses, physician assistants, nurse practitioners, and anyone else carrying an interest in this field. While textbooks will always lag behind journals, experienced otolaryngologists will find both the traditional and contemporary otolaryngology in this handbook a useful confirmation of what they know or a tool for maintaining certification in areas that are beyond their expertise. For the medical student, the basics of otolaryngology are included and further detail helps to build a better understanding of the pathophysiology and treatment.

There are many tools used in a good head and neck examination that are not routinely used to capture photographs. For example, the ear exam requires an otoscope. The nasal examination requires a good light and a nasal speculum. The oral exam often requires a headlight and two free hands. The laryngeal examination requires a head mirror. Instead of photographs taken in conjunction with any of these tools, these images are typically captured with an endoscope or microscope. An endoscope is often needed for a complete nasal and sinus examination and pharyngeal or laryngeal examination but is also used in many cases for teaching purposes or capturing images. This should not deter the primary care provider from using this handbook. The main purpose of this book is to help the busy practitioner develop a differential diagnosis for the problems they encounter in the office, be it inpatient, outpatient, or acute care setting. It could also be useful for a primary care provider hoping to better understand the endoscopy examination performed by their otolaryngology consultants.

The scope of this book is broad enough to serve as a reference handbook for a variety of practitioners, but it is not inclusive of the entire field of otolaryngology. There are some areas within otolaryngology that are not conducive to this type of image-based reference learning. For example, the growing field of sleep medicine may seem lacking in this text, although it overlaps with areas such as tonsil hypertrophy.

While a handbook cannot replace clinical or surgical training, our hope is that this book will serve as a supplement to the clinical encounter and will help guide the critical steps of history taking, physical examination, and management. In many cases, it may serve as a limited surgical atlas as well. The objectives in this book vary somewhat by section, as per the following descriptions; however, they will generally include some normal anatomy followed by pathologies and/or surgical treatments. Each topic will generally include a definition and clinical features, differential diagnosis, suggestions for workup, and treatment. Treatment sections vary from minimal medical treatment options to extensive surgical descriptions. Providers from many fields may diagnose and/or treat head and neck diseases, but it is the skilled examiner, endoscopist, thinker, and surgeon that make the field of otolaryngology what it is. We hope that that is reflected in these pages.

Head and Neck

The head and neck section is arguably one of the most important areas in the study of otolaryngology. Resident rotations on an otolaryngology service are often divided in a similar manner as in the sections of this book, and it is often on the *head and neck* rotation that students learn the complex and fascinating anatomy of the head and neck and some of the worst pathology of the head and neck, such as malignant disease. This section explores the common pathologies of head and neck and surgical management and the management of complications.

Rhinology

When a rhinologist examines the nose, whether in the office, by computed tomography, or by endoscopy in the operating room, it is often with a different perspective than other providers. The rhinologist is able to navigate the "labyrinth" of the nose and sinuses from the easily visible mucosa to the depths of the sphenoid sinus and treat patients with both medical and surgical problems. This section is amenable to a classic photograph with a description of a disease and to an in-depth look at surgical techniques. Advances in endoscopy and digital imaging have greatly facilitated teaching rhinology and make this section robust.

Laryngology

In some subspecialties, such as laryngology, which is remarkably visual, a photograph can be helpful but cannot replace the active examination of the moving (or immobile) vocal folds nor can it replace the acoustic assessment of a patient's dysphonia. Nevertheless, a color handbook is a great way to teach laryngeal pathology. Digital laryngoscopy photographs are relatively easily captured. The addition of videostroboscopy to the physical examination is an invaluable tool for the subspecialist, student, and patient. A color handbook is an ideal way to showcase pathology and to teach laryngeal findings from examination. This book provides unique insights into surgical technique as well.

Otology and Neurotology

In otolaryngology, the physical examination is one of the most interesting aspects of the practice because it is so visually detailed and requires a well-trained, critical eye and often special instruments. This is especially true within the field of neuro-otology in which a novice and trained specialist may notice different findings on exam. The otoscope is one of the first tools that medical students are eager to obtain and learn to use; however, the beginner student examines the ear in a much different way from the neuro-otologist. When learning how to do an ear examination, adequately assessing the ear canal and tympanic membrane is the primary goal. However, the trained otologist is able to see beyond the tympanic membrane to identify nuances in the middle ear, from ossicular erosions to malignancy. The subspecialist may be adept at a cranial nerve examination or using a tuning fork and be able to identify inner ear disease on examination; however, the inner ear can often be difficult to assess by examination alone. The examination can be incredibly important or entirely unrevealing even in the presence of devastating disease. In the field of otology/neuro-otology, images of a patient may be helpful, but the audiogram, CT scan, or MRI can give the provider invaluable information. Otopathology is often located deep within the temporal bone, which is a challenging area for both the medical student and general otolaryngologist, and surgical management is difficult to capture intraoperatively as these images are often obtained after mastoidectomy or a skull base approach. These attributes make this section particularly challenging and interesting.

Facial Plastics

The subject of facial plastic surgery is important within the field of otolaryngology. It is extremely visual, which is excellent for a color handbook. However, it is not always conducive to the *differential* and *workup sections*. Also, treatment is primarily surgical. Subtitles vary purposefully by section to more appropriately address the unique issues in these subsections.

Pediatrics

A textbook on otolaryngology would not be complete without including a section on pediatric patients. Many primary care visits for children are related to ear, nose, and throat issues. Many general otolaryngology patients are children. Furthermore, many problems that are considered pediatric are common in adults as well, such as otitis media and tonsillitis. The pediatric subsections in this book reflect those of the adult sections but include problems that are more frequently diagnosed in childhood, whether congenital or acquired. Frequently, knowledge in a particular area can be supplemented with another chapter. For example, Chapter 26, on sinonasal disease, and Chapters 8 and 9 in the Rhinology section, are complementary. However, it is important to understand some key differences in children. The approach and differential may vary based on the patient's age. For example, the differential for a neck mass in a child is typically different than that of an adult. The surgical management for nasal obstruction in a child is usually different than that of an adult. At times, additional considerations in the workup may vary based on the patient's age, level of development, and level of cooperation. When children have multiple problems, it is important, of course, to consider systemic and syndromic causes of disease. Some syndromes commonly seen in an otolaryngology practice are discussed. This section is not comprehensive of the entire spectrum of congenital problems seen in a pediatric otolaryngology practice but encompasses the medical principles and surgical skills needed to diagnose and treat most problems.

Acknowledgments and Dedications

Thank you to all the authors for sharing your knowledge and wonderful photos with us. Thank you for your time and patience. Special thanks to Dr. Zdanski for sharing photos for several pediatric chapters and Dr. Gardner for sharing so much of his amazing library of laryngology photos. Thanks to Dr. Rose and Dr. Drake for their mentorship.

I would also like to thank my parents, who had helped me edit papers throughout my education—from elementary school through residency up until I wrote about the histopathology of radiofrequency ablation—and they said they did not think they could help me anymore.

Laura Rosenthal, MD

I dedicate this book to my family, especially my supportive husband Dipul, my "tae kwon do master" Rian, and my princess Reyna. Thank you for all your love and inspiration. You mean the world to me. Thank you also to all of my mentors who have instilled confidence in me and continue to inspire me to be better.

Mona Patadia, MD

I dedicate this book to the Department of Otolaryngology—Head and Neck Surgery at Loyola. I have been privileged to spend my career at Loyola and serve as department chair. Two of our excellent faculty edited this book, Drs. Rosenthal and Patadia. As you will see, they did a superb job! Much thanks to them for their hard work and effort.

James Stankiewicz, MD

Contributors

Oliver Adunka
Department of
    Otolaryngology—Head
    and Neck Surgery
The Ohio State University
    Wexner Medical Center
Columbus, Ohio

Muhamad A. Amine
Department of
    Otolaryngology—Head
    and Neck Surgery
Carle Foundation Hospital
Urbana, Illinois

and

College of Medicine
University of Illinois
    Urbana–Champaign
Champaign, Illinois

Pete S. Batra
Department of
    Otorhinolaryngology—
    Head and Neck Surgery
Rush University Medical
    Center
Chicago, Illinois

Mark J. Been
The Center for Facial Plastic
    Surgery
Barrington, Illinois

Michael S. Benninger
Head and Neck Institute
Lerner College of Medicine
The Cleveland Clinic
Cleveland, Ohio

Aditi Bhuskute
Department of
    Otolarygology—Head and
    Neck Surgery
The University of North
    Carolina at Chapel Hill
Sacramento, California

Anthony Chin-Quee
Henry Ford Health System
Detroit, Michigan

Amelia F. Drake
Department of
    Otolaryngology—Head
    and Neck Surgery
The University of North
    Carolina at Chapel Hill
Chapel Hill, North Carolina

Glendon M. Gardner
Department of
    Otolaryngology—Head
    and Neck Surgery
Henry Ford Medical Group
Detroit, Michigan

Celeste Gary
Department of
    Otolaryngology—Head
    and Neck Surgery
University of California,
    Davis Medical Center
Sacramento, California

Anand V. Germanwala
Department of Neurological
    Surgery
Loyola University Medical
    Center/Trinity Health
    Center
Maywood, Illinois

and

Edward Hines, Jr. VA Hospital
Hines, Illinois

Brent Golden
Division of Pediatric
    Craniomaxillofacial
    Surgery
Department of Children's
    Surgery
Arnold Palmer Hospital for
    Children
Orlando, Florida

Laura T. Hetzler
Department of
    Otolaryngology—Head
    and Neck Surgery
Louisiana State University
    Health Sciences Center
    New Orleans
New Orleans, Louisiana

Allison M. Holzapfel
Mangat, Holzapfel & Lied
 Plastic Surgery
and
Department of
 Otolaryngology—Head
 and Neck Surgery
University of Cincinnati
Cincinatti, Ohio

and

Northern Kentucky

and

Vail, Colorado

Jeffrey M. Hotaling
Department of
 Otolaryngology—Head
 and Neck Surgery
Thomas Jefferson University
Philadelphia, Pennsylvania

Neal M. Jackson
Department of
 Otorhinolaryngology
Louisiana State University
 Health Science Center
 New Orleans
New Orleans, Louisiana

Alice C. Lin
Kaiser Permanente
Los Angeles Medical Center
Los Angeles, California

Devinder S. Mangat
Department of
 Otolaryngology—Head
 and Neck Surgery
University of Cincinnati
Cincinnati, Ohio

Benjamin Marcus
Department of
 Otolaryngology—Head
 and Neck Surgery
University of
 Wisconsin–Madison
Madison, Wisconsin

Caitlin McLean
Department of
 Otolaryngology—Head
 and Neck Surgery
Lewis Katz School of
 Medicine
Philadelphia, Pennsylvania

Daniel W. Nuss
Department of
 Otolaryngology—Head
 and Neck Surgery
Louisiana State University
 Health Sciences Center
 New Orleans
New Orleans, Louisiana

and

Department of
 Otolaryngology
Children's Mercy
Kansas City, Missouri

Foluwasayo E. Ologe
Department of
 Otorhinolaryngology
University of Ilorin
and
University of Ilorin Teaching
 Hospital
Ilorin, Nigeria

Monica Oberoi Patadia
Department of
 Otolaryngology—Head
 and Neck Surgery
Loyola University Medical
 Center/Trinity Health
 Center
Maywood, Illinois

Krishna Patel
Department of
 Otolaryngology—Head
 and Neck Surgery
Medical University of South
 Carolina
Charleston, South Carolina

Urjeet A. Patel
Department of
 Otolaryngology—Head
 and Neck Surgery
Northwestern University
Chicago, Illinois

Lorien M. Paulson
Pediatric Otolaryngology—
 Head and Neck Surgery
Children's Mercy Hospital
University of Missouri
 Kansas City
Kansas City, Missouri

Blake Raggio
Department of
 Otolaryngology
Tulane University Medical
 Center
New Orleans, Louisiana

Austin S. Rose
Department of
 Otolaryngology—Head
 and Neck Surgery
The University of North
 Carolina at Chapel Hill
Chapel Hill, North Carolina

Laura H. Swibel Rosenthal
Department of
    Otolaryngology—Head
    and Neck Surgery
Loyola University Medical
    Center/Trinity Health
    Center
Maywood, Illinois

and

Department of
    Otolaryngology—Head
    and Neck Surgery
Northwestern University
Feinberg School of Medicine
and
Division of Otolaryngology
    Head and Neck Surgery
Ann & Robert H. Lurie
    Children's Hospital of
    Chicago
Chicago, Illinois

Kristin Seiberling
Department of
    Otolaryngology—Head
    and Neck Surgery
Loma Linda University
    Medical Center
Loma Linda, California

Michael D. Seidman
Otologic/Neurotologic/
    Skull Base Surgery,
    Wellness
Florida Hospital Celebration
    Health
University of Central
    Florida
Orlando, Florida

Lane D. Squires
Department of
    Otolarygology—Head and
    Neck Surgery
University of California,
    Davis
Sacramento, California

James Stankiewicz
Department of
    Otolaryngology—Head
    and Neck Surgery
Loyola University Medical
    Center/Trinity Health
    Center
Maywood, Illinois

Kevin Swong
Department of Neurological
    Surgery
Loyola University Medical
    School
Maywood, Illinois

Jonathan Sykes
Department of
    Otolaryngology—Head
    and Neck Surgery
University of California,
    Davis Medical Center
Sacramento, California

Bradford Terry
Department of
    Otolaryngology—Head
    and Neck Surgery
Louisiana State University
New Orleans, Louisiana

Christopher Tran
Department of
    Otorhinolaryngology
Louisiana State University
    Health Science Center
    New Orleans
New Orleans, Louisiana

Christopher Vanison
Department of
    Otolaryngology
University of California,
    Davis Medical Center
Sacramento, California

Sean Weiss
Department of
    Otolaryngology—Head
    and Neck Surgery
and
Department of General
    Surgery
Louisiana State University
New Orleans, Louisiana

Peter-John Wormald
Department of
    Otolaryngology—Head
    and Neck Surgery
The University of Adelaide
Adelaide, South Australia,
    Australia

Carlton Zdanski
Department of
    Otolaryngology—Head
    and Neck Surgery
The University of North
    Carolina at Chapel Hill
Chapel Hill, North Carolina

SECTION 1

HEAD AND NECK

CHAPTER 1

Diseases of the Oral Cavity

Urjeet A. Patel, Alice C. Lin, and Christopher Vanison

- **Angioedema**
- **Ameloblastoma**
- **Keratocyst odontogenic tumor**
- **Lip cancer**
- **Mucosal melanoma**
- **Oral cancer**
- **Ranula**

Angioedema

DEFINITIONS AND CLINICAL FEATURES
Angioedema is a rapid swelling or edema of the dermis, mucosa, or submucosa. It is usually associated with allergy and is frequently seen as a drug reaction, particularly to antihypertensive ACE inhibitors. The skin of the face and lips may become rapidly swollen over the course of minutes to hours. More concerning, however, is the edema that often occurs in the oral and oropharyngeal mucosa resulting in dramatic tongue and pharynx edema. In such cases, inspiratory stridor can develop with imminent airway obstruction (Figures 1.1 and 1.2).

Angioedema can be classified as acquired or hereditary. Patients with acquired angioedema generally have a history of allergy, and episodes may occur in conjunction with other allergic findings such as urticaria. Hereditary angioedema is caused by a genetic mutation that is

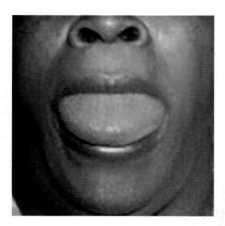

Figure 1.1 Angioedema involving the oral tongue.

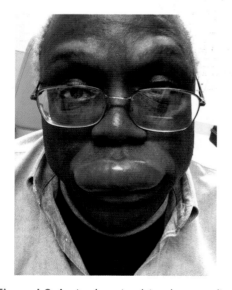

Figure 1.2 Angioedema involving the upper lip.

inherited in an autosomal dominant fashion. This results in diminished levels of the C1-inhibitor protein, which then leads to abnormal activation of the complement cascade as the trigger for clinically apparent angioedema.

DIFFERENTIAL DIAGNOSIS
Urticaria, allergic reaction, anaphylaxis.

WORKUP
The diagnosis of angioedema is based largely on the clinical picture. Testing may include routine blood tests in addition to complement levels.

TREATMENT
Since the acute episode may be life threatening, early treatment involves acute administration of steroids and antihistamines. If a drug history demonstrates a likely culprit, such medications are of course discontinued. In life-threatening cases, the airway must be stabilized by either elective intubation or urgent/emergent tracheotomy or cricothyrotomy placement. In less critical patients, airway observation may be sufficient as medical therapy is instituted and the angioedema resolves.

Ameloblastoma

DEFINITION AND CLINICAL FEATURES
Ameloblastoma is a benign tumor arising from the odontogenic epithelium and is more commonly seen in the mandible compared to the maxilla (Figure 1.3). They are most commonly associated with unerupted teeth and are generally seen in the posterior aspect of the maxilla or mandible. These tumors are rarely malignant or metastatic; however, they are progressively enlarging lesions that can be locally destructive to the native bone and surrounding soft tissue. Accordingly, they can cause significant facial deformity and functional difficulties with mastication if left untreated.

DIFFERENTIAL DIAGNOSIS
Other benign tumors of the mandible and maxilla including dentigerous cyst, odontogenic keratocyst, odontogenic myxoma, giant cell granuloma.

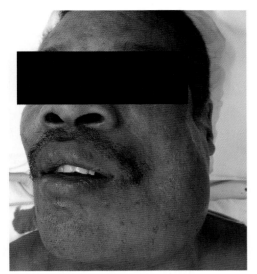

Figure 1.3 Facial deformity caused by underlying ameloblastoma of the left mandible.

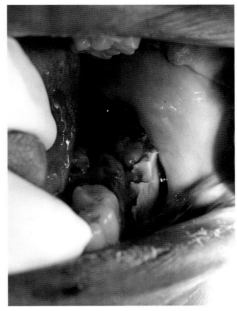

Figure 1.5 Intraoral appearance of soft tissue extension to the gingival and buccal mucosa.

WORKUP

Imaging is recommended for workup of ameloblastoma. This begins with either plain films or panorex imaging, followed by CT scan if ameloblastoma is considered (Figure 1.4). Given the slow-growing nature of this lesion, the bone is often expanded and remodeled with a thin layer of new bone deposited and the leading edge of growth.

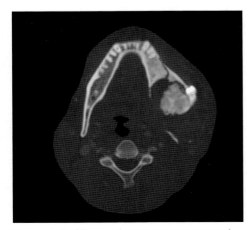

Figure 1.4 CT scan demonstrating expansile lesion of the mandible.

This can often be seen as an expansile lesion on imaging studies. Biopsy is recommended, often transoral, to make the definitive diagnosis to guide further treatment (Figure 1.5).

TREATMENT

The mainstay of treatment is surgical excision. Given the locally aggressive nature of this disease, curettage is considered insufficient and proper treatment requires wide surgical excision. Curettage has been attempted, though often results in recurrence of disease. Accordingly, wide surgical margins are required for definitive treatment and may result in segmental resection of the jawbones to optimize prognosis.

Keratocyst odontogenic tumor

DEFINITION AND CLINICAL FEATURES

Keratocystic odontogenic tumor (KCOT) is a developmental cystic lesion arising from remnants of the dental lamina, most often in the posterior mandible. Previously referred to as "odontogenic keratocyst," this lesion was recently reclassified as a neoplasm due to its aggressive clinical course and high propensity for recurrence. KCOTs are typically unilocular cysts that are lined with epithelium and filled with keratinaceous material. Patients with basal cell nevus syndrome (Gorlin syndrome) may have multiple KCOTs. These tumors may grow rapidly and can be locally destructive. Many prove difficult to eradicate and recurrence is common. Rarely, KCOTs may transform to other benign odontogenic tumors such as ameloblastomas or even malignant tumors such as squamous cell carcinoma. Patients most commonly present with enlarging facial mass or swelling in the second through fourth decades.

DIFFERENTIAL DIAGNOSIS

Ameloblastoma, dentigerous cyst, giant cell granuloma, radicular cyst, metastasis.

WORKUP

KCOTs are typically first noted on plain film or panorex. CT and MRI are typically not necessary. Imaging alone is insufficient for diagnosis as the radiographic appearance frequently mimics that of a variety of odontogenic cysts and tumors. Because KCOTs behave aggressively, they must be differentiated from these other lesions. Therefore, histologic diagnosis is important for both patient counseling and treatment choices. Biopsy including the epithelium should be performed transorally, if feasible (Figure 1.6).

TREATMENT

Surgery is the mainstay of treatment for KCOT. The removal of the epithelial lining is imperative for successful eradication. For this reason, simple marsupialization and curettage are considered less effective than more aggressive methods. Enucleation is performed and is typically

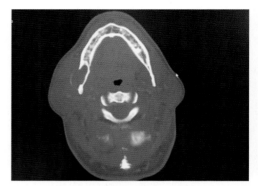

Figure 1.6 CT scan of keratocystic odontogenic tumor involving the right mandible posteriorly.

accompanied by removal of a peripheral margin or bone or by cryotherapy. In cases of extensive or recurrent disease, more radical resections such as segmental mandibulectomy or partial maxillectomy may be required.

Lip cancer

DEFINITION AND CLINICAL FEATURES

Lip cancer is considered the most common form of oral cancer, though it has its own dedicated staging system separated from other oral cavity tumors. It can occur on either the upper or lower lip, though the lower lip is more common and slow growing. The vast majority are squamous cell carcinomas that arise from the normal squamous cells of the lip epidermis. While squamous cell carcinoma is the most common, basal cell carcinoma and minor salivary gland carcinoma may also arise in the lip. Risk factors include cigarette smoking, pipe smoking, thermal or traumatic injury, and UV light exposure. Lesions may arise as small ulcers at the vermillion border of the lip that are most often painless. Lesions continue to grow and may ultimately invade deeper structures such as the mandible or may metastasize to regional lymph nodes in the submental and submandibular regions (Figures 1.7 and 1.8).

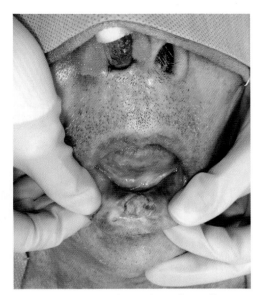

Figure 1.7 Lip cancer involving the midline lower lip.

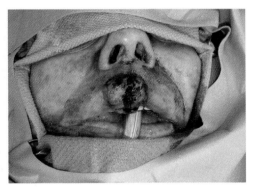

Figure 1.8 Lip cancer involving the midline upper lip.

DIFFERENTIAL DIAGNOSIS

Like other forms of oral cancer, lip carcinoma must be distinguished from other benign or infectious lesions. These include aphthous ulcer, herpes infection, leukoplakia, and lichen planus.

WORKUP

The workup of a concerning lip lesion begins with incisional biopsy. If the lesion is very small, the entire lesion may be removed at time of biopsy with an adequate margin. For larger lesions, incisional bx yields the diagnosis, and definitive treatment can then be planned. For small lip carcinomas, CT scan is recommended to assess for deeper invasion and assess regional lymph nodes. For small lesions, CT scan may not be required.

TREATMENT

Lip cancer is most often treated with surgical excision. Lip lesions measuring several centimeters may be resected with good reconstructive options that offer good functional and cosmetic results. Lesions are generally resected with a 1 cm margin, though smaller margins may be possible. Moh's surgery can also be considered for recurrent cases or aggressive variants such as morpheaform basal cell carcinoma. After resection, primary closure can be attempted; otherwise, there are a variety of local flaps that can be performed to achieve good results. Radiation therapy is also effective for treatment of lip cancer. For lesions that require sacrifice of the majority of the lip, radiation therapy offers good local control and cure while maintaining normal lip appearance and function. Accordingly, a multidisciplinary approach is ideal to offer each patient a treatment plan that is well suited to the particular lesion at hand (Figures 1.9 and 1.10).

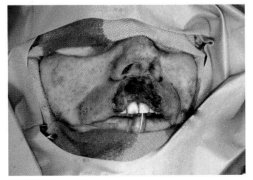

Figure 1.9 The tumor is resected from the midline upper lip.

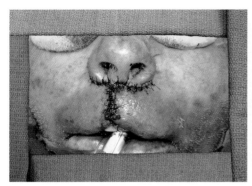

Figure 1.10 Given the relatively modest size of the defect, primary closure is achieved after minimal advancement is performed from each side toward the midline.

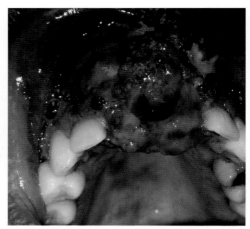

Figure 1.11 Mucosal melanoma involving the midline maxilla and anterior incisors.

Mucosal melanoma

DEFINITION AND CLINICAL FEATURES

A small subset of melanomas arises from mucosal surfaces, and about 50% occur in the head and neck. Of these, the nasal cavity is the most common location. In the oral cavity, mucosal melanoma (MM) most commonly arises from the hard palate and gingiva overlying the maxillary alveolus. While exceedingly rare, MM may also occur in the pharynx, larynx, and esophagus. Lesions, particularly those in the sinonasal region, are often missed on exam and do not initially cause symptoms. Appearance ranges from small, flat hyperpigmented lesions to large, destructive, ulcerative tumors. It is not uncommon for MM to be amelanotic. A subset of patients is noted to have hyperpigmentation of mucosal surfaces (i.e., the palate) preceding diagnosis; however, it is unclear if this represents a premalignant state (Figure 1.11).

While MM can occur at any age, patients are usually diagnosed in the seventh to ninth decades. Currently there are no clear risk factors, although cigarette smoking has been implicated. Recently, a subset of MM tumors has been shown to carry c-KIT mutations. MM is aggressive and most tumors present at late stages with regional lymphatic spread. Treatment failure is unfortunately common. Overall, the prognosis is poor with few patients surviving at 5 years after diagnosis.

DIFFERENTIAL DIAGNOSIS

Metastasis from cutaneous melanoma, minor salivary tumors, head and neck squamous cell carcinoma, benign melanosis, sinonasal cancers.

WORKUP

Hyperpigmented lesions and frank tumors should be biopsied. When melanoma is suspected, staining for melan-A and S-100 and genetic testing for b-RAF and c-KIT mutations should be considered. When a diagnosis of melanoma is confirmed, it is imperative to distinguish between primary MM and metastatic spread from a cutaneous site. This includes comprehensive skin and ocular exams. When MM is favored, the patient should be assessed for metastatic spread regardless of stage. This includes imaging of the primary site and neck; this is typically with contrast-enhanced CT, although MRI may also be useful in its ability to distinguish tissue planes and detect perineural invasion. A thorough workup

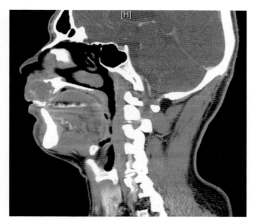

Figure 1.12 CT scan demonstrates the infiltrative nature of this tumor with extension into bone of the maxilla.

for distant metastases includes CT scanning of the chest and abdomen and MRI of the brain (Figure 1.12).

TREATMENT

As with cutaneous melanomas, treatment of MM is primarily surgical. Given the location of these tumors, this often includes oral cavity resection or maxillectomy and may involve radical procedures such as craniofacial resection for larger sinonasal tumors. Even so, negative margins are often hard to achieve, and there is a high rate of recurrence despite seemingly adequate resection. Neck dissection is performed for clinically node-positive disease but is not recommended for clinical N0 necks. Unlike in cutaneous disease, sentinel lymph node biopsy is not routinely performed in cases of MM. The benefit of radiation therapy is questionable, and currently radiotherapy is usually used in cases where there are positive surgical margins or for palliation. Chemotherapy may be used as an adjunct to surgery or for palliation. When MM is metastatic or unresectable, patients may benefit from inclusion in clinical trials. Given the recent finding of c-KIT mutations in some MM tumors, some have recommended

the use of imatinib based on its success in treating other c-KIT-positive tumors such as gastrointestinal stromal tumor. This, however, is still experimental.

Oral cancer

DEFINITION AND CLINICAL FEATURES

Oral cancer is one of the major categories of head and neck cancer and is defined as any cancerous tissue within the oral cavity. Over 90% of such cancers are squamous cell carcinomas arising from the mucosal surfaces of the oral cavity. This includes the tongue, floor or mouth, buccal surface, hard palate, and alveolar ridges of the mandible and maxilla. Cancer may arise from different cell types including minor salivary glands, bone tumors from the mandible or maxilla, sarcoma from mesenchymal tissues, and also MM (Figure 1.13).

Oral cancers generally start as small lesions or ulcers in the mouth. These lesions range from asymptomatic to causing significant pain with chewing and swallowing. Any oral lesion that does not resolve after 2–3 weeks should be assessed to rule out malignancy. Lesions may demonstrate bleeding and may be associated with ear pain depending on the depth of invasion of the tumor with referred otalgia.

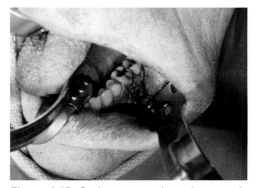

Figure 1.13 Oral cancer involving the gingival of the left lateral mandible and adjacent buccal mucosa.

There are a number of independent risk factors for oral cancer. The two most prominent risk factors are tobacco and alcohol use. Tobacco use can take the form of smoking, chewing tobacco, or snuff. Betel nut use, which is common in India and Asia, is also a significant risk factor, where oral cancer comprises 40% of all new cancers. Alcohol consumption is an independent risk factor, though synergistic when combined with the carcinogenic effects of tobacco. Finally, human papilloma virus infection, particularly type 16, is associated with both oral and oropharyngeal cancer. HPV types 16 and 18 are the most common sexually transmitted diseases in the United States and are a leading cause of both cervical and oral cancers. Oral cancers that arise from HPV infection occur in younger patients ages 30–50 often with no significant smoking or drinking history. Prognosis in this cohort of oral cancer patients is actually more favorable than what is seen in the HPV(–) oral cancer population.

DIFFERENTIAL DIAGNOSIS

Oral cancers must be distinguished from the myriad abnormalities that can occur in the mouth. Nonneoplastic ulcers, infectious process such as fungal infection, and benign abnormalities of the minor salivary glands should be considered. Benign papilloma as well as fibroma and neuroma can also occur on the tongue or buccal mucosa, sometimes related to previous trauma in the biteline. In addition, there are a number of premalignant lesions that occur in the mouth. Cancers may begin as leukoplakia, erythroplakia, or lichen planus (Figure 1.14).

WORKUP

The initial step toward workup of the suspicious lesion is biopsy. This can often be done in the office with topical or local anesthetic. Tissue biopsy is used to distinguish oral cancer from other benign and infectious processes on the differential diagnosis list. If biopsy does confirm carcinoma, complete

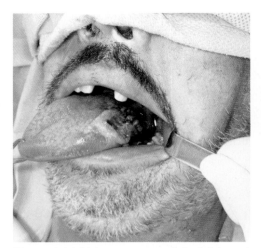

Figure 1.14 Malignant tumor of the left lateral tongue.

staging of the tumor is needed. This includes contrasted CT scan of the neck to assess depth of the primary lesion and also muscle or bone invasion. The neck CT also is used to identify if pathological node is present. Chest CT scan is also needed to rule out distant metastasis to the lungs and also to assess for second primary lesion in the esophagus or the bronchial tree. PET scan may be obtained but is not required in the workup of oral cancer (Figures 1.15 and 1.16).

TREATMENT

The mainstay of treatment of oral cancer is surgical resection. A wide local excision is performed, with attempt to achieve a 1 cm margin of normal tissue surrounding the lesion. The details governing what is resected depend on the anatomical location of the tumor and its depth of invasion. Resection may include partial glossectomy, floor-of-mouth resection, buccal resection, or palate and mandible resection in the case of bone invasion. Most regions of the oral cavity are amenable to surgical reconstruction with local, regional, or free flaps. Prosthetic rehabilitation is also a consideration after bone resection in effort to restore mastication.

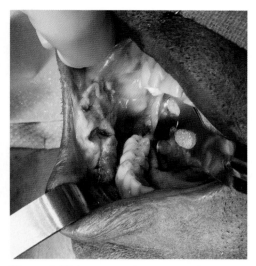

Figure 1.15 Larger carcinoma over the majority of the right buccal mucosa.

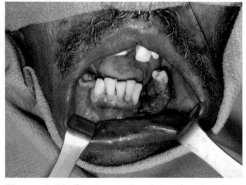

Figure 1.16 Carcinoma involving the alveolar ridge, extending down to the floor of mouth just posterior to the lateral incisor.

In the event that there is clinical evidence of cervical metastasis, neck dissection is recommended on one or both sides of the neck. In the event of an N0 neck, there may still be great enough risk of occult metastasis to recommend staging or prophylactic neck dissection depending on the size and depth of the primary lesion. Radiation therapy can be considered as a primary mode of therapy, though there are significant risks associated

with oral radiation including mucositis, xerostomia, and osteoradionecrosis of the mandible or maxilla. Finally, in cases of oral cancer where the entire tongue is involved and total glossectomy is needed, many patients and surgeons will consider chemotherapy and radiation therapy as a primary treatment choice given the significant morbidity of total glossectomy.

Ranula

DEFINITION AND CLINICAL FEATURES

A ranula is a mucous retention cyst of the floor of the mouth associated with the sublingual gland or duct. The etiology is typically trauma resulting in either injury to or blockage of the sublingual duct. The sublingual gland continuously secretes mucous that, in the setting of such trauma, extravasates into surrounding tissues. Most are not lined by true epithelium and thus should be classified as pseudocysts, although some may be partially lined. Ranulas may be classified as simple or plunging. Simple ranulas are limited to the sublingual space. These present as soft, compressible intraoral swelling that cause elevation of the tongue; they may appear blue in color. Plunging ranulas, which are less common, extend through the mylohyoid muscle into the submandibular space, either due to iatrogenic injury to the muscle or via a preexisting dehiscence. Plunging ranulas may present as a mass involving both the floor of the mouth and neck or solely as a neck mass. Ranulas are often asymptomatic but may grow rapidly and cause airway compromise if they become infected. Ranulas may occur in both children and adults but most commonly arise during the second and third decades with a slight female predominance.

DIFFERENTIAL DIAGNOSIS

Lymphatic malformation, cystic hygroma, benign or malignant salivary tumor, dermoid cyst, thyroglossal duct cyst.

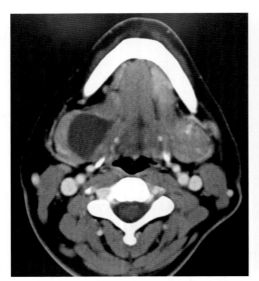

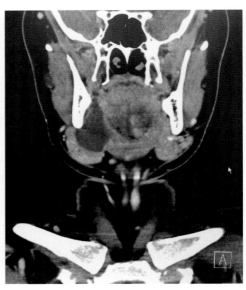

Figure 1.17 CT scan demonstrating a ranula of the right neck. It displaces the submandibular gland laterally.

Figure 1.18 Coronal view CT scan showing the typical location of a ranula between the tongue and the submandibular gland. The lesion extends right up to the floor of the mouth on the right side.

WORKUP

Physical exam is often sufficient for diagnosis of simple ranulas. Plunging ranulas, particularly those without an obvious intraoral component, may be confused with many other cystic neck lesions and therefore imaging may be warranted. Both ultrasound and CT scan may be employed. Ranulas appear as homogenous cysts in the sublingual and/or submandibular space. A submandibular space cyst with a tail entering into the sublingual space is highly suggestive of a plunging ranula. Tissue biopsy is not required for diagnosis (Figures 1.17 and 1.18).

TREATMENT

Ranulas may be observed if they are asymptomatic. Gold standard treatment is surgical excision of the affected sublingual gland. Marsupialization of the ranula may be associated with recurrence. Excision of the ranula and associated gland is performed intraorally for simple ranulas and should also be attempted for plunging ranulas. Occasionally, an additional neck incision must be performed to address large plunging ranulas.

Diseases of the Salivary Glands

Urjeet A. Patel, Alice C. Lin, and Christopher Vanison

- **Sialolithiasis and sialoadenitis**
- **Benign parotid masses**
- **Parotid malignancy**
- **Submandibular malignancy**
- **Minor salivary gland malignancy**

Sialolithiasis and sialoadenitis

DEFINITION AND CLINICAL FEATURES
Sialolithiasis is a condition where salivary calculi or stones form in the salivary glands, usually in the duct. It is much more common in the submandibular gland than the parotid, sublingual, or minor salivary glands. The presentation of sialolithiasis is often with sialoadenitis or inflammation of the salivary gland. Blockage of the drainage system causes stasis and ensuing inflammation and infection of the gland. Sialoadenitis can also occur without sialolithiasis, and is caused by poor oral hygiene and other causes of decreased salivary flow or autoimmune disease (Figure 2.1).

DIFFERENTIAL DIAGNOSIS
Benign and malignant tumors of the salivary glands including pleomorphic adenoma, mucoepidermoid carcinoma, and adenoid cystic carcinoma can also present with hardening or enlargement of the gland. Blockage of the ductal system by tumors such as salivary ductal carcinoma, trauma with scarring or interruption of the duct, or oral cavity lesions can also mimic sialolithiasis and cause sialoadenitis.

WORKUP
A thorough physical exam is essential in the workup. Culture of any purulent drainage will help dictate antibiotic therapy. Imaging is recommended to determine the location and

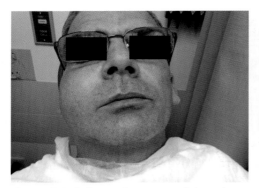

Figure 2.1 Diffuse enlargement of the right face due to obstruction of Stensen's duct by a salivary gland stone.

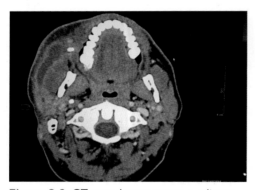

Figure 2.2 CT scan demonstrates a salivary gland stone anterior to the masseter at the distal aspect of Stensen's duct where it meets the buccal mucosa.

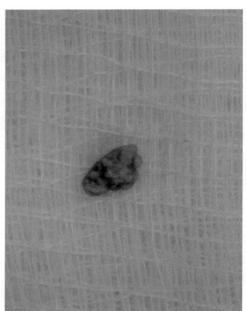

Figure 2.3 Typical appearance of a salivary gland stone.

character of the stone and rule out other pathologies. This can be performed as a CT scan or an ultrasound. Sialoendoscopy can also be performed diagnostically although this is usually done in conjunction with an attempt at therapeutic removal endoscopically. Laboratory studies such as a complete blood panel and electrolytes are helpful. Autoimmune studies may be obtained if an autoimmune process is suspected (Figures 2.2 and 2.3).

TREATMENT
The immediate treatment is with hydration, gentle massage, analgesics, and sialogogues.

Antibiotics may be used if there is evidence of an infection. Small stones are sometimes expulsed with this therapy and observation. As stones increase in size, the likelihood of spontaneous expulsion decreases. Stones near the opening of Wharton's duct may be removed intraorally with ductal cannulation, dilation, and retrieval of the stone. Stones near the hilum or multiple stones require a submandibular gland excision transcervically. Sublingual stones can be removed transorally. Parotid sialolithiasis can be managed expectantly or via sialoendoscopy. Parotidectomy for recurrent sialolithiasis or sialoadenitis is rarely indicated and is associated with a high complication and recurrence rate.

Benign parotid masses

DEFINITION AND CLINICAL FEATURES
Of all parotid neoplasms, roughly 80% are benign. Of those, the most common histologic types include pleomorphic adenomas,

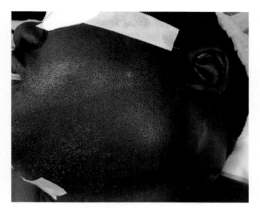

Figure 2.4 Benign parotid gland tumor with gross distortion of the left inferior face extending to the neck.

Warthin's tumors (papillary cystadenoma lymphomatosum), oncocytomas, and monomorphic adenomas. In children, hemangioma is the most common benign parotid tumor. These tumors are typically unilateral; however, a small percentage of Warthin's tumors are bilateral. Benign lymphoepithelial lesions are commonly found in parotid glands of individuals with HIV or Sjögren syndrome, and these often occur bilaterally. Benign parotid tumors typically present as slow-growing, painless upper cervical or preauricular masses. If located in the deep lobe, they may present as an oropharyngeal mass. Risk factors include ionizing radiation or silica dust exposure. Smoking is thought to be a risk factor for Warthin's tumors. Although uncommon, certain benign salivary tumors may metastasize or undergo malignant transformation if left untreated (Figures 2.4 and 2.5).

DIFFERENTIAL DIAGNOSIS

Malignant parotid tumor, intraparotid lymphadenopathy, metastatic tumor, sialolithiasis, sialoadenitis, odontogenic infection, odontogenic neoplasm, congenital neck cyst, autoimmune disease (Sjögren syndrome, scleroderma, sarcoidosis).

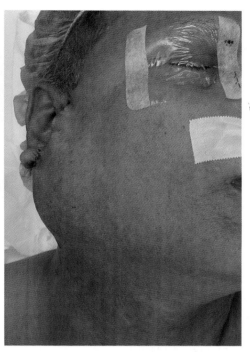

Figure 2.5 Right-sided parotid tumor showing diffuse enlargement of the right face.

WORKUP

Patients presenting with a parotid mass typically first undergo contrast-enhanced CT scan of the neck. This can provide useful information about location (superficial vs. deep lobe; intra- vs. extra-parotid), size, presence of lymphadenopathy, and tumor characteristics (solid vs. cystic). MRI is recommended for imaging of tumors in the deep lobe as it can better delineate tumor from salivary gland, fat, and various neurovascular structures of the parapharyngeal space. Fine needle aspiration (FNA) can be an accurate, sensitive, and specific method for diagnosing salivary neoplasms, although it is still considered to be controversial by some. It is highly dependent upon the experience of the pathologist. FNA is not typically feasible for deep lobe tumors.

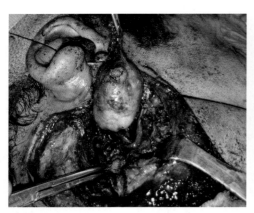

Figure 2.6 Benign parotid tumor dissected away from the right facial nerve and its distal branches.

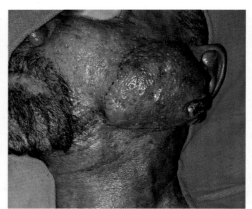

Figure 2.7 Parotid malignancy involving the left parotid gland extending to the skin.

TREATMENT

Surgical resection is typically recommended to prevent complications associated with continued tumor growth and malignant transformation. Benign lymphoepithelial lesions are usually observed unless they are symptomatic. Because simple enucleation has been associated with unacceptable rates of recurrence, superficial or deep lobe parotidectomy is performed. This ensures that a cuff of normal parotid is also removed. The facial nerve should be preserved for benign disease. Occasionally, more extensive approaches such as mandibular swing may be required for access to deep lobe lesions. Occasionally, in poor surgical candidates or those with recurrent disease, radiation therapy may be used (Figure 2.6).

Parotid malignancy

DEFINITION AND CLINICAL FEATURES

While the majority of parotid tumors are benign, roughly 20% are malignant. This includes a diverse group of tumors with mucoepidermoid carcinoma arising most commonly, followed by adenoid cystic carcinoma, adenocarcinoma, and acinic cell carcinoma. There are several lymph nodes contained within the parotid, and these may

harbor lymphoma, regional metastases from head and neck skin cancers, or even distant metastases. Behavior of these lesions ranges from indolent and highly treatable (low-grade mucoepidermoid carcinoma, acinic cell carcinoma) to highly aggressive (high-grade mucoepidermoid, salivary ductal carcinoma, adenocarcinoma). A unique feature of some salivary malignancies (particularly adenoid cystic carcinoma) is the propensity for local and distant recurrence after long disease-free intervals. A parotid mass that grows rapidly, causes pain, is fixed to or breaks through the skin or is associated with facial weakness should raise concern for malignancy (Figure 2.7). Radiation exposure is thought to be a risk factor for malignant and benign parotid tumors. Smoking and alcohol abuse are not thought to be risk factors.

DIFFERENTIAL DIAGNOSIS

Benign parotid tumor, intraparotid lymphadenopathy, metastatic tumor, sialolithiasis, sialoadenitis, odontogenic infection, odontogenic neoplasm, congenital neck cyst.

WORKUP

As with benign parotid tumors, contrast-enhanced CT is most often performed and is important in the evaluation of potential metastasis to cervical lymph nodes. MRI may

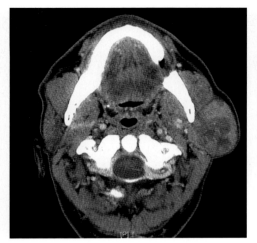

Figure 2.8 CT scan of left parotid gland malignancy.

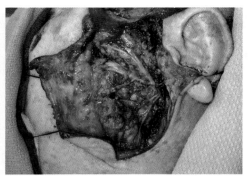

Figure 2.9 Surgical field after resection, with preservation of the facial nerve tree.

be helpful in identifying gross perineural invasion or extraglandular invasion. While certain features may be suggestive, characterization of a tumor as benign or malignant should not be based solely on radiographic workup. FNA is often diagnostic, but there is overlap of features between certain malignant and even benign tumors and diagnosis is heavily reliant on pathologist experience (Figure 2.8).

TREATMENT
Parotidectomy (superficial or total depending on extent and location of the disease) is the treatment of choice. Attempts should be made to preserve the facial nerve; however, disease involvement may necessitate sacrifice of some or all of its branches. Neck dissection should be performed if there is evidence of metastatic lymphadenopathy. This is more controversial in the setting of a clinically node-negative neck. In the absence of gross lymphadenopathy, neck dissection is performed in the setting of more aggressive histologic subtypes (e.g., adenocarcinoma, salivary ductal carcinoma) or when there are high-risk features of the primary tumor (high grade, high T-stage, extraparotid extension).

Indications for adjuvant radiation therapy include advanced stage, aggressive histologic subtype, positive resection margins, and perineural invasion. Chemotherapy is used only for palliation (Figure 2.9).

Submandibular malignancy

DEFINITION AND CLINICAL FEATURES
Submandibular tumors, both benign and malignant, are relatively rare. Unlike in the parotid gland, where the majority of neoplasms are benign, about 40% of submandibular tumors are malignant. Adenoid cystic carcinoma is diagnosed most commonly, followed by adenocarcinoma and mucoepidermoid carcinoma. The submandibular gland does not contain lymph nodes, and thus, lymphomas are very rare. As with other salivary gland tumors, features concerning for malignancy include rapid growth, pain, cutaneous involvement, and cranial nerve palsies (e.g., lower lip weakness, ipsilateral tongue numbness, ipsilateral tongue weakness). For unclear reasons, prognosis appears to be worse for salivary malignancies arising from the submandibular gland compared to the parotid gland.

DIFFERENTIAL DIAGNOSIS
Benign submandibular tumor, submandibular triangle lymphadenopathy, sialolithiasis, sialoadenitis, deep neck space infection, plunging ranula.

WORKUP

Workup of a persistent or enlarging submandibular mass usually begins with contrast-enhanced CT, although ultrasound may be useful in ruling out certain benign pathologies such as sialolithiasis. As with other salivary lesions, MRI may be employed when there is concern for perineural invasion. In addition to providing information about the tumor, imaging should also evaluate for the presence of any suspicious adenopathy. CT of the chest is often performed when malignancy is suspected or confirmed, to evaluate for distant metastases. FNA may be performed to identify malignancy or specific tumor type, although false-negative results are a risk.

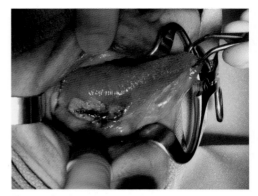

Figure 2.10 Minor salivary gland cancer involving the right lateral tongue.

TREATMENT

Other than lymphomas, which are treated medically, the treatment modality of choice for submandibular gland malignancies is surgery. This includes removal of the submandibular gland and other locally involved structures. Neck dissection should be considered for high-risk tumors, such as those with high histologic grade, high T-stage, and extraglandular extension. Adjuvant radiation therapy is typically employed for high-risk lesions. Chemotherapy is largely palliative at this time. Given the risk of late recurrence with certain salivary malignancies, patients should be followed long term.

Minor salivary gland malignancy

DEFINITION AND CLINICAL FEATURES

Individuals have up to 1000 minor salivary glands that are found in submucosal tissue throughout the oral cavity as well as in the paranasal sinuses, pharynx, and upper airways. Of these anatomic locations, the highest distribution is in the soft tissues covering the hard palate. Each gland is small, measuring only 1–2 mm in diameter. Tumors involving these glands are relatively rare; of

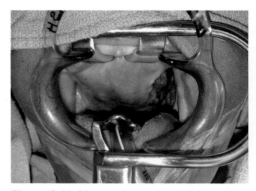

Figure 2.11 Minor salivary gland of the palate that had grown large and occupies the entire roof of the mouth.

those, approximately one half to two thirds are malignant. While these tumors can arise in any location containing minor salivary glands, the most common location is the hard palate. The most common tumor type is adenoid cystic carcinoma, followed by mucoepidermoid carcinoma and adenocarcinoma (Figures 2.10 and 2.11).

Tumors located in the oral cavity present as fixed, enlarging masses that are frequently ulcerated. Pain and cranial neuropathies are worrisome symptoms. Sinonasal tumors are often discovered at late disease stages due to lack of early symptoms. Initial signs and symptoms are nonspecific and may include nasal obstruction, epistaxis, nasal pain, epiphora (tearing), and headaches—these are typically unilateral. Later signs and symptoms include changes in facial appearance, orbital proptosis or telecanthus, hyposmia/anosmia, extraocular palsies, CSF leak, and altered mental status.

DIFFERENTIAL DIAGNOSIS
Benign minor salivary gland tumor, autoimmune disease (Sjögren syndrome), head and neck squamous cell carcinoma, odontogenic tumor, benign sinonasal lesion (e.g., antrochoanal polyp, inverting papillomas), other malignant sinonasal tumors (SNUC, olfactory neuroblastoma), encephalocele.

WORKUP
Targeted physical exam should be performed according to tumor site. Workup of sinonasal tumors includes nasal endoscopy. Cranial nerves and regional lymph nodes should be assessed. Oral cavity and pharyngeal and upper airway lesions should be biopsied if feasible. Biopsy of sinonasal tumors should be done only after encephalocele or vascular lesions are ruled out by imaging. Contrast-enhanced CT is typically the first imaging modality employed. Because workup of nasal obstruction is geared toward more common benign pathologies such as chronic sinusitis, sinonasal CT scans are often performed without the use of contrast material. CT is useful for evaluating size and location of tumors, assessing regional lymph node basins and ruling out boney invasion. MRI is useful for assessing perineural invasion. For sinonasal tumors, MRI may be warranted to investigate extent of orbital or intracranial extension. Additionally, the chest should be imaged to evaluate for possible distant metastatic spread. Unlike major salivary gland tumors that have their own staging system, minor salivary cancers are staged according to their location (e.g., oral cavity, paranasal sinus) (Figure 2.12).

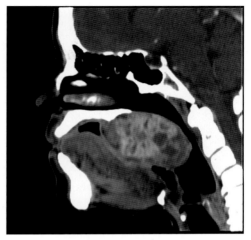

Figure 2.12 CT scan demonstrates the large size of this lesion and its placement on the dorsal tongue at rest.

TREATMENT
As with other salivary malignancies, the primary treatment modality for minor salivary malignancies is surgery. En bloc resection may require radical surgical approaches such as maxillectomy with orbital exenteration or craniofacial resection for large sinonasal tumors.

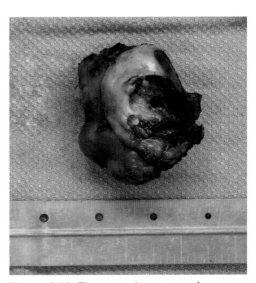

Figure 2.13 The surgical specimen after resection.

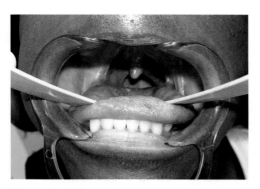

Figure 2.14 Postoperative appearance of the patient at 6 months. Note the preservation of the soft palate and uvula.

These surgeries occasionally require assistance from neurological surgeons or ophthalmologists. Reconstruction, frequently requiring free tissue transfer, is performed for both cosmetic and functional reasons. Neck dissection is performed for high-grade tumors or when aggressive histologic features are present. Similarly, adjuvant external beam radiation is employed for more aggressive disease. Some salivary malignancies have shown good response to fast neutron beam radiation; however, the toxicities of this treatment are often severe, making it an unpopular choice (Figures 2.13 and 2.14).

CHAPTER 3

Masses of the Head and Neck

Urjeet A. Patel, Alice C. Lin, and Christopher Vanison

- **Carotid body tumor**
- **Deep neck space abscesses**
- **Glomus vagale**
- **Lymphangioma**
- **Necrotizing fasciitis**
- **Schwannoma**

Carotid body tumor

DEFINITION AND CLINICAL FEATURES

Carotid body tumor is the most common benign lesion arising from the paraganglia, and generally presents as a slowly enlarging painless neck mass. It derives from the glomus cells at the carotid body and falls under the classification of neuroendocrine tumor. The majority of these lesions are sporadic, though 25% may follow a hereditary pattern of inheritance: 1%–3% may be metabolically active and secrete catecholamines. Given the highly vascular nature of this lesion, it may have a pulsatile quality on physical exam.

DIFFERENTIAL DIAGNOSIS

This includes other causes of neck mass, such as cervical adenopathy, schwannoma, glomus vagale, and glomus jugulare.

WORKUP

Being vascular lesions, once a pulsatile nature is confirmed by physical exam, needle biopsy is frowned upon. Instead, imaging studies are recommended, beginning with a contrast-enhanced neck computed tomography (CT) scan or magnetic resonance imaging (MRI). CT imaging will show a lesion that splays the internal and external carotid arteries and carries a "salt/pepper" appearance (Figure 3.1). Once the diagnosis is suspected, a vascular

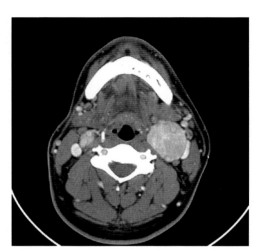

Figure 3.1 CT scan demonstrating large carotid body tumor of the left neck, encasing the external carotid artery and abutting the internal carotid artery. A smaller carotid body tumor is seen on the contralateral side.

study such as MRA or formal angiography is recommended to confirm the diagnosis. A characteristic blush is noted on angiography, and not tissue sampling is needed to proceed with treatment (Figure 3.2).

TREATMENT

Definitive treatment of a carotid body tumor requires surgical excision. Generally, the tumor can be readily dissected free of the carotid artery system as dissection proceeds through the arterial adventitia. Preoperative embolization is recommended for larger lesions to minimize blood loss during surgery. Radiation therapy may be a consideration, though it is generally reserved for patients who refuse surgery or for patients that are suboptimal surgical candidates. Recent studies do support the option of observation, given the slow-growing nature of this tumor and its relatively limited risk of malignancy (Figures 3.3 and 3.4).

Deep neck space abscesses

DEFINITION AND CLINICAL FEATURES

Deep neck space abscesses involve the deep layers of the neck. The presenting symptoms include fever, sore throat, neck stiffness, and neck swelling. The majority of cases are caused by pharyngitis, but other etiologies such as odontogenic infections, foreign body ingestion, postoperative infections, and trauma should be considered. There is a high mortality associated with deep neck space infections due to potential complications related to its proximity to other important structures and delay in diagnosis. These complications include airway obstruction, mediastinitis, epidural abscess, jugular vein thrombosis, sepsis, and necrotizing fasciitis.

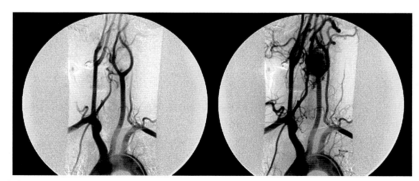

Figure 3.2 Angiography showing the vasculature nature of these tumors, both sitting at the carotid bifurcation.

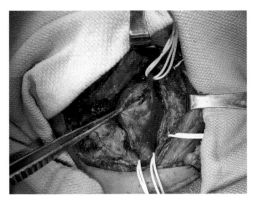

Figure 3.3 The left-sided tumor is dissected away from surrounding structures after first gaining vascular control of the arterial tree.

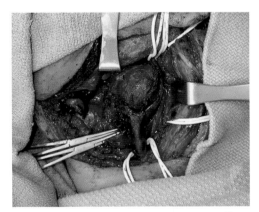

Figure 3.4 The tumor is now dissected off the common carotid artery and then off the internal and external arteries in sequence.

DIFFERENTIAL DIAGNOSIS

The differential diagnosis of deep neck space abscess includes phlegmon, pharyngitis, peritonsillar abscess, pharyngeal foreign body, epiglottitis, epidural abscess, and esophagitis.

WORKUP

The workup starts with a thorough physical exam. The status of the airway should be a part of the early assessment. Other signs include neck edema, erythema, or stiffness. However, the exam can often be unremarkable as the infection and abscess is located deep in the neck far from the surface. Laboratory studies such as a complete blood count, blood chemistries, clotting profile, and blood cultures are helpful. Lateral neck x-rays showing prevertebral thickening may suggest a retropharyngeal abscess. Imaging with CT is important to determine the extent of the abscess and its location in proximity to important neurovascular structures. MRI can show great soft tissue detail, but the increased detail usually does not warrant the increased expense and difficulty in obtaining the scan.

TREATMENT

Empiric antibiotic therapy should be initiated early, covering gram-positive, gram-negative, and anaerobic organisms. Early assessment of the airway in deep neck space abscesses is paramount. In patients with airway compromise, an awake tracheostomy may be the safest way to establish an airway. The presence of the abscess may make endotracheal intubation difficult and complicated. In patients with small abscesses and without airway compromise, a period of observation with antibiotic therapy may be sufficient. In patients who do not improve within 48 hours with antibiotic therapy, surgical intervention with drainage of the abscess should be strongly considered. In the majority of patients, a transcervical approach is safest to protect neurovascular structures. In select patients with retropharyngeal abscesses, a transoral approach may be sufficient. Cultures of the fluid are important to direct antibiotic therapy. In patients who are unable to undergo general anesthesia, a needle aspiration may be performed and the aspirate can be cultured to direct antibiotic therapy.

Glomus vagale

DEFINITION AND CLINICAL FEATURES

Glomus vagale is another benign lesion arising from the paraganglia, and also presents as a slow-growing painless neck mass.

Like the carotid body tumor, it also derives from glomus cells, though in from cells associated with the vagus nerve in this setting. The lesion may occur anywhere along the course of the vagus nerve. Accordingly, it may be first noticed in the mid-neck, though it can also extend up toward the skull base. Depending on its location with respect to the superior laryngeal nerve, the patient may notice difficulty with motor function of the larynx or both sensory and motor functions with higher lesions. This may manifest as hoarseness, shortness of breath, or aspiration symptoms.

DIFFERENTIAL DIAGNOSIS

This includes other causes of neck mass, such as cervical adenopathy, schwannoma, carotid body tumor, and glomus jugulare.

WORKUP

Imaging studies are recommended, beginning with a contrast-enhanced neck CT scan or MRI. CT imaging will show a neck mass that likely enhances with contrast given its vascular nature. The lesion may separate the jugular vein from the common or internal carotid artery but does not typically separate the internal from external arteries as is seen with carotid body tumors. Once the diagnosis is suspected, an MRI can be obtained to better distinguish this from a schwannoma, which might otherwise have a similar anatomic location (Figure 3.5).

TREATMENT

Definitive treatment of a glomus vagale requires surgical excision. Generally, the tumor can be readily dissected away from other carotid sheath structures. Unlike schwannoma, however, the nerve fibers themselves are involved with the lesion and can rarely be dissected free of the mass. As such, resection does often require sacrifice of the vagus nerve with accompanying larynx dysfunction depending on the location of the lesion. Preoperative embolization may be recommended for larger lesions. Radiation

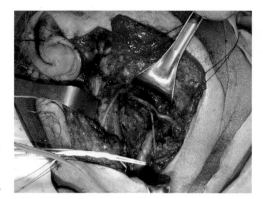

Figure 3.5 Glomus tumor is seen in the right neck, lying between the jugular vein and carotid artery, deep to the hypoglossal nerve that runs obliquely over it.

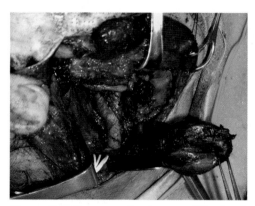

Figure 3.6 The tumor has been mobilized and now remains attached only by the vagus nerve inferiorly. This will be severed to complete the resection.

therapy and observation may also be a reasonable alternative for management depending on the age and comorbidities of the patient and their ability to tolerate surgery (Figure 3.6).

Lymphangioma

DEFINITION AND CLINICAL FEATURES

Lymphangiomas are malformations of the lymphatic system, which is a network of vessels that carries lymph or tissue fluid back

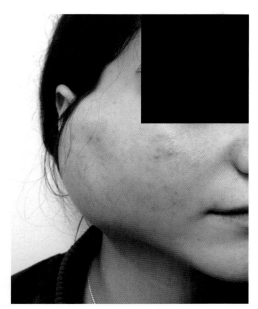

Figure 3.7 Large lymphangioma involving the right lateral neck and face causing significant cosmetic deformity.

to the venous system. They can occur anywhere throughout the body, but are most common in the head and neck. Most present under the age of 2, though they can present later in life as well. These lesions are benign, and typically present as slow-growing doughy masses in the neck, though they can also grow rapidly. Also known as cystic hygroma, the lesions can be collections of large, cystic areas and are often soft and ballotable to palpation (Figure 3.7).

DIFFERENTIAL DIAGNOSIS

Other cystic neck masses, branchial cleft cyst, thyroglossal duct cyst, arteriovenous malformation.

WORKUP

Imaging studies such as ultrasound or CT scan are most often the initial study in the diagnosis of lymphangioma. With demonstration of fluid-containing cystic structures, MRI can help further differentiate this from other vascular and congenital lesions.

TREATMENT

Given that these are benign collections of malformed vessels, there is no malignant potential. Consequently, treatment is focused on cosmetic outcomes or possible functional concerns if the size of lesion is causing symptoms. Surgical excision is the preferred method of definitive treatment if this can be performed with low morbidity and if surgery improves rather than worsens cosmetic appearance. In many instances, the lesion can be locally infiltrative, and complete surgical excision may not be possible. In other cases, revision surgery is needed to address portions of the lesion that are not excised at the initial attempt. For lesions with large cystic areas, injection with sclerosing agents such as OK-432, ethanol, or tetracycline can be effective in controlling the lesion without surgery. With this approach, the sclerosing agent ablates the endothelial cells that contribute lymphatic fluid to the malformation.

Necrotizing fasciitis

DEFINITION AND CLINICAL FEATURES

Necrotizing fasciitis is a severe life-threatening infection of the deep layers of the skin and subcutaneous tissues and spreads easily across fascial planes. The progression can be rapid and involve a large surface area in a short amount of time. As the infection begins in the deep layers, the infection may not be clinically obvious until the process has spread substantially. Necrotizing fasciitis may occur postoperatively, posttraumatically, or be completely idiopathic.

DIFFERENTIAL DIAGNOSIS

The differential diagnosis of necrotizing fasciitis includes cellulitis or infection/inflammation of other deep structures such as parotitis, myositis, thyroiditis, etc.

WORKUP

The diagnosis of necrotizing fasciitis should be based on high clinical suspicion followed by prompt surgical exploration. Laboratory studies can help with raising the clinical suspicion such as CRP, a complete blood count, and serum chemistry. Radiographic workup can be obtained as either a CT scan or an MRI scan. Radiography can validate the presence of an infection, show subcutaneous air in gas forming infections, and indicate the extent of the subcutaneous spread of infection. Cultures of the tissue and infectious fluid reveal aerobic, anaerobic, or mixed flora, but superficial cultures are usually not indicative of the pathogens, and these cultures should be obtained intraoperatively or via a needle aspiration. The most common isolates are *Clostridium*, group A *Streptococcus*, or polymicrobial. While studies for the workup may help raise or lower clinical suspicion, they should not delay movement to the operating room in a critically ill patient.

TREATMENT

Early initiation of empiric broad-spectrum intravenous antibiotic therapy is paramount. These antibiotics can be switched to culture-directed therapy after operating room cultures are resulted. Surgical exploration should be initiated as soon as possible based on the index of suspicion. Intraoperatively, the diagnosis is made by the appearance of the tissues, the pattern of spread of the infection, and pathologic evaluation. The mainstay of treatment is aggressive surgical debridement of necrotic tissue to clear and stop the spread of infection. Wounds are left open as repeat examinations and repeat debridement in the operating room may be needed until the necrotizing portion of the infection has cleared. Intensive care monitoring is also required as the patients often have cardiovascular instability mediated by a systemic inflammatory response to toxins or sepsis. Once the infection is cleared, reconstruction with skin grafts or free flaps for coverage of major structures and to prevent contracture is often required.

Schwannoma

DEFINITION AND CLINICAL FEATURES

Schwannoma, also known as neurinoma or Schwann cell tumor, is a benign tumor that originates from the nerve sheath composed of Schwann cells that normally produce myelin that insulates peripheral nerves. They are slow-growing tumors that tend to push the nerve fibers to the side as they grow, and may not cause nerve dysfunction until quite large. They generally occur as solitary tumors, though they may also present as multiple lesions. Schwannomas may arise from any peripheral nerve that contains Schwann cells, including the cranial nerves. This is most commonly seen with the vestibular nerve (vestibular or acoustic neuroma) and is also often seen with the vagus nerve or the sympathetic chain in the neck (Figure 3.8).

These lesions generally present as a slow-growing painless mass, or may frequently be asymptomatic and only present as an incidental finding on imaging for other medical problems. As they enlarge, they may cause nerve dysfunction, which may be sensory or motor depending on the nerve of origin.

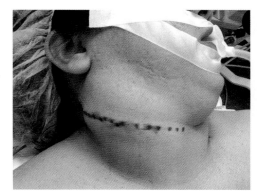

Figure 3.8 Right neck showing diffuse enlargement due to right vagal schwannoma.

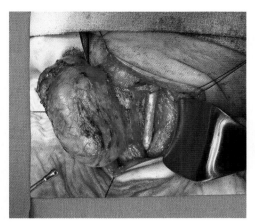

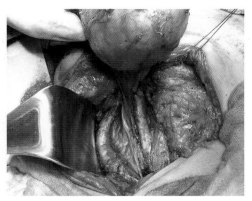

Figure 3.10 The specimen is mobilized superiorly, with the internal jugular vein preserved lateral to the mass.

Figure 3.9 Schwannoma dissected away from surrounding neck structures with preservation of the common carotid artery medially.

DIFFERENTIAL DIAGNOSIS

This includes other causes of neck mass, such as cervical adenopathy, paraganglioma, and branchial cleft cyst.

WORKUP

When these lesions are detected in the neck, initial workup begins with a neck CT with contrast. Imaging characteristics will raise suspicion for schwannoma, though paraganglioma may have similar enhancement characteristics on CT scan. MRI may then be obtained to further distinguish schwannoma from other soft tissue neoplasms that are commonly found in the neck.

TREATMENT

Definitive treatment of a schwannoma requires surgical excision. Since the tumor originates from the nerve sheath, it is often possible to dissect the schwannoma away from the actual nerve fibers and thus preserve function. This is commonly attempted for schwannoma of the vagus nerve to prevent vocal cord dysfunction that would otherwise arise if the vagus nerve is sacrificed with tumor removal. Radiation therapy may also be an option for schwannoma in the neck, if surgery is not feasible. For vestibular neuroma, stereotactic radiation therapy is often the first line of treatment recommended, depending on the anatomic details of the lesion and the approach that would be required if surgery were undertaken (Figures 3.9 and 3.10).

CHAPTER 4

Malignancy of the Pharynx and Larynx

Urjeet A. Patel, Alice C. Lin, and Christopher Vanison

- **Hypopharyngeal cancer**
- **Laryngeal cancer**
- **Nasopharyngeal cancer**
- **Oropharyngeal cancer**

Hypopharyngeal cancer

DEFINITION AND CLINICAL FEATURES

The hypopharynx extends from the level of the hyoid bone superiorly to the pharyngoesophageal junction inferiorly. The larynx is located anterior and medial to the hypopharynx. It can be divided into subsites, including the pyriform sinus, posterior pharyngeal wall, and postcricoid region. The overwhelming majority of hypopharyngeal cancers are squamous cell carcinomas (SCCs), and most arise in the pyriform sinus. Men in their sixth and seventh decades with heavy tobacco use and alcohol consumption histories are most commonly affected. In a small subset of younger female patients, postcricoid carcinoma may be associated with Plummer–Vinson syndrome.

Many hypopharyngeal cancers go undetected at early stages and tumors often must grow to larger sizes in order to produce symptoms. In about half of the patients, neck mass secondary to nodal metastasis is the presenting sign. Early symptoms are nonspecific and include sore throat and dysphagia. Otalgia is a worrisome symptom. Larger tumors may invade the larynx or recurrent laryngeal nerve, causing vocal cord paralysis and resulting hoarseness and stridor. Airway obstruction may occur with larger tumors. Nearly two-thirds will have nodal spread at the time of diagnosis and about 10% will already have distant metastases. Compared to other head and neck sites, cancers of the hypopharynx have a poorer prognosis and only one-quarter to one-third of patients are alive 5 years after diagnosis.

DIFFERENTIAL DIAGNOSIS

Lymphoma, pharyngitis, neck abscess, laryngopharyngeal reflux, laryngeal cancer.

WORKUP

Patients with a neck mass or aforementioned symptoms should undergo comprehensive head and neck exam including flexible laryngoscopy. If possible a mass should be biopsied in clinic; if not possible, biopsy can be performed in the OR. Contrast-enhanced CT of the neck should be performed to evaluate location and extent of disease as well as to evaluate for nodal metastases. CT of the chest should be obtained to evaluate for metastatic spread or for secondary malignancy (Figure 4.1). Similarly liver function tests and either esophagoscopy or esophagography should be performed, to evaluate for metastatic spread and second primary malignancies respectively. If patients are to undergo radiation, thyroid function tests should be done.

TREATMENT

To prevent airway obstruction and to maintain nutrition, patients may need to undergo tracheostomy and/or gastrostomy tube placement prior to treatment. Treatment may include surgical and/or medical therapy. Traditionally, surgical treatment of larger tumors has involved total laryngopharyngectomy. For smaller lesions, partial laryngopharyngectomy may be possible. Neck dissection is typically performed as well. To select smaller lesions, transoral robotic surgery (TORS) may be performed. In extensive cases, partial or total esophagectomy may also be required. Based on staging and pathologic features of the tumor, radiotherapy or chemoradiotherapy may still be needed postoperatively. Patients may also choose chemoradiotherapy as primary treatment, particularly those wishing to preserve their voices when given an option of laryngectomy. Early lesions can be treated with radiation alone, whereas later-stage disease requires the addition of chemotherapy. Given the risk of radiation-induced osteonecrosis of the mandible, patients may require dental extractions prior to treatment.

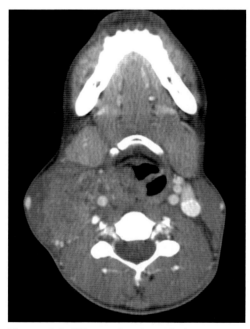

Figure 4.1 CT scan showing right hypopharynx cancer medial to the right carotid artery. Large cervical adenopathy is also seen on the same side of the neck, lateral to the carotid artery.

Laryngeal cancer

DEFINITION AND CLINICAL FEATURES

The larynx can be divided into three parts: supraglottis (epiglottis, aryepiglottic folds, false vocal folds, ventricle, arytenoids), glottis (true vocal folds), and subglottis (beneath vocal folds). The most common malignancy involving the larynx is SCC, and in most cases, a history of tobacco and/or alcohol abuse is implicated as the main causal factor. The distribution of primary sites is as follows: glottis, 50%–60%; supraglottis, 30%–40%; and subglottis, 1%–2%. For the remainder, the origin is difficult to determine. Early symptoms of laryngeal cancer include hoarseness, throat pain, hemoptysis, and dysphagia/odynophagia. As disease progresses, vocal folds may become fixed and patients may experience aspiration or develop stridor and airway compromise, occasionally necessitating emergent tracheostomy.

Based on differences in embryologic origin and lymphatic drainage patterns, cancers of supraglottic origin are far more likely to spread to regional lymph nodes than tumors of glottic origin. Nodal metastases are often bilateral. Prognosis is typically better in tumors of glottic origin compared to those of supra- or subglottic origin. Laryngeal cancer is nearly four times more common in men than women. The average age at time of diagnosis is about 65 years.

DIFFERENTIAL DIAGNOSIS

Laryngitis, laryngopharyngeal reflux disease, vocal fold nodules/polyps, respiratory papilloma, Reinke's edema.

WORKUP

Patients presenting with hoarseness or neck mass should undergo head and neck exam including in-office laryngoscopy. This will almost always reveal the tumor except for small subglottic tumors, which may be difficult to visualize on endoscopy. Biopsy should be performed but is difficult and dangerous to perform on an awake patient, so most will be taken to the OR for direct laryngoscopy and biopsy under general anesthesia. This allows for better characterization of origin and extent of the tumor. CT of the neck and chest with contrast should be obtained along with liver function tests. Esophagoscopy or esophagogram should be performed to investigate for esophageal second malignancy (Figure 4.2).

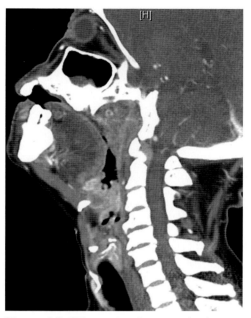

Figure 4.2 CT scan showing supraglottic larynx cancer. The enhancing mass is seen extending up to the level of the tongue base.

TREATMENT

Treatment options vary based on disease stage. For early T-stage lesions, patients are typically treated with single modality therapy. Patients with early glottic lesions may choose to undergo radiation therapy or surgical therapy, with comparable results. Surgical therapy for these lesions typically involves transoral laser resection (Figure 4.3). Early-stage supraglottic lesions require more radical surgeries such as partial laryngectomy, which may be performed open or transorally using a surgical robot. Even so, many patients opt for radiation therapy as it may be less morbid in these cases. Neck dissection is not necessary for early-stage glottic cancers but should be performed bilaterally for early-stage supraglottic lesions given the propensity for nodal spread. For later-stage diseases, surgical

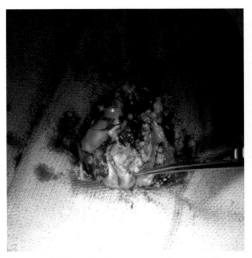

Figure 4.3 Surgical specimen of resected larynx showing extensive involvement of the larynx.

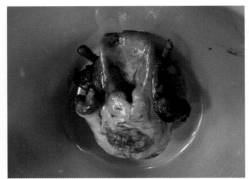

Figure 4.4 Surgical specimen of resected larynx, where the disease is located more inferiorly at the level of the cricoid cartilage.

therapy is more radical and often results in total laryngectomy. In a select subset of late-stage supraglottic cancers without significant tongue base involvement or transglottic extension, partial laryngectomy may be feasible. These patients must first undergo pulmonary function tests as they will likely have some degree of aspiration and must be able to expectorate adequately. In later-stage disease, bilateral neck dissections are performed for tumors of both glottic and supraglottic origin. Patients undergoing laryngectomy lose the ability to speak but typically have good functional swallow, although there are options for postlaryngectomy speech (electrolarynx, tracheoesophageal puncture). Some patients with late-stage disease choose primary chemoradiotherapy as it is voice-sparing. However, many of these patients suffer from radiation-induced dysphagia. Patients with recurrent disease who have failed radiation therapy or conservation surgeries are most often treated with salvage total laryngectomy. Those who have previously been radiated also often undergo either pectoralis major flap or free flap reconstruction to minimize the risk of postoperative fistula formation (Figure 4.4).

Nasopharyngeal cancer

DEFINITION AND CLINICAL FEATURES

The nasopharynx is the superior most region of the pharynx, bordered superiorly by the skull base, inferiorly by the superior surface of the soft palate, and anteriorly by the choanae, or posterior opening of the nasal cavities. The Eustachian tube orifices and adenoids are found in this region. The majority of nasopharyngeal cancers (NPCs) are SCCs. Other less common tumors include nasopharyngeal undifferentiated carcinoma and lymphomas. Significant risk factors include tobacco and alcohol abuse. NPC is also associated with Epstein–Barr virus. There are particularly high incidences in southern China and Greenland. There is a bimodal incidence, with a small peak in the second and third decades and a larger peak in the sixth and seventh decades. NPC tends to be about three times more common in males than females.

Early-stage NPC may cause few or no symptoms, and diagnosis is more often made at later disease stages. In fact, the most common presenting sign of NPC is an enlarging neck mass, indicating nodal metastatic spread. Early signs and symptoms are nonspecific and may include epistaxis, nasal obstruction and unilateral ear fullness, conductive hearing loss, or serous otitis media. As the disease progresses, cavernous sinus or intracranial extension may result in cranial neuropathies. Orbital extension may cause visual changes, diplopia, or proptosis.

DIFFERENTIAL DIAGNOSIS
Lymphoma, minor salivary tumor, sinonasal tumor, sarcoma, angiofibroma, encephalocele.

WORKUP
Since most patients present with a neck mass, contrast-enhanced CT of the neck is often the first step in workup. Detection of a nasopharyngeal tumor on scanning should prompt endoscopic exam. Biopsy should be taken as long as encephalocele can be ruled out. CT of the chest and liver function tests should be performed to evaluate for metastatic spread. While CT provides useful information, MRI may provide more detail regarding intracranial extension, cavernous sinus invasion, perineural invasion, and extent of tumor infiltration into the parapharyngeal space or pterygopalatine and infratemporal fossae (Figure 4.5).

TREATMENT
The nasopharynx is difficult to access surgically without significant morbidity. Thus, the mainstay of treatment for NPC is chemoradiotherapy. For early T-stage disease, single modality therapy may be used; this is typically external beam radiation. For later-stage disease, chemotherapy is added. Based on individual protocols, pre- or posttreatment selective neck dissection(s) may be performed or, similarly, the neck(s) may be radiated. Radiation-induced Eustachian tube dysfunction may necessitate myringotomy tube placement. Recurrent disease presents a treatment challenge—both reirradiation or salvage surgery may be used

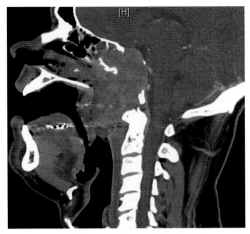

Figure 4.5 CT scan showing large nasopharyngeal cancer. The tumor erodes into the sphenoid sinus and extends intracranially to the pituitary. It also extends inferiorly to the free edge of the soft palate.

on a case-by-case basis. Both radiation and chemotherapy may be used to palliate symptoms such as bleeding, pain, and dysphagia.

Oropharyngeal cancer

DEFINITION AND CLINICAL FEATURES
The oropharynx (OP) is bordered superiorly by the inferior surface of the soft palate and inferiorly at the level of the hyoid bone. The OP contains the palatine tonsils as well as the tongue base and lingual tonsils. By far, the most common cancer arising from the OP is SCC, followed distantly by lymphomas and minor salivary tumors. Traditionally, the main risk factors for oropharyngeal SCC were tobacco and alcohol abuse. That remains true in much of the world. However, in more developed countries, the human papilloma virus (HPV), particularly type 16, is now arising as the predominant cause of oropharyngeal SCC. Higher numbers of lifetime sexual partners and oral sex partners are risk factors for HPV-related OP SCC. Compared to those

with tobacco- and alcohol-related disease, patients with HPV-related disease are typically younger and are less likely to have smoked or abused alcohol. HPV-related cancers tend to present at later stagers, yet survival is better when compared to that of non-HPV-related disease.

Early signs and symptoms may include sore throat, otalgia, dysphagia, voice changes, and neck mass. Tonsillar and palatal tumors are more easily visualized on physical exam than tongue base tumors, and typically appear as friable, ulcerated masses. Up to two-thirds of patients may have neck metastases at the time of diagnosis and these are often bilateral with more midline primary lesions. Larger tumors may cause airway obstruction or significant difficulties with feeding. Whereas OP SCC was historically associated with the poorest survival rates among head and neck SCC, survival is now improving, likely in part due to the rise in incidence of HPV-related disease.

DIFFERENTIAL DIAGNOSIS

Lymphoma, minor salivary tumor, metastatic tumor, pharyngitis, deep neck space abscess.

WORKUP

Patients with concerning histories and symptoms should undergo comprehensive head and neck exam including fiber-optic laryngoscopy. Tumors should be biopsied, and this is often easy to perform in clinic. CT with contrast of the neck and chest is performed to evaluate extent of local-regional disease, to asses for pulmonary metastases and second primary lesions. Liver function tests should be obtained. Patients should undergo esophagoscopy or esophagography to evaluate for second primaries. Thyroid function tests are included if radiation therapy is planned. MRI may be useful to assess perineural invasion, parapharyngeal space invasion, or intracranial extension.

TREATMENT

Traditionally, surgical access to the OP has required procedures with high morbidity, such as mandibulotomy. In certain early-stage tonsillar lesions, transoral approach and radical tonsillectomy may be sufficient. More recently, the advent of TORS has allowed for the surgical treatment of a greater number of OP SCCs with greatly reduced morbidity. Because of the high likelihood of metastatic spread to regional lymph nodes, neck dissection is usually performed. For small tonsillar lesions, ipsilateral dissection is typically sufficient. For larger tonsillar lesions, base of tongue lesions, and other midline lesions, bilateral neck dissection is performed. Chemoradiotherapy is commonly used as a primary treatment method and has similar outcomes when compared to surgical therapy. In early-stage disease, single modality radiation may be used. Chemoradiotherapy is the indicated treatment in surgically unresectable disease. As with other upper aerodigestive lesions, patients with OP cancers may need to undergo temporary tracheostomy and or gastrostomy tube placement. Unlike with SCC, treatment of lymphoma is nonsurgical; chemotherapy and/or radiotherapy is typically employed (Figure 4.6).

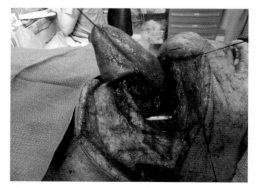

Figure 4.6 Surgical approach where the tongue has been dropped to the neck, and large left tongue base oropharyngeal tumor has been resected.

CHAPTER 5

Thyroid and Parathyroid Disease

Urjeet A. Patel, Alice C. Lin, and Christopher Vanison

- ## Multinodular goiter
- ## Papillary thyroid carcinoma
- ## Parathyroid adenoma

Multinodular goiter

DEFINITION AND CLINICAL FEATURES

Multinodular goiter is a clinical disease of diffuse or nodular overgrowth of the thyroid gland. Multinodular goiter can be further divided into two clinical entities: nontoxic and toxic goiter. Nontoxic goiters do not secrete an abnormal amount of thyroid hormone. Toxic goiters can be inflammatory or neoplastic and secrete an elevated amount of thyroid hormone. The growth of multinodular goiters is hereditary or sporadic in the majority of cases in the United States. Since the iodinization of salt, endemic goiters related to iodine deficiency are rarely seen. However, internationally, regions of iodine deficiency have an increased incidence of goiters that is proportionally related to the rate of iodine deficiency.

DIFFERENTIAL DIAGNOSIS

Thyroid nodule, thyroid malignancy, lymphoma, reactive lymphadenopathy, metastatic disease to the thyroid, Hashimoto's thyroiditis, Reidel's thyroiditis, subacute thyroiditis.

WORKUP

Physical exam may reveal an enlarged thyroid with multiple palpable nodules or cysts. All patients should be assessed for thyroid function studies. Thyroid ultrasound will reveal an enlarged thyroid with multiple nodules and/or cysts and should be used to look for suspicious characteristics of malignancy. Fine needle aspiration of suspicious thyroid nodules may be used to investigate possible thyroid malignancy. CT and MRI scans are useful to determine the relationship between the goiter and other structures such as substernal extension, tracheal compression, or relationship with the esophagus. Pulmonary function tests may also reveal airway obstruction from the goiter. Nuclear scintigraphy with radioactive iodine-123 or technetium-99m is useful in toxic multinodular goiters as they can reveal the cause of hyperthyroidism.

TREATMENT

Treatment for toxic multinodular goiters is controversial. Treatment for nontoxic multinodular goiters is only indicated for symptomatic relief. For goiters that cause no symptoms, observation alone is sufficient. Any nodules will need to be followed as multinodular goiter has the same risk of malignancy as a solitary thyroid nodule. Surgery is the definitive treatment of multinodular goiter that is causing compressive symptoms or thyrotoxicosis. In most cases, a total thyroidectomy should be performed to prevent regrowth of the remaining thyroid. Studies have shown that there is no increased risk, but there is increased benefit of a total thyroidectomy over subtotal thyroidectomy. Risks of the procedure include bleeding, recurrent laryngeal nerve injury, persistent hypoparathyroidism, or very rarely chyle leak. Most goiters with substernal extension do not require median sternotomy for removal. In patients who have a contraindication to surgery or who are older, radioactive iodine can be used. The majority of patients will experience a decrease in goiter size after radioactive iodine and the effect is dose dependent. Complications include transient hyperthyroidism and thyroiditis. The use of thyroid hormone (T4) to reduce the size of goiters is controversial in a euthyroid patient. The efficacy is disputed and the risks of creating a chronic hyperthyroid state are weighed against the benefit of shrinking the goiter. In patients with toxic goiters, thioamides and beta-adrenergic receptor antagonists can be used as a short-term treatment especially while rendering the patient euthyroid prior to radioactive iodine or surgery (Figures 5.1 and 5.2).

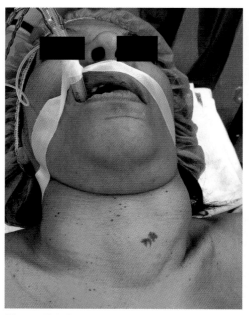

Figure 5.1 External appearance of the neck demonstrating a large multinodular goiter prior to planned resection.

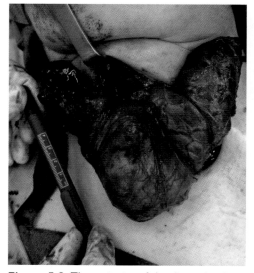

Figure 5.2 The majority of the dissection is complete, showing the bilateral gland being delivered from the surgical bed.

Papillary thyroid carcinoma

DEFINITION AND CLINICAL FEATURES

Papillary thyroid carcinoma (PTC) is the most common malignancy of the thyroid gland. Patients are most commonly diagnosed in the third to sixth decades of life and females are three times as likely as males to develop PTC. The most common presentation is a palpable thyroid nodule. Occasionally, these tumors may be detected incidentally during radiographic workup for other conditions. Rarely, PTC is discovered when a patient presents for evaluation of enlarged cervical lymph nodes. Risk factors for developing PTC include history of radiation exposure, Hashimoto's thyroiditis, low iodine diet, family history of thyroid cancer, and certain genetic conditions such as familial adenomatous polyposis (FAP). Overall, survival is excellent. Characteristics associated with poorer outcomes include male gender, age >45 years, larger tumor size, extrathyroidal spread, vascular invasion, and aggressive histologic subtype (see the following text).

The majority of PTCs are well differentiated. Poorly differentiated tumors are rare but behave more aggressively. There are several histologic subtypes of PTC, some of which behave more aggressively than typical PTC. These include Hurthle cell, tall cell, and columnar cell variants.

DIFFERENTIAL DIAGNOSIS

Benign thyroid nodule, multinodular goiter, thyroid lymphoma, medullary thyroid carcinoma, reactive lymphadenopathy, head and neck squamous cell carcinoma.

WORKUP

When a thyroid nodule is detected on exam, ultrasound will provide excellent information and can be used to guide fine needle aspiration biopsy (FNAB). Findings related to malignancy on ultrasound include hypoechogenicity and microcalcifications. MRI and CT scans are of limited use for evaluating the thyroid gland. CT may be useful to determine extent of cervical or mediastinal nodal metastasis or presence of distant metastatic disease. FNAB is safe and easily performed by experienced physicians with very high diagnostic accuracy. After treatment, surveillance for recurrence may include monitoring of serum thyroglobulin levels, serial ultrasound examination, or radionucleotide scanning. Poorly differentiated tumors may fail to produce thyroglobulin and may have decreased radioiodine avidity. In these cases, PET-CT may be very useful for detecting residual or recurrent disease.

TREATMENT

Surgery is the mainstay of treatment for PTC. In most cases, total thyroidectomy should be performed. In select cases, hemithyroidectomy or subtotal thyroidectomy is sufficient when only microscopic disease exists. Elective central neck dissection is typically performed when primary tumors are >1 cm. When lateral cervical adenopathy is present, selective or modified radical neck dissection should be performed, based on the extent of metastatic nodal involvement. Rarely, partial sternotomy must be performed to adequately resect large tumors, which have grown into the mediastinum. Major risks of thyroidectomy include recurrent laryngeal nerve injury and hypoparathyroidism and hypocalcemia. Postoperatively, patients may undergo radioactive iodine treatment when high-risk disease or residual disease is present. These patients must first become hypothyroid. Occasionally, the burden of residual disease is too great and radioiodine alone is insufficient. In these cases, external beam radiation may be offered (Figures 5.3 through 5.5).

Parathyroid adenoma

DEFINITION AND CLINICAL FEATURES

A parathyroid adenoma is a benign hypercellular neoplasm that secretes excess parathyroid hormone (PTH). An increased serum PTH causes an increase in serum calcium.

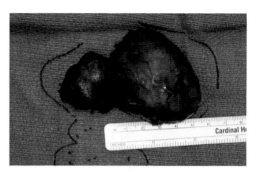

Figure 5.3 Surgical specimen of total thyroidectomy demonstrating thyroid carcinoma throughout the left lobe of the thyroid gland.

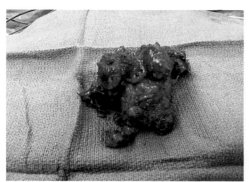

Figure 5.5 Surgical specimen of total thyroidectomy for papillary thyroid carcinoma.

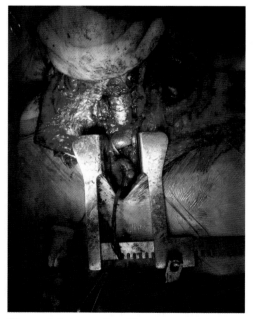

Figure 5.4 Large thyroid cancer requiring sternotomy for resection of the intrathoracic component.

In the majority of cases of primary hyperparathyroidism, a single adenoma is the source. However, a double adenoma may exist in about 10% of cases. Many cases are asymptomatic and are only discovered after a patient is incidentally noted to have elevated serum calcium on routine blood work. When

symptomatic, patients may experience joint or muscle pains, kidney stones, depressed mood, or memory loss. Most cases of parathyroid adenoma are sporadic in nature. Parathyroid hyperplasia is a rarer cause of primary hyperparathyroidism. In these cases, multiple parathyroid glands are enlarged. This is seen in multiple endocrine neoplasia (MEN) types 1 and 2a. These conditions are usually hereditary, with autosomal dominant transmission. Parathyroid adenomas are rarely palpable or visible. Normal parathyroid glands are about 3–5 mm in size. The mass of an adenoma is, on average, 10 times that of a normal gland, although there is great variation. Adenomas are about 2.5 times more common in females. They occur in all age groups, although the average age is around 60 years old.

DIFFERENTIAL DIAGNOSIS
Parathyroid hyperplasia, thyroid nodule, paraneoplastic hypercalcemia, lymphadenopathy, parathyroid carcinoma (extremely rare).

WORKUP
Hypercalcemia should prompt serum PTH testing. Phosphate and vitamin-D levels should also be tested. In cases when underlying malignancy is suspected, PTH-related protein (PTHrP) testing may be considered. For primary hyperparathyroidism,

preoperative imaging is necessary for localization purposes. While a wide array of imaging methods can be employed, the most common are ultrasound and nuclear scintigraphy (most commonly ^{99m}Tc-sestamibi scan). Nuclear scanning is fairly sensitive for locating the offending parathyroid gland; this is helpful in planning surgical intervention. Sestamibi scanning may not be as accurate in multiglandular disease and false-positives may occasionally occur in the setting of thyroid disease. SPECT imaging may be more sensitive but is less commonly used. It is common for both ultrasound and nuclear imaging to be used before treatment.

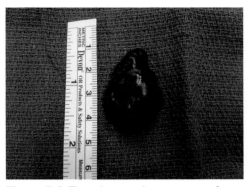

Figure 5.6 Typical size and appearance of a parathyroid adenoma, after resection for primary hypoparathyroidism.

TREATMENT

The primary treatment modality for parathyroid adenoma is surgery. Indications include symptomatic disease, severe hypercalcemia, renal failure, decreased bone mineral density, or younger age (<50). Surgery is usually performed under general anesthesia, although select cases may be performed with just local anesthetic. Traditionally, bilateral neck exploration was performed via a horizontal incision, similar to that made for a thyroidectomy. Minimally invasive approaches using smaller incisions and endoscopic resection are now being used. These approaches rely more heavily on preoperative localization. In certain cases, radiotracer material can be injected preoperatively, and the surgeon may use a handheld gamma probe for better intra-op

localization. Rarely, if an offending gland cannot be found, the surgeon must extend the approach to include areas known to contain ectopic parathyroid tissue including the superior mediastinum, carotid sheath, thyroid gland, and retroesophageal soft tissues. The use of intraoperative PTH testing is common, and rapid assays are available. Typically, a baseline PTH level is drawn prior to manipulation of any glands. When the offending gland is removed, another level is drawn about 10–20 minutes later. If the PTH level falls by at least half, it is generally considered that the abnormal tissue has been removed. Surgery is commonly performed on an outpatient basis, although occasionally, placement of a surgical drain and inpatient observation is required for a brief period (Figure 5.6).

CHAPTER 6

Reconstructive Surgery of Head and Neck Defects

Urjeet A. Patel, Alice C. Lin, and Christopher Vanison

- **Anterolateral thigh flap**
- **Fibula free flap**
- **Latissimus dorsi flap**
- **Radial forearm free flap**

Anterolateral thigh flap

DEFINITION AND CLINICAL FEATURES

The anterolateral thigh (ALT) flap is commonly used to reconstruct large head and neck defects. This is a free flap that requires reestablishment of its blood supply via microvascular anastomosis to recipient vessels in the head and neck. The ALT may be composed of skin, fat, and fascia lata, or may be used solely as a fascial flap. In some instances, the vastus lateralis muscle may be included in the flap. Its blood supply is based off the descending branch of the lateral femoral circumflex artery. On occasion, the flap can be made sensate by including the lateral femoral cutaneous nerve (Figures 6.1 through 6.3). A large skin paddle can be harvested, typically up to 8 cm × 25 cm or more in some cases, making this a good flap for reconstruction of larger wounds. The ALT has a wide array of applications in the head and neck, including reconstruction of scalp, midface, sinonasal, skull base, oral cavity, and laryngopharyngectomy defects (Figure 6.4). Contraindications to using this flap include prior injury to donor blood vessels and morbid obesity. In many cases, the donor site may be closed primarily. However, occasionally skin grafting is required. As with other free flaps, patients undergoing ALT flap reconstruction will require

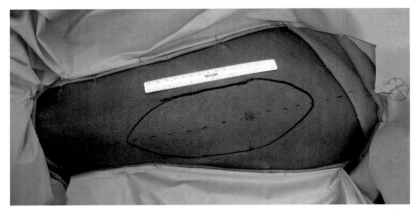

Figure 6.1 The flap is marked in the upper thigh.

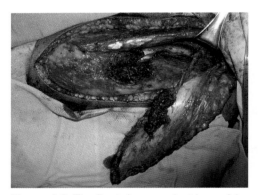

Figure 6.2 The flap is harvested with careful dissection of the vascular pedicle between the rectus and vastus lateralis.

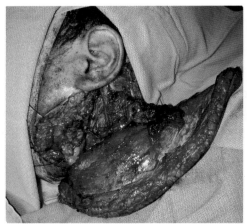

Figure 6.3 The flap is brought to the recipient bed where microvascular anastomosis is performed.

frequent flap monitoring in an intensive care unit in the immediate postoperative period. Patients can typically ambulate on the donor leg after surgery and physical therapy is rarely required. In general, very little donor site morbidity is encountered after ALT flap reconstruction (Figure 6.5).

Fibula free flap

DEFINITION AND CLINICAL FEATURES

The fibular free flap (FFF) is most commonly used to reconstruct mandibular defects. It has also been used to reconstruct skeletal midface defects after extensive trauma or maxillectomy. The flap contains bone (up to about 25 cm), a portion of the soleus muscle and a skin paddle, though skin is not always needed. In most cases, the fibula bone is adequate to support dental implants (Figures 6.6 and 6.7). The FFF blood supply is from the peroneal artery. During or after flap harvest, osteotomies can be made in the donor fibula in order to create appropriate bone contours for the recipient site (Figure 6.8). As with other free flaps, the donor vessels must undergo

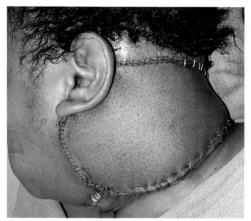

Figure 6.4 The flap is tailored to appropriate dimensions and is inset to the defect.

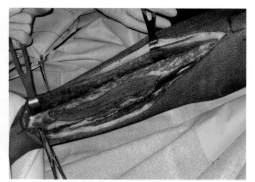

Figure 6.6 The left leg, in surgical position, with the fibula bone and skin paddle dissected from surrounding tissue in the leg.

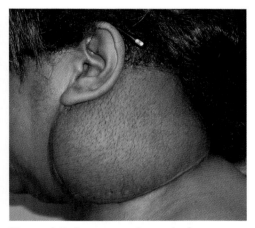

Figure 6.5 Appearance 1 month after surgery.

microvascular anastomosis to recipient vessels (Figure 6.9). During harvest, some bone is left proximally in order to avoid injuring the common peroneal nerve and distally to preserve stabilization of the ankle mortis. A contraindication to harvesting the fibula is a history of significant peripheral vascular disease. In the setting of PVD, sacrificing the peroneal artery may lead to inadequate blood supply to the foot. This is a significant concern in head and neck patients, many of whom are smokers and have comorbidities

such as diabetes and coronary artery disease. Preoperatively, patients should undergo CT angiography of the lower extremities to assess adequacy of the infrapopliteal blood vessels. Although the fibula contributes about 10% to weight-bearing capabilities of the lower extremity, patients are typically able to regain normal mobility with a short course of physical therapy. If a skin paddle is harvested with the flap, a skin graft is often required to close the donor site.

Latissimus dorsi flap

DEFINITION AND CLINICAL FEATURES

The latissimus dorsi flap (LDF) is occasionally used to reconstruct large soft tissue defects in the head and neck. It can be used as a free flap, requiring microvascular anastomosis, or as a pedicled flap, keeping it attached to its native blood supply. This is a muscle and fascia flap that can be harvested with skin, if necessary (Figure 6.10). In advanced applications, a portion of serratus anterior and underlying rib may be included. Its blood supply is based off the thoracodorsal artery, a branch of the subscapular artery. In the head and neck, the LDF is often used to reconstruct large scalp defects, although it has a broad range of applications including reconstruction of the

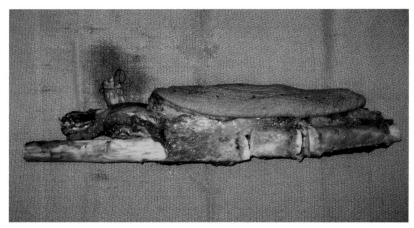

Figure 6.7 The vascular pedicle has been ligated and the flap harvested for planned reconstruction.

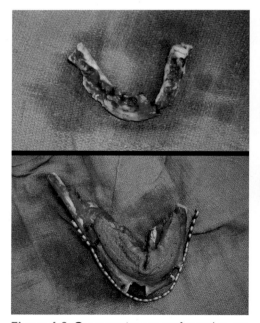

Figure 6.8 Osteotomies are performed to cut the fibula bone and shape the reconstruction to match the resected mandible and the metal reconstruction plate.

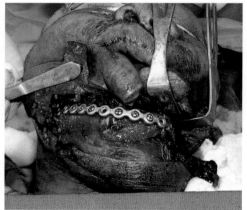

Figure 6.9 The flap and plate are positioned and secured to the native mandible to restore mandibular continuity. The microvascular anastomosis is then performed to restore blood flow.

oral cavity and oropharynx (Figure 6.11). Flaps of up to 20 cm × 40 cm can be used, making the LDF ideal for reconstructing large soft tissue defects. Primary closure of the donor site is feasible with skin paddles

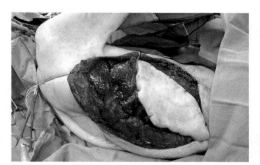

Figure 6.10 The flap is harvested from the right posterolateral trunk, with the patient in a lateral decubitus position.

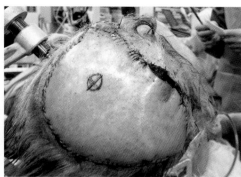

Figure 6.12 The flap is then tailored to the appropriate size and inset to the defect.

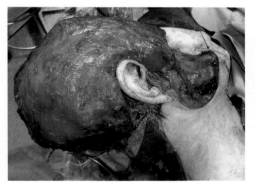

Figure 6.11 The flap is brought to the head/neck where microvascular anastomosis is performed to vessels in the right lateral neck.

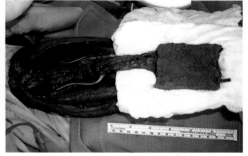

Figure 6.13 Harvest of the radial forearm flap from the left arm. The vascular pedicle is dissected toward the antecubital fossa.

up to about 10 cm. Despite the latissimus dorsi's size, harvesting this flap results in little to no functional deficit. The only contraindication to using this flap is prior damage to the donor thoracodorsal vasculature (Figure 6.12).

Radial forearm free flap

DEFINITION AND CLINICAL FEATURES

The radial forearm free flap (RFFF) is an extremely versatile flap used quite commonly in the reconstruction of head and neck defects. The flap is composed of skin and fascia, although in some instances the palmaris longus tendon and a rim of the radius bone may also be included. RFFF is harvested from the distal aspect of the volar surface of the forearm (Figure 6.13). Its blood supply is from the radial artery. As with other free flaps, its vessels must be anastomosed to recipient vessels in the head and neck using microvascular techniques. The most common application of the RFFF in the head and neck is in the reconstruction of oral cavity defects including tongue, floor of mouth, and buccal mucosal surfaces.

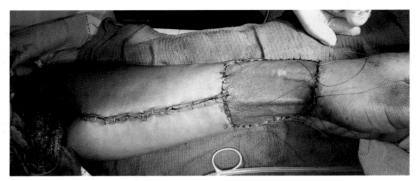

Figure 6.14 The donor site is closed with a split thickness skin graft.

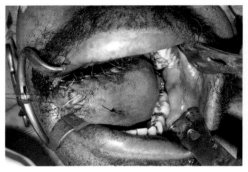

Figure 6.15 The flap is inset to the left lateral tongue and floor of the mouth following surgical resection of an oral tongue cancer.

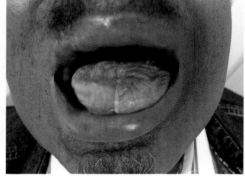

Figure 6.16 Appearance of the flap 6 months after surgery.

However, it is also utilized to reconstruct many other defects including those of the palate, pharynx, cervical esophagus, skull base, and skin. It is a thin flap and thus not a good choice in reconstructing areas that require significant soft tissue bulk. Because of its pliability, RFFF can be used to reconstruct complex 3D defects. Use of this flap may be contraindicated when there is prior radial artery trauma or if there is insufficient collateral blood flow to the hand from the ulnar arterial system. The latter may be assessed preoperatively with an Allen's test. It is possible, during harvest, that the superficial branches of the radial nerve can be injured, resulting in numbness in the lateral digits. For this reason, the nondominant hand is often chosen. If bone is harvested, there is a risk of pathologic fracture of the donor radius. Closure of the donor site requires skin grafting (Figure 6.14). There is usually little to no donor site morbidity and postoperative physical therapy is rarely required (Figures 6.15 and 6.16).

SECTION 2

RHINOLOGY

CHAPTER 7

General Rhinology

Jeffrey M. Hotaling and Monica Oberoi Patadia

Normal nasal anatomy: Turbinates, septum, and paranasal sinuses

The nasal cavity can be conceptualized as a triangle divided sagittally in half by the nasal septum, which is composed of cartilage anteriorly and bone posteriorly. Each nasal cavity is bounded superiorly by the cribriform plate of the anterior cranial fossa, inferiorly by the hard and soft palate, and laterally by the orbit and maxillary sinus.[1] The nasal cavity's anterior limit is the bony pyriform aperture, and it is continuous with the nasopharynx posteriorly via the posterior nasal aperture or choana. The lateral wall of each nasal cavity typically has three bony turbinates (or conchae) projecting inferomedially into the nasal cavity: the inferior turbinate, middle turbinate, and superior turbinate. The spaces confined below each of these turbinates are referred to as the inferior, middle, and superior meatuses, corresponding with the turbinate defining each space. These turbinates increase the surface area of the nose and serve to humidify and clean the inhaled air.[2] The inferior turbinate is the largest of these projections and can be easily visualized on anterior rhinoscopy.

The paranasal sinuses are paired, mucosa-lined structures contiguous with the nasal cavity, consisting of pneumatized spaces within the maxillary, ethmoid, frontal, and sphenoid bones. The frontal sinus consists of two paired air cells within the frontal bone separated by an intersinus septum, which drain inferiorly into the middle meatus. The frontal sinus is the last to develop and is typically not present at birth; full development continues into early adulthood although 10%–12% of frontal sinuses remain underdeveloped and hypoplastic.[3] The ethmoid sinuses are actually a complex of two large groups of cells that are separated by the basal or ground lamella of the middle turbinate: the anterior ethmoid air cells that drain into the middle meatus and the posterior ethmoid cells that drain into the superior meatus. These air cells are the most mature of the paranasal sinuses at birth, reaching adult dimensions by about 12 years of age. Importantly, ethmoid air cells can expand beyond the boundaries of the ethmoid bone, pneumatizing superolaterally into the sphenoid bone (sphenoethmoidal or Onodi cells) or laterally into the maxillary bone (infraorbital ethmoid or Haller cells).[2]

The maxillary sinuses are large, paired air cells that lie between the orbit and hard palate that drain medially into the middle meatus. The maxillary sinuses are hypoplastic at birth, typically reaching adult dimensions around 12 years of age. The maxillary sinuses drain into the middle meatus, contributing to form the osteomeatal complex, which is a common channel linking the drainage pathways of the maxillary, frontal, and anterior ethmoid sinuses. The osteomeatal complex is an anatomically constricted area that is prone to obstruction.[4] A concha bullosa, which is an air cell within the middle turbinate, may often contribute to narrowing of this osteomeatal complex. The sphenoid sinus is the most posterior and medial of the paranasal sinuses, situated between the cavernous sinuses at the central skull base. The sphenoid sinuses are intimately related to the optic nerves and carotid artery and are divided into right and left by an irregular intersinus septum.

The sphenoid sinus typically begins to develop at age 1, reaching adult size by approximately 12 years of age. The sphenoid sinuses drain anteriorly into the sphenoethmoidal recess located above the superior turbinate (Figures 7.1 through 7.3).[1,2]

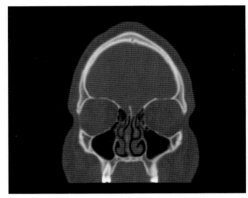

Figure 7.1 CT sinus scan, coronal view showing a patient with normal sinuses. Note the slight deviation of the septum to the right and the paradoxic curvature of each middle turbinate.

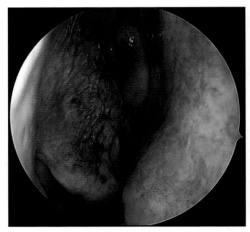

Figure 7.2 Endoscopic view of the right nasal cavity showing the inferior turbinate (anatomic right), middle turbinate (center), and nasal septum (anatomic left).

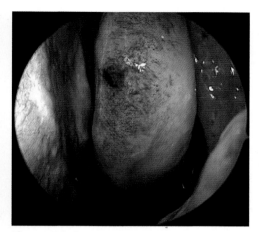

Figure 7.3 Endoscopic view of the left nasal cavity showing the middle turbinate (center), uncinate process (anatomic left), and nasal septum (anatomic right). The turbinate appears pale because this photo was taken intraoperatively after injection with 1% lidocaine with epinephrine, 1:100,000.

Allergic rhinitis

DEFINITIONS AND CLINICAL FEATURES
Allergic rhinitis is an IgE-mediated clinical hypersensitivity of the nasal mucosa to inhaled substances with a prevalence of 10%–20% in the United States. Although individuals of any age can be affected, onset is most frequently in adolescents with a decreasing incidence with advancing age.[5] Patients classically present with recurrent episodes of sneezing, rhinorrhea, nasal congestion, pruritus, and lacrimation. Pruritus is the symptom most suggestive of an allergic etiology and can be nasal, orbital, pharyngeal, or even palatal. Patients with perennial allergies may not have the classic symptoms of pruritus and sneezing and are more likely to present with nasal congestion only. In contrast to the purulent rhinorrhea in bacterial rhinosinusitis, rhinorrhea in allergic rhinitis is typically clear. The rhinorrhea can

be anterior, resulting in sniffing and nose-blowing, or posterior, leading to postnasal drip and symptoms of laryngopharyngeal reflux. The nasal congestion associated with allergic rhinitis is most usually episodic and may be unilateral, bilateral, or even on alternate sides in a cyclical fashion. Ocular symptoms including pruritus, lacrimation, and conjunctival injection are common.

On examination, patients may have conjunctival injection, generalized edema of the eyelids, and, particularly in children, so-called allergic shiners (periorbital cyanosis). Anterior rhinoscopy will classically demonstrate pale, boggy, and/or bluish inferior turbinates with diffusely edematous nasal mucosa coated with thin, clear secretions (Figures 7.4 and 7.5). In severe allergic rhinitis, nasal endoscopy may also demonstrate polypoid degeneration of the middle and inferior turbinates.

Allergic rhinitis can be seasonal or perennial and may be a combination of both. As its name suggests, seasonal allergic rhinitis

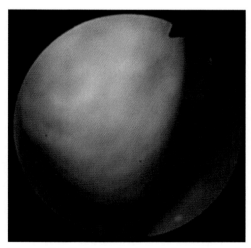

Figure 7.4 Endoscopic view of the right nasal cavity demonstrating a pale, hypertrophic, and boggy inferior turbinate consistent with allergic rhinitis.

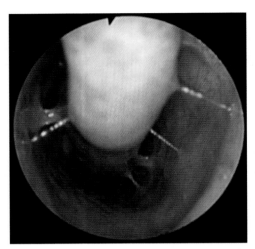

Figure 7.5 Endoscopic view of the right nasal cavity demonstrating an inferior turbinate with clear mucoid secretions, often an exam finding consistent with allergic rhinitis.

varies by season, with symptoms occurring or exacerbated by the seasonal pollination of plants to which the individual is allergic. While allergens vary by geographic location, trees usually pollinate in the spring, grass pollinates in the summer, and weeds pollinate in the fall. In contrast, perennial allergic rhinitis is more likely to present with only nasal symptoms and is frequently due to indoor allergens including dust mites, indoor molds, and animal dander, which is present year-round.

DIFFERENTIAL DIAGNOSIS

Infectious rhinitis (bacterial or viral), nonallergic rhinitis (vasomotor rhinitis), mechanical nasal obstruction (deviated nasal septum), rhinitis medicamentosa, granulomatous rhinitis (Wegener's granulomatosis, sarcoidosis), and neoplastic rhinitis (nasal polyposis, malignant nasal tumors).

WORKUP

Although clinical examination and history often point to the diagnosis of allergic rhinitis, allergy testing remains an important means of differentiating between allergic and nonallergic rhinitis. The two most common tests used to confirm the diagnosis of allergic rhinitis are skin-prick testing and in vitro immunoassays, more appropriately known as serum specific IgE testing. Skin testing is performed by injecting antigen extracts into the dermis with a subsequent wheal reaction indicating hypersensitivity to that antigen. Although fast and inexpensive, skin testing has relative contraindications including uncontrolled asthma, dermatographism, and prior history of anaphylaxis. Skin testing is safe, but there is always a risk of local or systemic reaction, especially in a *brittle* patient that is tested during peak allergy season. In order for skin testing to be accurate, patient must be off antihistamine medications for at least 5 days and must have a positive histamine control and negative control wheal. There is an increased risk of false-positives compared to blood testing, and sensitivity declines in patients older than 50.

In contrast, although in vitro testing for specific serum IgE levels to specific allergens eliminates the risk of anaphylaxis and the need for multiple skin pricks, it is more expensive and often less sensitive than skin-prick testing.[5–7] It remains a good option for patients with contraindications noted earlier and is a highly specific test.

TREATMENT

The treatment triad for allergic rhinitis includes environmental control/avoidance, pharmacotherapy, and immunotherapy. Simple avoidance of allergens and decreased exposure should always be emphasized, but is often not sufficient for symptom control and near impossible when a patient owns pets they are allergic to, for example.

The mainstay of pharmacotherapy is intranasal steroids. Multiple studies have demonstrated the effectiveness of these agents in reducing all nasal symptoms in patients with allergic rhinitis within 7–8 hours of dosing although maximal efficacy requires days of administration.[8]

Synergistic effects have been noted with the addition of intranasal antihistamine sprays. Second-generation antihistamines are also commonly employed, and are rapidly efficacious in controlling histamine-induced symptoms such as rhinorrhea, itching, and sneezing. Leukotriene modifiers can be used to modulate the allergic pathway aside from histamine control. Adjunctive therapies including anticholinergic nasal sprays are employed especially for patients with vasomotor or nonallergic rhinitis. The first FDA-approved sublingual grass and ragweed immunotherapy tablets have hit the market in the spring of 2014. These pills require administration of the first dose in the doctor's office and have relative contraindications similar to allergy testing and subcutaneous immunotherapy.

Allergen-specific immunotherapy is an option and involves the repeated subcutaneous administration of progressively increasing doses of antigen extract with the goal of altering the patient's immunologic responses to the allergen. Indications for this include patients who fail medication management, patients who wish to avoid medications, patients who have symptoms >6 months of the year or are looking for a cure to allergies.

Adjunctive surgical maneuvers including septoplasty and turbinate reduction remain options for patients with underlying anatomic obstruction and persistent congestion with treatment failure.

Turbinate hypertrophy

DEFINITIONS AND CLINICAL FEATURES
The nasal turbinates are projections extending inferomedially from the lateral walls of the nasal cavity. There are three turbinates or conchae on each side, named based on their position on the lateral nasal wall: the superior turbinate, middle turbinate, and inferior turbinate, respectively. In some individuals, there is a fourth turbinate above the superior turbinate, the supreme turbinate. Each turbinate is composed of a thin, central layer of bone with overlying, adherent mucoperiosteum. These turbinates, particularly the inferior and middle turbinates, serve to increase the total mucosal surface of the nose, thereby increasing the nasal cavity's ability to humidify and warm inspired air.[9]

Hypertrophy of these turbinates can be classified as either bony or mucosal and is a common cause of symptomatic nasal obstruction. Bony hypertrophy refers to a congenitally large turbinate, often with a broad inferolateral osseous turn. Mucosal hypertrophy is much more common, often secondary to conditions such as allergic rhinitis, causing chronic mucosal inflammation.[10] This hypertrophy most commonly affects the inferior turbinate and is typically seen bilaterally. As physiologic studies have demonstrated that 50% of nasally inspired air passes along the nasal floor, inferior turbinate hypertrophy, in particular, can have a dramatic effect on nasal breathing. Clinically, patients with turbinate hypertrophy will present with nasal obstruction, which is most often bilateral, although there may be some asymmetric variation in tune with the nasal cycle (see Figure 7.4).

While bony turbinate hypertrophy can cause a unilateral obstruction, persistent unilateral nasal obstruction is more commonly due to a deviated nasal septum. Anterior rhinoscopy will demonstrate large inferior or middle turbinates, which may completely obstruct the nasal cavity and prohibit endoscopic examination. These patients may also have signs and symptoms of allergic or nonallergic rhinitis, including rhinorrhea and pruritus, and may give a history of seasonal variation of symptoms.

DIFFERENTIAL DIAGNOSIS
Deviated nasal septum, allergic rhinitis, nonallergic (vasomotor) rhinitis, internal or external nasal valve collapse, nasal polyposis, nasal mass including inverted papilloma versus malignancy.

WORKUP

Physical examination including anterior rhinoscopy and endoscopy remains the mainstay of diagnosis of turbinate hypertrophy. CT scans will elucidate any bony component to the turbinate hypertrophy but are not required to make the diagnosis. It is also important to identify any narrowing or dynamic collapse of nasal structures with nasal breathing as this suggests underlying nasal valve collapse rather than obstruction purely from enlarged turbinates. A thorough history is also important in detecting any seasonal variation or accompanying allergic symptoms, which would point to a diagnosis of allergic rhinitis. Relief of nasal congestion and obstruction with topical decongestants also indicates mucosal turbinate hypertrophy and can easily be performed in the doctor's office. Nasal obstruction may also be assessed objectively by means of acoustic or airflow rhinometry, although this is rarely necessary and usually not performed in the clinical setting.

TREATMENT

Most important in the treatment of turbinate hypertrophy is elucidation of the underlying cause of the hypertrophied turbinate(s). Primary treatment consists of an intranasal topical steroid, possibly with the addition of an antihistamine nasal spray in those patients with an allergic component. Surgery is reserved for patients who fail medical management and surgical intervention is frequently limited to the inferior turbinate. Soft tissue submucous reduction or resection of the turbinates remains the mainstay of surgical management and may be performed using electrocautery, radiofrequency techniques, or a microdebrider. Simple lateralization of the inferior turbinate is often performed in conjunction with turbinate reduction in order to change the position of the turbinate within the nasal cavity and thereby improve airflow.[11] While submucous resection of the bony turbinate may be indicated if this bony component is a large contributor to overall turbinate hypertrophy, full-thickness turbinate resection is limited to patients with recalcitrant disease and extensive resection may lead to the paradoxical nasal obstruction of so-called empty nose syndrome.[12]

Septal deviation

DEFINITIONS AND CLINICAL FEATURES

The nasal septum is a sagittally oriented structure composed of bone and cartilage, which divides the nose into two separate nasal cavities and serves as the main support for the external nose. More specifically, the nasal septum is composed of septal cartilage (the quadrangular cartilage) anteriorly, the perpendicular plate of the ethmoid bone posterosuperiorly, and the bony vomer posteroinferiorly.[1,13] Deviation of the nasal septum is a very common cause of unilateral nasal obstruction and patients may give a history of trauma to the nose. In many cases, however, there is no clear history of facial trauma, and the deviation may be secondary to either birth trauma or microfractures sustained in early life leading to asymmetric growth of the cartilage.[14] Interestingly, several studies have demonstrated that a nondeviated septum is present in only 7.5%–23% of patients, making septal deformity extremely common.[10]

Paradoxically, patients with a deviated nasal septum will often present with subjective nasal obstruction on the side contralateral to the deviation, which is secondary to a compensatory hypertrophy of the inferior turbinate on the unobstructed side. Septal deviations can involve the bony or cartilaginous nasal septum and can take the form of a single septal spur or a C- or even S-shaped deviation of the entire septum. These septal irregularities can even result in aesthetic deformity including columellar irregularities, twisting of the nasal dorsum, and underprojection of the nasal tip.[15] However, it is important to note that septal deviation is not always symptomatic, and studies have indicated that the degree of septal deviation has little correlation with a patient's level of symptoms.[14]

DIFFERENTIAL DIAGNOSIS

Allergic rhinitis, nonallergic rhinitis, nasal polyposis, internal or external nasal valve collapse, turbinate hypertrophy.

WORKUP

Anterior rhinoscopy and nasal endoscopy both allow visualization of the nasal septum. However, while anterior septal deviations are easily visualized on anterior rhinoscopy, more posterior deviations and spurs may only be visualized via endoscopic evaluation. This examination should be performed both before and after decongestion in order to evaluate the contribution of mucosal edema of the turbinates and septum to the patient's obstruction. It is also important to rule out any dynamic narrowing of the nostrils, nasal vestibule, and nasal lumen with inhalation, as this would suggest nasal valve compromise as playing a role in the patient's obstruction. Imaging is rarely necessary unless concomitant paranasal sinus disease is suspected. Acoustic and airflow rhinometry may be used to provide objective measures of nasal obstruction.

TREATMENT

Prior to any surgical intervention, patients with symptomatic deviations of their nasal septums are started on a topical nasal steroid spray, antihistamines, and even decongestants. Patients with persistent nasal obstruction despite medical treatment may be offered a septoplasty, a procedure in which deviated septal cartilage and bone is either removed or realigned to straighten the nasal septum. Patients with very anterior or caudal deviations of their nasal septum, however, may require an open rhinoplasty approach to correct their septal deviation.[15] Additionally, as patients with septal deviations often have hypertrophy

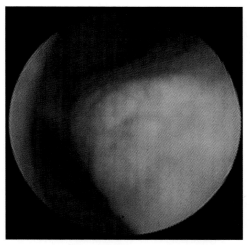

Figure 7.6 Endoscopic view of the right nasal cavity demonstrating a significant nasal septal deviation to the right abutting the inferior turbinate. Note the flattened appearance of the inferior turbinate due to the septal spur.

of the inferior turbinate on the side opposite the deviation, turbinate reduction/resection is often performed concurrently (Figures 7.6 and 7.7).

Septal perforation

DEFINITIONS AND CLINICAL FEATURES

Nasal septal perforations are defined as a direct communication (or fistula) between the two nasal cavities across the nasal septum and are relatively common, affecting almost 1% of the general population.[16] While these perforations may occur as the result of inflammatory, neoplastic, or autoimmune processes, the overwhelming majority are either secondary to trauma or are iatrogenically produced. Iatrogenic causes include surgery, septal cauterization, and intranasal packing. While illegal drugs including cocaine may cause septal perforations, prescription and over-the-counter medications including intranasal steroids and topical vasoconstrictors can

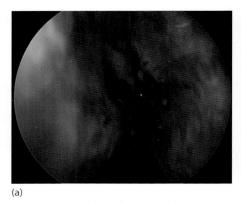

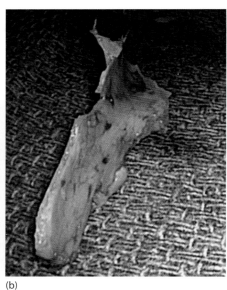

(a)   (b)

Figure 7.7 (a) Endoscopic view of the left nasal cavity demonstrating left septal deviation. (b) Intraoperative view of the deviated quadrangular cartilage after a septoplasty.

also produce perforations when used in high doses. Because the mucoperichondrium of the nasal septum is responsible for the blood supply to the relatively avascular septal cartilage, disruption of this mucosal covering on opposing locations via mechanical or chemical trauma can lead to ischemic necrosis of the cartilage, producing an ulceration and, ultimately, a perforation. The turbulent airflow over the edges of the perforation leads to crusting and bleeding, which may also lead to progressive enlargement of the perforation.[17]

Patients with larger and more anteriorly located perforations will often complain of epistaxis, nasal crusting, nasal obstruction, and rhinorrhea. Smaller perforations may actually cause whistling with nasal breathing due to the turbulent airflow across the perforation.[17] Extremely large perforations can eventually result in changes to the external nose including loss of septal support ("saddle nose") and nasal tip collapse. As up to 92% of nasal septal perforations are located anteriorly, septal perforations are often easily recognized on anterior rhinoscopy.[18] Perforations located more posteriorly or superiorly may require nasal endoscopy for visualization (see Figures 7.8 through 7.10).

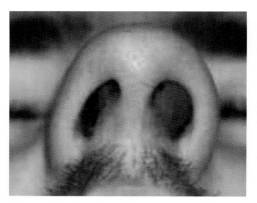

Figure 7.8 Anterior rhinoscopy revealing a widened and soft nasal septum, indicative of a septal hematoma. This patient was involved in a nasal trauma. If left untreated, a septal hematoma can ultimately lead to a septal perforation and/or saddle nose deformity.

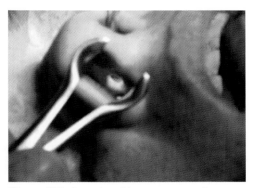

Figure 7.9 Anterior rhinoscopy revealing a caudal septal perforation. This can result in a bothersome whistling or drying sensation to the nose and must either be repaired or monitored such that it does not enlarge.

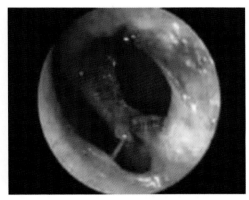

Figure 7.10 Large septal perforation with surrounding friable edges and crusting.

DIFFERENTIAL DIAGNOSIS

Nasal septal ulceration, history of nasal septal fracture, history of prior nasal surgery or nasal trauma, history of prior prolonged nasal spray use, autoimmune disease process, drug abuse, malignancy, and infection.

WORKUP

A careful history is the most important component in the workup with patients with septal perforations as it is prudent to determine the cause of the perforation prior to undertaking any sort of repair. Pertinent inquiries regarding prior nasal procedures (including nasal cauterization and packing), nasal trauma, and cocaine or excessive vasoconstrictor use will reveal the etiology for the majority of patients. Chronic infections and autoimmune disease can also lead to septal perforation, which can be investigated by means of laboratory tests, radiographs, biopsies, and cultures. Endoscopic examination of the septum is the best means of evaluation, as it enables visualization of the entire perforation and the anatomic details including location, size, and status of the edges of the perforation. Patients with inflamed or actively ulcerating lesions of the septum should undergo biopsy of the posterior edge of the perforation with tissue sent both for pathology and culture.[19] Imaging is rarely required except when a more systemic process or coexisting sinus disease is suspected.

TREATMENT

Asymptomatic nasal septal perforations or those giving rise to only intermittent symptoms may be treated conservatively with nasal saline sprays, regular humidification, and lubricating ointments to help prevent crusting. Patients with large perforations or more regular symptoms may undergo placement of a septal button, which is a silastic disk that straddles the perforation to close the perforation. Septal buttons are easily placed in the doctor's office under local anesthesia and may remain in place for over a year. Septal buttons have been demonstrated to improve the rates of epistaxis, nasal airway obstruction, and whistling in patients with septal perforations.[17] Surgical repair is typically reserved for symptomatic patients without underlying chronic infection or autoimmune diseases. It should also be considered for those with an anteriorly located perforation where concern for collapse or saddle nose exists. Depending on the size and location of the perforation, surgical closure may be attempted via an endonasal or external rhinoplasty approach, often employing some form of interposition graft (cartilage, fascia, dermal allografts) layered in between intranasal mucosal flaps.[20] Large defects (>2 cm) may require regional or free microvascular flaps for closure.

Epistaxis

DEFINITIONS AND CLINICAL FEATURES

Epistaxis is extremely common with an estimated lifetime incidence of 60%.[21] Despite this high incidence, there is a large range in severity of episodes with only 6% requiring medical attention.[22] This disparity between incidence and severity is in large part due to the vascular anatomy of the nasal cavity, which has many anastomoses and receives contributions from both the internal and external carotid systems. While epistaxis is frequently idiopathic in nature, it may result from myriad local and systemic causes. Common local causes including nasal trauma, nasal neoplasms, septal deviations, and chemical irritation; systemic causes including coagulopathies, renal/liver failure, and vascular abnormalities are less common but often more difficult to manage.[23] Importantly, anticoagulants including warfarin, enoxaparin, clopidogrel, and NSAIDs have also been linked with epistaxis.[22]

Clinically, epistaxis is typically divided into anterior and posterior bleeding based upon the anatomic location of the bleeding and the clinical severity. Anterior bleeding is defined as that which is easily visible and controlled via anterior rhinoscopy. Anterior epistaxis most commonly arises from a plexus of vessels on the anterior septum referred to as Little's or Kesselbach's area, which is a site of anastomosis between the internal and external carotid systems. Posterior epistaxis, which is more difficult to visualize and often more profuse, typically emanates from branches of the sphenopalatine and posterior ethmoid arteries.[23] While some patients may present with minor unilateral bleeding, more severe epistaxis may result in bilateral arterial hemorrhaging with hemoptysis and the potential for airway compromise or exsanguination.

DIFFERENTIAL DIAGNOSIS

Neoplasm, vascular malformation, juvenile nasopharyngeal angiofibroma, allergic rhinitis, coagulopathy, hereditary hemorrhagic telangiectasia.

WORKUP

In patients with minor bleeds who are hemodynamically stable, a patient history should be taken to distinguish recurrent bleeding versus a solitary episode, unilateral versus bilateral bleeding, and any history of recent nasal trauma or surgery. Also important to elucidate are any underlying medications or medical conditions that may predispose the patient to bleeding as well as a family history of epistaxis and death. Physical examination is often challenging in patients with epistaxis and should include a full head and neck exam to evaluate for vascular lesions as well as examination of the oropharynx for any bleeding or clots. Nasal examination should initially consist of anterior rhinoscopy, with nasal endoscopy necessary for evaluation of more posterior sources. Laboratory evaluation is typically necessary only in patients with recurrent epistaxis and those on anticoagulation therapy. Similarly, radiographic evaluation is rarely necessary except in cases of facial trauma and concern for nasal neoplasms.

TREATMENT

Paramount in the management of epistaxis is establishment of both the site and the cause of bleeding. In any nosebleed, application of topical vasoconstrictors such as 1% phenylephrine or 0.05% oxymetazoline is the first line of treatment with the goal of stopping the bleeding and improving visualization. In patients with anterior bleeds, the addition of external nasal compression for 10–30 minutes may actually control the bleeding. Once the site origin of the bleeding has been identified, it can be cauterized with silver nitrate. Care should be used to only perform unilateral cautery to prevent occurrence of a septal perforation. Electrocautery can also be used, but typically requires application of an anesthetic. If local therapy fails or the bleeding cannot be pinpointed, nasal packing is required. Importantly, patients should be on antistaphylococcal prophylaxis while packing remains in place, which is typically 3–5 days. If recalcitrant or recurrent, epistaxis may require surgical ligation of the affected arterial distribution, namely, the sphenopalatine or ethmoidal arteries. This may be done endoscopically or via open approaches with reported success rates of endoscopic sphenopalatine artery ligation as high as 75%–100%.[24] Selective arterial embolization is another viable option for control of epistaxis, particularly in cases where surgery fails or the patient is unable to tolerate general anesthesia. Success rates of embolization are on par with that of surgical ligation, but embolization carries the additional risks of tissue necrosis, blindness, and cerebrovascular accidents.[21]

References

1. Wiggins RH, III. 2006. Sinonasal overview. In: Harnsberger, HR and Macdonald, AJ (eds.), *Diagnostic and Surgical Imaging Anatomy: Brain, Head & Neck, Spine*. Salt Lake City, UT: Amirsys, pp. 104–113.
2. Wise SK, Richard RO, John MD. 2012. Sinonasal development and anatomy. In: David, WK and Peter, HH (eds.), *Rhinology: Diseases of the Nose, Sinuses, and Skull Base*. New York: Thieme, pp. 1–19.
3. McLaughlin RB, Jr., Rehl RM, Lanza DC. 2001. Clinically relevant frontal sinus anatomy and physiology. *Otolaryngologic Clinics of North America* 34:1–22.
4. Wiggins RH, III. 2006. Ostiomeatal unit (OMU). In: Harnsberger, HR and Macdonald, AJ (eds.), *Diagnostic and Surgical Imaging Anatomy: Brain, Head & Neck, Spine*. Salt Lake City, UT: Amirsys, pp. 114–117.
5. Baroody FM, Robert MN. 2010. Immunology of the upper airway and pathophysiology and treatment of allergic rhinitis. In: Flint, PW (ed.), *Cummings Otolaryngology: Head & Neck Surgery*. Philadelphia, PA: Mosby Elsevier, pp. 597–623.
6. Corriveau MN, Bachert C. 2012. Allergic and nonallergic rhinitis. In: Kennedy, DW and Hwang, PH (eds.), *Rhinology: Diseases of the Nose, Sinuses, and Skull Base*. New York: Thieme, pp. 82–91.
7. Hamilos DL. 2012. Principles of allergy skin testing and immunotherapy. In: Kennedy, DW and Hwang, PH (eds.), *Rhinology: Diseases of the Nose, Sinuses, and Skull Base*. New York: Thieme, pp. 92–103.
8. Meltzer EO. 2011. The role of nasal corticosteroids in the treatment of rhinitis. *Immunology and Allergy Clinics of North America* 31:545–560.
9. Nurse LA, Duncavage JA. 2009. Surgery of the inferior and middle turbinates. *Otolaryngologic Clinics of North America* 42:295–309.
10. Neskey D, Eloy JA, Casiano RR. 2009. Nasal, septal, and turbinate anatomy and embryology. *Otolaryngologic Clinics of North America* 42:193–205.
11. Larrabee YC, Kacker A. 2014. Which inferior turbinate reduction technique best decreases nasal obstruction? *Laryngoscope* 124:814–815.
12. Goyal P, Hwang PH. 2012. Surgery of the septum and turbinates. In: Kennedy, DW and Hwang, PH (eds.), *Rhinology: Diseases of the Nose, Sinuses, and Skull Base*. New York: Thieme, pp. 444–456.
13. Stamm AC, Cassol A, Pignatari SSN. 2010. Transnasal endoscopic-assisted surgery of the anterior skull base. In: Flint, PW (ed.), *Cummings Otolaryngology: Head & Neck Surgery*. Philadelphia, PA: Mosby Elsevier, pp. 2471–2485.

14. Fettman N, Sanford T, Sindwani R. 2009. Surgical management of the deviated septum: Techniques in septoplasty. *Otolaryngologic Clinics of North America* 42:241–252.

15. Haak J, Papel ID. 2009. Caudal septal deviation. *Otolaryngologic Clinics of North America* 42:427–436.

16. Oberg D, Akerlund A, Johansson L et al. 2003. Prevalence of nasal septal perforation: The Skovde population-based study. *Rhinology* 41:72–75.

17. Lanier B, Kai G, Marple B, Wall GM. 2007. Pathophysiology and progression of nasal septal perforation. *Annals of Allergy, Asthma and Immunology* 99:473–479.

18. Diamantopoulos JNS, II. 2001. The investigation of nasal septal perforations and ulcers. *Journal of Laryngology and Otology* 115:541–544.

19. Watson D, Barkdull G. 2009. Surgical management of the septal perforation. *Otolaryngologic Clinics of North America* 42:483–493.

20. Kim SW, Rhee CS. 2012. Nasal septal perforation repair: Predictive factors and systematic review of the literature. *Current Opinion in Otolaryngology & Head and Neck Surgery* 20:58–65.

21. Vaughan W, Khanna K, Fong K. 2012. Epistaxis. In: Kennedy, DW and Hwang, PH (eds.), *Rhinology: Diseases of the Nose, Sinuses, and Skull Base*. New York: Thieme, pp. 491–502.

22. Simmen DB, Jones NS. 2010. Epistaxis. In: Flint, PW (ed.), *Cummings Otolaryngology: Head & Neck Surgery*. Philadelphia, PA: Mosby Elsevier, pp. 682–693.

23. Gifford TO, Orlandi RR. 2008. Epistaxis. *Otolaryngologic Clinics of North America* 41:525–536.

24. Barnes ML, Spielmann PM, White PS. 2012. Epistaxis: A contemporary evidence based approach. *Otolaryngologic Clinics of North America* 45:1005–1017.

CHAPTER 8

Sinusitis

Muhamad A. Amine and Monica Oberoi Patadia

- **Acute rhinosinusitis**
- **Chronic rhinosinusitis**
- **Nasal polyposis**
- **Allergic fungal sinusitis**
- **Subperiosteal abscess**
- **Suggested reading**

Acute rhinosinusitis

DEFINITION AND CLINICAL FEATURES

Acute rhinosinusitis (ARS) is defined as symptoms due to inflammation of the sinonasal cavities for less than a 4-week duration. Diagnostic criterion is defined as the presence of three cardinal symptoms lasting up to 4 weeks—purulent nasal discharge (Figure 8.1) plus nasal obstruction, facial pain–pressure–fullness, or both. In addition, ARS can be characterized by fever, cough, fatigue, hyposmia, dental pain, or ear fullness or pressure; however, these symptoms are less sensitive and specific. ARS can be divided into viral and bacterial. Viral ARS is more common and often preceded by an upper respiratory infection in which nasal contents are blown into the sinuses. Rhinovirus followed by influenza and parainfluenza viruses was the most commonly aspirated virus from sinus puncture studies of patients with acute community-acquired rhinosinusitis. The most common bacterial isolates include *Streptococcus pneumoniae, Haemophilus influenzae,* and *Moraxella catarrhalis.* Viral ARS is complicated by secondary bacterial ARS 0.5%–2% of the time. In order to truly distinguish between viral and bacterial ARS, one must obtain a culture; however, this is not practical given the incidence in the general population. Therefore, in order to distinguish between the two, one must rely on illness pattern and duration. Bacterial ARS is suspected if symptoms last more than 10 days, if there is worsening after an initial period of improvement, or if symptoms are severe with fevers >39°C/102°F, facial pain and purulent drainage that lasts for at least three consecutive days.

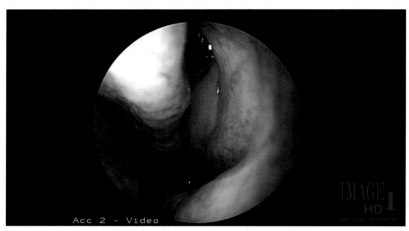

Figure 8.1 Thick yellow purulence emanating from the left osteomeatal complex.

DIFFERENTIAL DIAGNOSIS

Upper respiratory infection, viral ARS, bacterial ARS, chronic rhinosinusitis (CRS), allergic rhinitis, nasal foreign body, migraine headaches, dental infection.

WORKUP

Diagnosis is based on history and physical. Routine imaging is not recommended unless a complication is suspected such as orbital, intracranial, or soft tissue involvement. When a complication is suspected, CT imaging with contrast of the sinuses is preferred. MRI can also be obtained if more information is needed to evaluate the extent of disease, especially if there is concern for a mass or intracranial involvement. Cultures can be considered in the setting of complications or treatment failure in order to provide culture-directed antibiotic therapy.

TREATMENT

Treatment consists of symptomatic relief when treating viral ARS. These symptoms will usually resolve within 7–10 days and treatment will not shorten the duration of the viral infection. Analgesics or antipyretics are provided for pain relief. Decongestants in the topical or systemic form may be used in order to reduce nasal congestion and drainage. However, patients should be cautioned on the limited duration of use (no more than three consecutive days for topical decongestants such as neosynephrine) in order to prevent tachyphylaxis and rebound congestion. Nasal steroids are often recommended. There is data showing symptomatic improvement in viral and bacterial ARS; however, studies show it is mostly helpful in patients with an underlying allergic component. Mechanical irrigation of the nasal lining and sinus passageways with nasal saline irrigations may improve quality of life, decrease nasal congestion, and reduce medication use for bacterial ARS although the data are limited. Only distilled, sterile, or bottled water should be used given rare but serious reports of amoebic encephalitis from use of tap water. Antibiotic use is not indicated in viral ARS; however, it is debated in the setting of noncomplicated bacterial ARS. Antibiotics have some modest proven benefit at the cost of adverse side effects. Therefore, their benefits must be weighed against their potential risks. Clinical practice guidelines used to recommend amoxicillin as the first-line treatment if a decision is made to treat with antibiotics. However, there is increased resistance, especially for *H. influenzae* and pneumococci. Therefore, the Infectious Disease Society of America (IDSA) 2012 guidelines recommends amoxicillin/clavulanate as first-line therapy. Culture-directed therapy is most optimal, although this requires the availability of endoscopes or an antral puncture. There is no proven benefit for various treatment lengths and doses.

Chronic rhinosinusitis

DEFINITION AND CLINICAL FEATURES
CRS is defined as the inflammation of the sinonasal cavities lasting at least 12 weeks and resulting in a combination of symptoms and physical findings. Guideline definitions require the presence of at least two of the following symptoms:

- Mucopurulent drainage (anterior, posterior, or both)
- Nasal obstruction (congestion)
- Facial pain, pressure, or fullness
- Decreased sense of smell

In addition, documentation of inflammation is required by one or more of the following:

- Purulent (not clear) mucus or edema in the middle meatus or ethmoid region
- Polyps in nasal cavity or the middle meatus
- Radiographic imaging showing inflammation of the paranasal sinuses

As opposed to ARS, etiology is debated. Theories include superantigens, biofilms, osteitis, immune-related deficiencies, and a dysfunctional host–environment interaction. There is an association between atopic diseases, such as asthma and allergic rhinitis, and CRS. Patients' symptoms tend to be low grade and chronic compared to ARS; hence, patients or physicians may overlook symptoms prior to finally seeking treatment.

CRS is broken down into two main categories: chronic rhinosinusitis without nasal polyposis (CRSsNP) and chronic rhinosinusitis with nasal polyposis (CRSwNP). An additional category includes allergic fungal sinusitis (AFS). CRSsNP is the most common type.

DIFFERENTIAL DIAGNOSIS
ARS, allergic rhinitis, migraines, sinonasal neoplasms, rhinitis medicamentosa, antrochoanal polyp, intranasal drug abuse.

WORKUP
The workup begins with a history and physical. This includes eliciting a history of sinonasal complaints that may confirm or lead to an alternate diagnosis. Comorbid conditions must also be elicited as treatment of comorbidities may be adjunctive, especially in the case of allergic rhinitis. A history of asthma, allergies to nonsteroidal anti-inflammatories and aspirin, and a finding of nasal polyps may clue the physician to a diagnosis of aspirin-exacerbated respiratory disease/Samter's triad. A history of frequent sinus, respiratory, and ear infections may prompt the initiation of an immune deficiency workup. The exposure to chemicals, especially smoke, cannot be ignored, as this has been shown to increase the incidence of CRS. A full head and neck exam is needed including endoscopy, which allows for the objective documentation of inflammation. CT imaging can be helpful to confirm the diagnosis of CRS as endoscopy can often be negative (Figure 8.2).

TREATMENT
Treatment begins with medical therapy, which is directed at the underlying or exacerbating factor. This includes antibiotics, corticosteroids, immune-modulating drugs, and nasal irrigations. Antibiotics are commonly used; however, no consensus guidelines exist regarding their use. The strongest of evidence exists for macrolide use specifically in patients with a

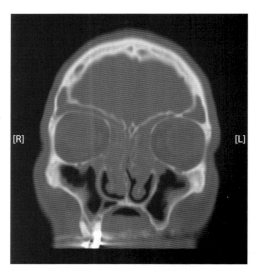

Figure 8.2 This is a coronal CT sinus scan obtained of a patient with CRSwNPs. Near-complete opacification of the frontal sinuses and ethmoid sinuses is noted. The maxillary sinus lining is thickened and the nasal cavity is filled with soft tissue, which in this case is nasal polyps.

lower serum IgE; however, even these reviews state that treatment is *optional*. Corticosteroids are the mainstay of treatment including both topical and systemic therapy. Corticosteroids are the most well studied with proven benefits as shown from randomized clinical trials. Corticosteroid use has many benefits including symptom relief, objective improvements, reduced bleeding intraoperatively, and, in some studies, improved long-term outcomes. Topical intranasal corticosteroid use has the most amount of evidence that show reduced polyp sizes and improved symptoms. They have also been shown to reduce polyp recurrence following surgery. Antileukotrienes may be helpful in patients with leukotriene-mediated inflammatory disease such as allergic rhinitis, asthma, and nasal polyposis and aspirin-sensitive patients. Irrigation using saline has been shown to reduce symptoms and is a low-cost and low-risk

adjunct, assuming sterile or bottle water is used. Surgical treatment is reserved for patients who fail medical management but has been shown to be very effective. Goals of surgery include removal of gross disease, preservation of mucosa, restoration of natural drainage sinus pathways, and access for future topical drug delivery. Patients who demonstrate CRS consistent with an eosinophilic or systemic process must continue with medical management postoperatively in order to prevent recurrence of symptoms.

Nasal polyposis

DEFINITION AND CLINICAL FEATURES
Nasal polyposis is a manifestation of inflammation seen in CRS. Polyps appear as benign, smooth, and edematous pedunculated masses either in isolation or in clusters. Polyps can form anywhere in the nose and sinuses but most commonly are seen in the middle meatus and sphenoethmoid recess. Histologically, they demonstrate a thickened basement membrane, damaged epithelium, and massive tissue edema. Nasal polyps can be seen in asymptomatic patients. Patients with CRS and polyps more commonly complain of nasal congestion and hyposmia than CRS patients without polyps (Figure 8.3).

DIFFERENTIAL DIAGNOSIS
Inverted papilloma, sinonasal neoplasm, aspirin-exacerbated respiratory disease, allergic fungal rhinosinusitis (AFRS), CRS, allergic rhinitis, encephalocele.

WORKUP
Polyps can sometimes be visualized on anterior rhinoscopy; however, endoscopic visualization provides a superior view of the sinonasal cavity particularly in the postsurgical setting. It is important to note that polyps should be bilateral. If a unilateral polyp is noted, imaging must be pursued and the differential diagnosis must be

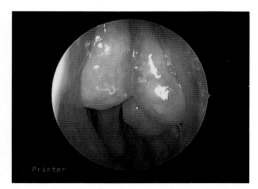

Figure 8.3 Nasal endoscopy of the left side of the nose. Polyps are noted in the left middle meatus. They are obstructing the osteomeatal complex. Behind the polyps, a normal anatomic structure known as the head of the middle turbinate can be seen.

reconsidered. Endoscopically, polyps can be graded using the Lund–Kennedy grading system as follows:

- 0 = no polyps
- 1 = polyps confined to the middle meatus
- 2 = polyps extending beyond the middle meatus
- 3 = polyps obstructing the nasal cavity

There are other similar grading systems as well. CT imaging is not necessary to document inflammation when diagnosing CRS if polyps are visualized on exam. However, imaging is helpful when polyps are not visualized and inflammation is present within the sinuses. On CT, polyps cannot be distinguished from hypertrophic or thickened mucosa. CT allows for evaluation of the extent of disease and is helpful for preoperative planning. MRI is discouraged for the routine diagnosis of CRS with nasal polyposis. However, MRI is helpful when a neoplastic process is suspected and when more soft tissue detail is desired. Allergy testing is used to rule out comorbid allergic disorders. Nasal polyps in children may suggest cystic fibrosis and mandates a proper workup.

TREATMENT

As nasal polyps are found in the setting of CRS, treatment is essentially the same. It consists of medical management first, followed by surgery for failure. Mainstay medical management consists of topical and systemic corticosteroids that have the most proven benefits. Antibiotic use is debated as the majority of nasal polyps are eosinophilic in nature. Steroid injections have been shown to reduce polyp size temporarily. Surgery is used to eradicate the majority of disease while preserving mucosa, to provide natural drainage pathways and ventilation, and to allow for medication delivery into the sinonasal cavities. It must be emphasized that surgery is followed by continued medical management, as these patients require management of a chronic disease lifelong.

Allergic fungal sinusitis

DEFINITION AND CLINICAL FEATURES

AFRS falls within the family of eosinophilic diseases and is characterized by thick allergic mucin with necrotic inflammatory cells, eosinophils, and Charcot–Leyden crystals. It occurs in immunocompetent and atopic individuals and accounts for ~5% of cases of CRS in the United States with the highest incidence occurring in the southern states. AFRS tends to occur in the younger population. Classically, AFRS is diagnosed by the Bent–Kuhn criteria: nasal polyposis, fungi on staining, eosinophilic mucin without fungal invasion into sinus tissue, type I hypersensitivity to fungi, and characteristic radiological findings with soft tissue differential densities on CT scanning. The pathophysiology is thought to be related to a hypersensitivity reaction to fungal antigens, which leads to obstruction of the sinuses and prevents elimination of the provoking fungal antigens resulting in a perpetual cycle. The presentation is typically gradual in onset where patients may complain of thick discolored discharge, hyposmia, nasal

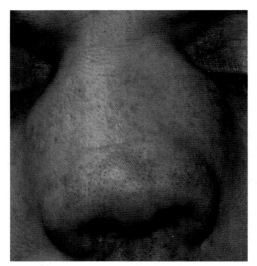

Figure 8.4 Note the widened bony nasal dorsum of this patient due to extensive bony expansion. (Photo courtesy of Jay Dutton, MD.)

obstruction, or other sinonasal-related complaints. On exam, patients may have external signs of bony expansion and facial dysmorphia (Figure 8.4).

DIFFERENTIAL DIAGNOSIS

Acute invasive fungal rhinosinusitis, fungal ball, sinonasal neoplasm, aspirin-exacerbated respiratory disease, chronic invasive fungal rhinosinusitis.

WORKUP

The workup is similar to other forms of CRS and starts with a detailed history and physical. Imaging is called for as part of the diagnostic criteria, which tends toward unilateral or asymmetric complete opacification of contiguous sinuses. On CT imaging, classic findings of AFRS include dramatic bony expansion or erosion and signal heterogeneity due to accumulation of heavy metals. On MRI, T1 weighted images have a variable appearance. On T2 weighted images, there is peripheral mucosal hyperintensity with a hypointense

signal within the sinus due to the high protein and low water content of the allergic mucin. Laboratory findings include elevated IgE and peripheral eosinophilia. Skin or in vitro allergy testing is indicated and must demonstrate fungal-specific hypersensitivity, which commonly shows a broad sensitivity to fungal and nonfungal antigens. Histopathologic diagnosis is obtained typically from the surgical specimen and reveals fungal hyphae without evidence of invasion and a prominent eosinophilic infiltrate with necrotic and degranulating eosinophils.

TREATMENT

Treatment consists of surgery in order to eradicate the bulk of disease and to create widely patent cavities to facilitate drainage and drug delivery (Figure 8.5). Continued medical management postoperatively is required in order to avoid recurrence. Medical management consists mainly of saline irrigations and topical corticosteroids. Immunotherapy may play

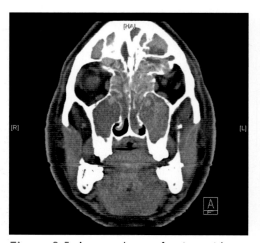

Figure 8.5 A coronal scan of patient with extensive pansinusitis. Again noted is bony expansion and thinning of the ethmoid sinuses as well as hyperdensities noted in the various sinuses. (Photo courtesy of Jay Dutton, MD.)

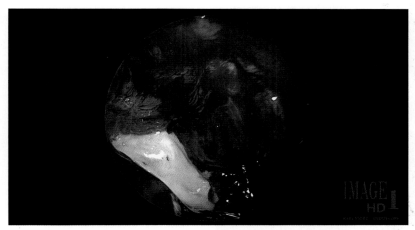

Figure 8.6 An intraoperative view of the left maxillary sinus after being surgically opened and irrigated. Note the remnant thick mucoid secretions. The maxillary sinus lining is inflamed and irritated.

a role in preventing recurrence, improving quality of life scores, and reducing the use of topical and systemic corticosteroids; however, these data are limited. Antifungals have been evaluated as potential therapy for AFRS. Systemic antifungal therapy has fallen out of favor due to its toxicity and lack of data supporting its efficacy. Topical antifungal therapy has the potential of delivering high doses of medications directly to sites of disease; however, the data is limited and this is not commonly used or recommended at this time (Figure 8.6).

Subperiosteal abscess

DEFINITION AND CLINICAL FEATURES
Orbital subperiosteal abscess is the collection of pus between the orbital periosteum and the bony orbital wall most commonly between the lamina papyracea and the medial periorbita. This occurs most commonly as a complication of acute sinusitis via direct extension. It is known as a *Chandler class III* within the Chandler classification of orbital complications. With progressive advancement of the infection, the periosteum may be penetrated and the orbit entered leading to an orbital abscess. Extraocular movement and visual acuity are affected with advancing disease. Chemosis and pain with eye movement may be present as well. Without prompt recognition and proper treatment, rapid progression may lead to devastating consequences such as blindness, meningitis, and even death.

DIFFERENTIAL DIAGNOSIS
Periorbital and orbital cellulitis, orbital abscess, cavernous sinus thrombosis, dacryocystitis.

WORKUP
After obtaining a history, clinical exam should assess for visual acuity, pupillary reactivity, and extraocular motion. An afferent pupillary defect is indicative of visual loss and is an ominous sign. A contrasted CT scan is the single best study to evaluate the extent of disease and can distinguish among cellulitis, subperiosteal abscess, and orbital abscess (Figure 8.7). Intraoperative cultures should be obtained in order to direct antibiotic therapy.

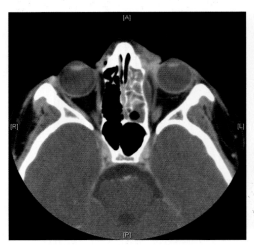

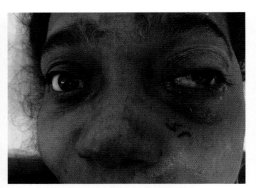

Figure 8.8 Note the orbital proptosis and cellulitis associated with this patient with a large medial subperiosteal abscess.

Figure 8.7 An axial CT sinus scan revealing left ethmoid sinusitis with a fluid collection between the lamina papyracea and the medial periorbita. As the collection enlarges, it would continue to displace the medial rectus laterally.

Treatment of a concomitant sinusitis should be done as well (Figure 8.8).

Suggested reading

Benninger MS, Ferguson BJ, Hadley JA et al. September 2003. Adult chronic rhinosinusitis: Definitions, diagnosis, epidemiology, and pathophysiology. *Otolaryngology: Head & Neck Surgery* 129(3 Suppl.):S1–S32.

Fokkens WJ, Lund VJ, Mullol J et al. March 2012. European position paper on rhinosinusitis and nasal polyps 2012. Rhinology Supplement.

Kennedy DW, Hwang PH. 2012. *Rhinology: Diseases of the Nose, Sinuses, and Skull Base.* New York: Thieme.

Rosenfeld RM, Andes D, Bhattacharyya N et al. September 2007. Clinical practice guideline: Adult sinusitis. *Otolaryngology: Head & Neck Surgery.* 137(3 Suppl.):S1–S31.

TREATMENT

A team-based approach should be considered including an otolaryngologist, ophthalmologist, infectious disease team, and radiologist. Prompt initiation of IV antibiotics is critical. Timing of surgical drainage is debated with regard to immediate versus an initial period of observation with a trial of antibiotics. This is dependent on many factors including the age of the patient (pediatric vs. adult), the size of the abscess, and location of the abscess. Visual acuity deficits are an absolute indication for immediate surgical exploration. Surgical drainage can be approached via an external Lynch incision, an endoscopic nasal approach, or both.

CHAPTER 9

Benign Sinonasal Masses

Kristin Seiberling and Peter-John Wormald

- **Mucocele**
- **Antrochoanal polyp**
- **Juvenile nasal angiofibroma**
- **Systemic disorders**
- **References**

Mucocele

DEFINITIONS AND CLINICAL FEATURES

Paranasal sinus mucoceles are expansile cystic lesions lined by respiratory epithelium. Mucoceles are thought to develop from the obstruction of the sinus ostium with resultant accumulation of mucus, which over time expands the sinus. Blockage of the sinus ostium may occur due to a variety of reasons including local trauma, previous surgery, repeated infections, polyps, and tumors. Although rare, they are the most common expansile lesions of the paranasal sinuses. Furthermore, while benign, local expansion may thin and destroy surrounding bone leading to extension into nearby structures such as the orbit and frontal lobe. Most mucoceles are sterile; however, if infected, a mucopyocele may develop, which has the potential to lead to meningitis or a brain abscess.

Mucoceles are most commonly located in the frontal sinus (77%) followed by the frontal/anterior ethmoids (14%), anterior ethmoids (5%), maxillary sinus (3%), and posterior ethmoids (1%).[1] The narrow anatomy of the frontal sinus drainage pathway likely contributes to its high propensity for mucocele development.

Presentation varies according to the location of the mucocele. Anterior mucoceles that push on the globe may present with proptosis, periorbital pain, and decreased mobility. Loss of the anterior table of the frontal sinus may lead to forehead swelling

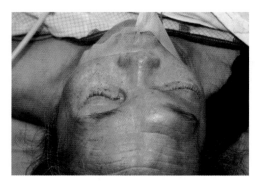

Figure 9.1 Right frontal sinus mucocele with visible expansion of the forehead and proptosis.

and headache (Figure 9.1). Localized oste-itis of the anterior table may result in Pott's puffy tumor (abscess), which in turn may form a chronic fistula connecting the fron-tal sinus mucocele with the skin. Maxillary sinus mucoceles may present with local-ized cheek discomfort, proptosis, and dental pain. Posterior ethmoid mucoceles may expand against the orbital apex lead-ing to blurred vision and decreased orbital mobility.

Histologically, mucoceles are lined with pseudostratified columnar epithelial cells with few ciliated cells and hypertrophic goblet cells. Reactive bone formation may be found adjacent to the mucocele as well as surrounding inflammatory infiltration. Inside the mucocele, there is sterile mucus with cholesterol crystals.

DIFFERENTIAL DIAGNOSIS

Differential diagnosis includes paranasal sinus tumors both benign and malignant, mucus retention cyst, antrochoanal polyp (ACP), and fungal ball. Tumors are easily differentiated by the presence of enhance-ment with contrast, while both mucus reten-tion cyst and ACP tend not to fill the entire sinus. A maxillary sinus fungal ball may cause bowing of the sinus wall; however, they can be differentiated by the presence of calcifications, which can be visualized on computed tomography (CT) scan.

WORKUP

CT is the imaging of choice for the diagnosis of mucoceles. Typical findings on CT scan include complete opacification of the sinus, low-density mucoid material, thinning of surrounding bone with bowing of the sinus wall, and sinus expansion (Figure 9.2). Over time, loss of surrounding bone may be seen with extension of the lesion into adjacent tissue. If contrast is administered, peripheral enhancement may or may not be seen. Magnetic resonance imaging (MRI) is not the modality of choice for diagnosis of mucocele. The MRI signal intensity is variable and depends on the concentration of water, protein, and mucus in the fluid. However, MRI may be beneficial to distin-guish mucoceles from solid tumors.

TREATMENT

Mucoceles are treated with surgical drain-age and marsupialization of the affected sinus (Figure 9.3). Medical therapy does not have a role in the management of mucoceles unless it becomes infected (mucopyelocele).

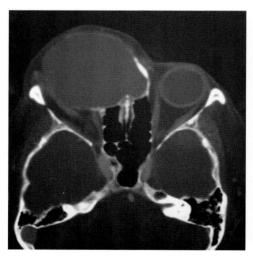

Figure 9.2 CT scan of patient pictured in Figure 9.1. Scan demonstrates the right frontal sinus mucocele with compression of the orbit. The mucocele appears as a smooth expansile mass.

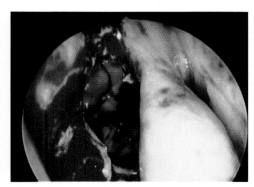

Figure 9.3 Intraoperative cavity of the right frontal sinus mucocele depicted in Figures 9.1 and 9.2.

In the case of the latter, surgery combined with antibiotics is appropriate. Surgery can be endoscopic (preferred), external, or a combined approach depending on the size and location of the lesion. The endoscopic approach allows for drainage and marsupialization of the mucocele without removal of the sinus mucosa, whereas the external approach involves complete extirpation of the lesion including the sinus mucosa. The treatment of choice for mucoceles is endoscopic drainage with close follow-up for recurrence.

Antrochoanal polyp

DEFINITIONS AND CLINICAL FEATURES
An ACP is a solitary polyp that arises from the maxillary sinus and extends into the choanae. Overall, ACPs account for 4%–6% of all intranasal polyps.[2,3] Although the etiologic causes of ACPs are yet to be determined, chronic sinusitis and allergic rhinitis have been implicated.[4,5] Etiologic factors may include allergic rhinitis and chronic sinusitis. They are more commonly found in children and young adults. ACPs are generally unilateral and typically present with nasal obstruction and drainage. Other symptoms may include snoring, mouth breathing, epistaxis, and anosmia. Pathologically,

ACPs are lined by respiratory epithelium with inflammatory infiltrates seen in the stroma much like inflammatory nasal polyps, however, with significantly less eosinophils.[6] Unlike nasal polyps, ACPs tend to be solitary and unilateral, although bilateral cases have been reported.[7,8] ACPs are pear shaped with two components: a large cystic component, which is found in the maxillary antrum, and a smaller solid part in the nasal cavity. The maxillary component originates from the posterior wall 85%–100% of the time.[9–11] Most ACPs leave the maxillary sinus thru an accessory ostium as reported in several studies.[11]

DIFFERENTIAL DIAGNOSIS
Inflammatory polyp, inverted papilloma (IP), mucus retention cyst, mucocele, malignant tumors of the sinonasal cavity and nasopharynx.

WORKUP
ACPs are diagnosed primarily by nasal endoscopy and CT scan. Nasal endoscopy typically reveals a large smooth polyp with extension into the nasopharynx (Figure 9.4). Larger polyps may be visualized through

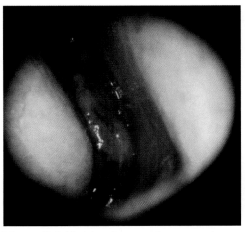

Figure 9.4 Nasal endoscopy demonstrating right antrochoanal polyp with obstruction of the nasal cavity.

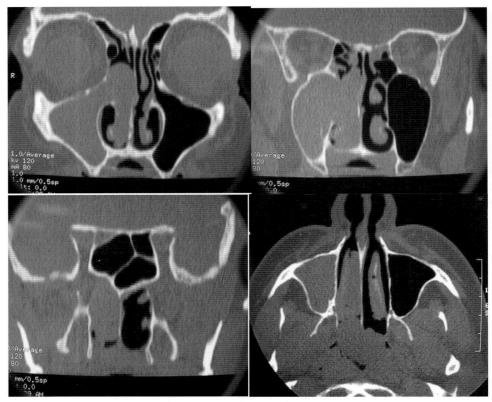

Figure 9.5 CT findings of a right ACP, which shows a smooth mass within the maxillary sinus with extension into the choana and nasopharynx.

the mouth as they hang down from the nasopharynx. On CT scan, ACP appears as a soft tissue mass that occupies the maxillary antrum with extension to the nasopharynx (Figure 9.5). There may be enlargement of the sinus without bony destruction.

TREATMENT

Complete surgical removal is the only treatment for ACP. Functional endoscopic sinus surgery with removal of the antral component is the preferred surgical technique. Recurrence rates are high with simple polypectomy without removal of the antral portion. A Caldwell–Luc procedure may be used in conjunction with FESS if there is concern that some of the antral component may be left behind.

Juvenile nasal angiofibroma

DEFINITIONS AND CLINICAL FEATURES

Juvenile nasal angiofibroma (JNA) is a benign highly vascular tumor found exclusively in males, usually in the adolescence years. Despite accounting for only 0.5% of all head and neck tumors, they are the most common of benign nasopharyngeal neoplasms.[12] JNAs originate from the superior lip of the sphenopalatine foramen at the junction of the pterygoid process of the sphenoid bone and the sphenoid process of the palatine bone. Although benign and

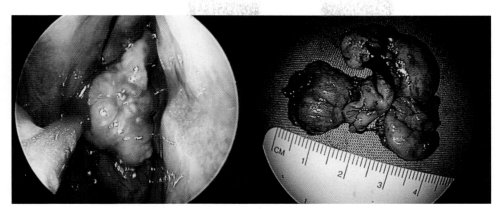

Figure 9.6 Nasal endoscopy and intraoperative specimen of a large JNA tumor.

slow growing, JNAs are locally aggressive and may invade critical surrounding structures if left untreated. JNAs initially expand intranasally into the nasopharynx and nasal cavity and then into the pterygomaxillary space. Over time, JNAs will eventually erode bone and invade the infratemporal fossa, orbit, and middle cranial fossa.

Patients commonly present with recurrent epistaxis and nasal obstruction. Other symptoms may include hearing loss due to chronic otitis media, nasal drainage, and soft palate deformity. In larger tumors facial swelling, cranial neuropathy, proptosis, and visual disturbances may occur. On endoscopy, a smooth lobulated mass is often noted in the nasopharynx and/or lateral nasal wall (Figure 9.6). The tumor may appear as a pale, purplish, red-gray, or beefy red mass. A patient presenting with these signs and symptoms should not undergo biopsy due to the risk of bleeding.

DIFFERENTIAL DIAGNOSIS
Malignancy of the nasopharynx or sinonasal cavity, IP, ACP, and nasal polyps.

WORKUP
Imaging is the key diagnostic modality in the workup of a suspected JNA. Biopsies are generally discouraged due to the risk of uncontrolled hemorrhage. CT is particularly effective at delineating bony changes, while MRI is useful in evaluating tumor extension into the orbit and intracranial compartments. MRI will also help delineate tumor from mucosal inflammation and sinus fluid. Extensive bony destruction is not a common feature; however, bone remodeling and resorbtion do occur with larger tumors. On imaging, a soft tissue mass is centered on the sphenopalatine foramen often causing it to be widened (Figure 9.7). There is typically bowing of the posterior wall of the maxillary antrum anteriorly (Holman–Miller sign) as the mass extends into the pterygopalatine fossa. Classically the Vidian canal is widened in the floor of the sphenoid and the tumor expands posteriorly. Angiography is helpful in defining the blood supply to the tumor and can be used to embolize the tumor prior to surgery (Figure 9.8). The supply of the tumor is mainly from branches of the external carotid artery, including the internal maxillary artery, ascending pharyngeal artery, and palatine artery.

TREATMENT
Surgical resection is the treatment of choice and is usually performed with preoperative embolization to help with hemostasis. Preoperative embolization has been shown to reduce intraoperative blood loss by up to 50% compared to those not treated with

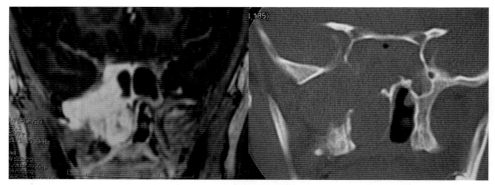

Figure 9.7 CT and MRI findings of a JNA centered on the sphenopalatine foramen with destruction of the sphenoid bone and pterygoid plate.

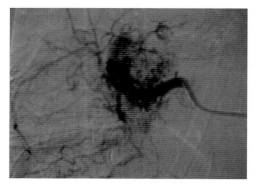

Figure 9.8 Angiography demonstrates large vascular tumor consistent with JNA.

embolization prior to surgery.[13] However, embolization does have its detractors with some studies noting that embolization may help obscure tumor extension and may increase the risk of leaving residual tumor behind.[14,15] Furthermore, the possible benefit of embolization must be weighed against known risks of the embolic material entering the internal carotid circulation.[16,17] Today embolization is routinely performed before endoscopic excision. The surgical approach chosen depends on the size, location, and extent of spread of the tumor. Transnasal endoscopic resection

is an established treatment of early-stage tumors and is associated with decreased morbidity (Figure 9.9).[18] Larger tumors may be resected with an external approach (transfacial, craniofacial resection) in less experienced hands; however, endoscopic-assisted resection of advanced JNAs has been reported with good success and minimal morbidity.[19] Surgical management of tumors that extend intracranially poses a significant challenge and usually requires a multidisciplinary team–based approach.

Nonsurgical treatment options include chemotherapy, radiation, and hormonal therapy. Oral antiandrogens may have a role as a neoadjuvant treatment in extensive tumors. Although clinical data are limited, antiandrogens have been shown to decrease tumor burden and may allow for a more conservative surgical resection.[20] Radiation is generally reserved for the treatment of advanced JNAs. Radiation has been shown to improve local control rates, but its use must be balanced by known complications such as cataracts, hypopituitarism, and malignant transformation.[21] Where complete tumor removal is not feasible, radiation is a viable postoperative option to help minimize the risk of recurrence.

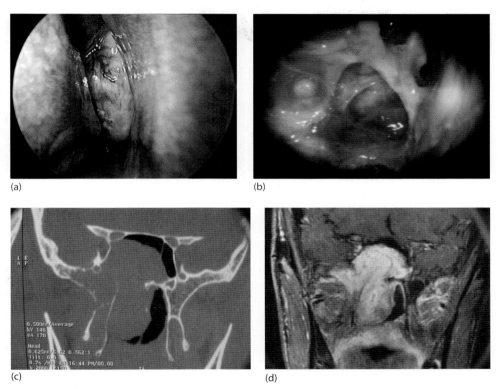

(a)

(b)

(c)

(d)

Figure 9.9 (a) Preoperative nasal endoscopy showing large vascular mass within the nasal cavity. (b) Postoperative nasal endoscopy after transnasal endoscopic removal. (c and d) CT and MRI findings of the vascular mass prior to surgical removal.

Systemic disorders

SARCOIDOSIS

Definitions and clinical features

Sarcoid is a multisystemic inflammatory disease of unknown etiology. In more than 90% of cases, it involves the lungs and intrathoracic lymph nodes, but it may involve virtually any organ in the body.[22] Sinonasal sarcoidosis is reported in about 1% of cases and tends to favor African-Americans and females. The most common site of involvement appears to be the septum and inferior turbinate. Sarcoid rhinosinusitis typically present with nasal obstruction, epistaxis, anosmia, and crusting.[23,24]

Failure to diagnosis sarcoid rhinosinusitis may lead to scarring and dysfunctional nasal epithelium and intractable symptoms similar to atrophic rhinosinusitis.

Differential diagnosis

Differential diagnosis includes other disease processes associated with granulomatous inflammation, including tuberculosis, Wegener's granulomatosis (WG), and fungal infection.

Workup

Diagnosis is made by clinical history, suitable x-ray findings, biopsy, and applicable laboratory findings. deShazo et al. proposed three

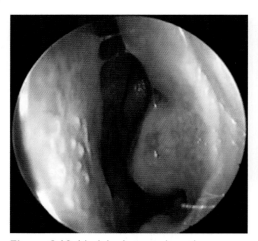

Figure 9.10 Nodular lesions along the septum and inferior turbinate in a patient with sarcoidosis.

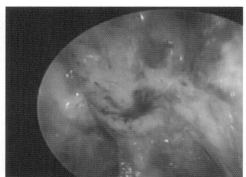

Figure 9.11 Septal perforation with adhesions between the septum and middle turbinate with diffuse nasal crusting seen in a patient with sinonasal sarcoidosis.

diagnostic criteria for sarcoid rhinosinusitis: (1) sinus mucoperiosteal thickening or opacification on imaging, (2) tissue biopsy from the upper respiratory tract consistent with noncaseating granuloma, and (3) data present to exclude other disease processes with granulomatous inflammation such as WG, tuberculosis, and fungal infection.[25] Angiotensin-converting enzyme (ACE) is commonly elevated in sarcoidosis; however, this finding is both nonspecific and insensitive.[26] Hypercalcemia is found in 10% of patients and hypercalciuria in 35% of cases.[27] On nasal endoscopy, nodules may be seen along the nasal septum and/or turbinates (Figure 9.10). The nasal mucosa may appear erythematous and granular with a polypoid appearance. Oftentimes, pale yellowish raised dots are visualized along the mucosa. In addition, crusting of nasal secretions may line the nasal cavity (Figure 9.11). CT imaging may reveal turbinate or septal nodularity, osteogenesis, and bone erosion.

Treatment

Treatment of sinonasal sarcoidosis is medical with saline irrigations and topical and/

or systemic corticosteroids. Steroid-sparing agents such as methotrexate are used as an alternative to long-term oral steroid use. Surgery is reserved for refractory cases.

WEGENER'S GRANULOMATOSIS
Definitions and clinical features

WG is a rare vasculitis disorder characterized by granulomatous inflammation and small vessel vasculitis that generally affects the kidneys and upper/lower respiratory tract. The majority of patients are Caucasians (97%) with a mean age of 40–50 years.[28] Up to 72%–99% of those diagnosed with WG will have head and neck manifestations with mostly sinonasal involvement.[29,30] Oftentimes, sinonasal complaints are the first symptoms of WG. In a study of 120 cases of WG, 89% exhibited sinonasal symptoms with the majority bothered by nasal crusting (69%) (Figure 9.12), chronic rhinosinusitis (61%), nasal obstruction (58%), and epistaxis (52%).[31] Other findings of sinonasal WG include smell loss, purulent rhinorrhea, mucocele formation, septal perforation, and saddle nose deformity (Figure 9.13). On endoscopy, diffuse crusting is typically seen with or without septal perforation and loss of normal visualized

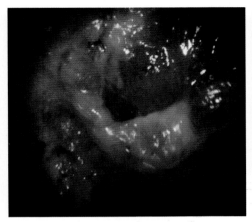

Figure 9.12 Nasal endoscopy showing granulomas on mucosa covered by extensive crusting in the nasal cavity.

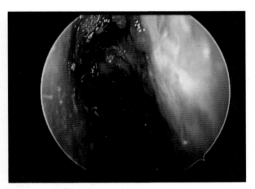

Figure 9.14 Complete loss of normal visualized structures in the nasal cavity of a patient with Wegener's granulomatosis. There is diffuse crusting seen lining the nasal cavity.

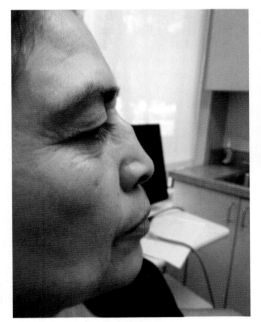

Figure 9.13 Saddle nose deformity from active Wegener's granulomatosis.

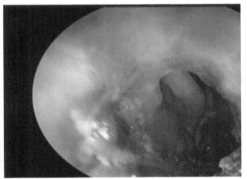

Figure 9.15 Dense adhesion between the septum and nasal wall with the middle turbinate seen posteriorly. Anteriorly, there is diffuse nasal crusting with scar tissue and loss of the normal appearance of the inferior turbinate in a patient with Wegener's granulomatosis.

structures (Figures 9.14 and 9.15). With advanced disease, there may be significant scarring with loss of normal visualized structures. Ophthalmologic symptoms include epiphora, dacryocystitis, orbital mass, and pseudotumor. Ocular manifestations usually occur in conjunction with sinonasal disease; however, this can represent an isolated manifestation of the WG (Figure 9.16).[32] Patients with WG are at risk of mucocele formation due to scarring of the sinus ostium. Figures 9.17 and 9.18 show a patient with orbital proposis and swelling due to a frontal

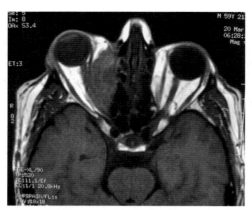

Figure 9.16 CT and MRI of Wegener's granulomatosis presenting as an orbital mass.

sinus mucocele, which eroded into the orbit. The patient underwent endoscopic marsupialization of the mucocele and responded well to the treatment (Figure 9.19).

Differential diagnosis

Differential diagnosis includes other granulomatous diseases as mentioned earlier.

Workup

Laboratory testing for antinuclear antibodies (c-ANCA) has become one of the primary diagnostic tools used to diagnose WG. Positive c-ANCA can be found in 96% of patients with severe and 83% of patients with limited disease.[33] Localized disease may be c-ANCA negative. As the disease progresses, the c-ANCA may convert to a positive finding. Localized disease may be c-ANCA negative and further testing with a biopsy may be indicated. Tissue biopsies typically demonstrate granulomatous inflammation, vasculitis, and necrosis.

Treatment

Conservative treatment is recommended before surgical intervention in these patients. For WG rhinosinusitis, long-term antibiotics paired with topical nasal steroids and aggressive saline irrigations are recommended. Endoscopic sinus surgery in the setting of WG is challenging due to ongoing inflammation, scarring, and crusting and distorted anatomy. Furthermore, complete surgical cure is uncommon and may contribute to additional scarring and lead to protracted sinonasal symptoms. For systemic manifestations, a combination of high-dose corticosteroids and immunosuppressants is used.

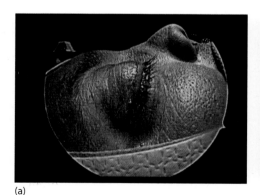

(a)

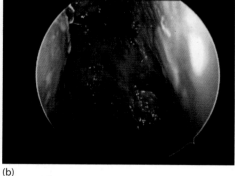

(b)

Figure 9.17 (a) Patient with Wegener's granulomatosis who presented with orbital proptosis secondary to frontal sinus mucocele, which eroded into the orbit. (b) Prior to endoscopic drainage, nasal endoscopy demonstrated scarring of the nasal cavity with crusts and no identifiable outflow track of the frontal sinus.

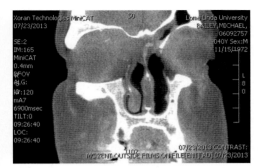

Figure 9.18 CT of patient with Wegener's granulomatosis who presented with orbital proptosis secondary to frontal mucocele with erosion into the orbit.

INVERTED PAPILLOMA
Definitions and clinical features

IP or Schneiderian papilloma is a benign neoplasm that represents 0.4%–4.77% of all sinonasal tumors.[34] There is a significant predilection for males and are most frequently seen in patients 40–60 years of age. IPs occur from localized attachment sites, most commonly the maxillary sinus (42%), ethmoid sinus (18%), nasal cavity (15%), middle/superior turbinate (12%), frontal sinus (10%), sphenoid sinus (1.5%), and cribriform plate (1.5%).[35] Presentation is similar to other sinonasal masses with the most common symptoms being that of nasal obstruction, sinus discomfort/pain, and epistaxis. IPs are locally aggressive, have a tendency for recurrence if not completely removed, and are associated with carcinoma in 11% of cases.[34] In a large analysis of the literature, IPs were found to be associated with carcinoma in situ 3.4% of the time, synchronous cases in 7.1%, and 3.6% with metachronous carcinoma.[12]

Differential diagnosis
Nasal polyps, sinonasal carcinoma, ACP, JNA, olfactory neuroblastoma, and paranasal sinus mucocele.

Workup
CT findings are generally nonspecific, demonstrating a soft tissue mass with some enhancement. The location of the mass may help with the diagnosis. IPs are typically found along the lateral nasal wall related to the middle turbinate and maxillary sinus ostium (Figures 9.19 and 9.20). Calcifications may be found as well as focal hyperostosis, which tends to occur at the site of tumor origin/attachment (Figure 9.21). As the IP enlarges, there may be bony resorption and destruction similar to that seen in malignant tumors. On both

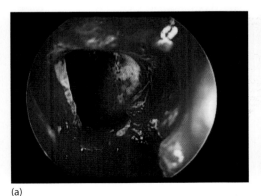

(a)

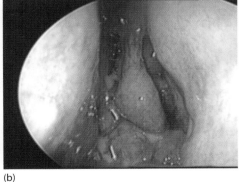

(b)

Figure 9.19 (a) Endoscopic view of the mucocele cavity after endoscopic drainage. (b) Inverted papilloma extending from the maxillary sinus ostium into the nasal cavity.

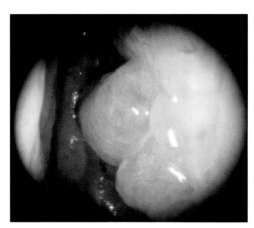

Figure 9.20 Nasal endoscopy demonstrating recurrent inverted papilloma extending through maxillary wall defect.

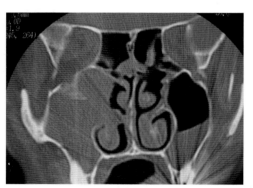

Figure 9.21 CT findings of right inverted papilloma. Hyperostosis along the superior maxillary wall may suggest the origin of the inverted papilloma.

T2- and contrast-enhanced T1-weighted images, a distinctive appearance termed convoluted cerebriform pattern may be visualized. This MRI finding is seen in 50%–100% of the cases and is uncommon in other sinonasal tumors.[36,37] On endoscopy, IP appears as irregular polypoid mass that tends to bleed with manipulation.

On histology, IPs demonstrate respiratory epithelium, which grows into the adjacent stroma in an inverted pattern with characteristic micromucus cysts.

Treatment

Due to the high association with malignancy and potential to recur, complete resection is advocated. Surgical approach depends on tumor origination and extent of spread. Historically, tumors located along the lateral nasal wall were removed using an open approach: most commonly a lateral rhinotomy incision with medial maxillectomy. With advances in endoscopic surgical technique, most tumors can now be removed endoscopically. Endoscopic medial maxillectomy with or without canine fossa puncture is now considered the gold standard treatment for maxillary sinus IP (Figure 9.22). Compared to open techniques, endoscopic resection appears to have similar outcomes with less morbidity.[38–40] Whether an open or endoscopic approach is used, the complete surgical resection is advised. For selected lesions, recurrence rates are similar between open and endoscopic approaches and range between 12% and 20%.[41] The presence of focal neo-osteogenesis on scan may

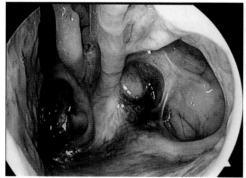

Figure 9.22 View into the maxillary sinus after endoscopic medial maxillectomy with removal of inverted papilloma.

be suggestive of tumor origin and site of attachment and may aid presurgical planning (Figure 9.21). The site of attachment should be drilled down to eradicate any fragments of the tumor that may lead to recurrence if not removed.

HEMANGIOMA
Definitions and clinical features
Lobular capillary hemangioma or pyogenic granuloma is a rare benign vascular tumor of the nasal cavity that is usually found along the anterior septum and nasal turbinates. Patients usually present with epistaxis and nasal obstruction. On examination, hemangiomas appear to be pedunculated red-to-purple hypervascularized mass with a predilection for the anterior nasal cavity (Figure 9.23). In a recent study of 38 cases, 66.7% were found on the septum, 18.2% on the vestibule, 12.1% on the nasal turbinate, and 3% in the ethmoid sinus.[42]

Differential diagnosis
JNA, hemangiopericytoma, angiomatous polyp, angiosarcoma, and hypervascular metastases.

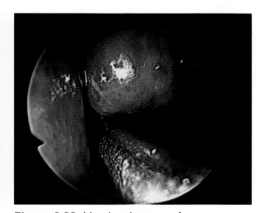

Figure 9.23 Nasal endoscopy of a pedunculated vascular nasal mass consistent with hemangioma.

Workup
Workup includes nasal endoscopy and imaging. Nasal endoscopy typically reveals a hypervascular mass located in the anterior nasal cavity. CT is the recommended imaging modality. Typical findings on imaging include an intensely enhancing mass usually without bony destruction or invasion into the paranasal sinuses.

Treatment
Complete surgical excision is recommended. Recurrence rates are increased if the lesion is not completely removed.

MENINGOCELE AND MENINGOENCEPHALOCELE
Definitions and clinical features
Intranasal meningoencephalocele is characterized by protrusion of cerebral tissue and meninges through a defect in the skull base into the nasal cavity. Meningocele is characterized by the protrusion of meninges without the presence of cerebral tissue. Most are formed as a result of a congenital anomaly where during development there is a discontinuity of the skull; however, others may occur following trauma or as a result of chronic elevated intracranial pressure. The majority of patients are diagnosed as infants with the suspicion raised in those with coexisting craniofacial anomalies and recurrent CNS infections.[43] Meningoencephalocele can be associated with Chiari malformations, holoprosencephaly, Dandy–Walker syndrome, and agenesis of the corpus callosum.[44,45] Cases diagnosed as adults are rare.[46,47] Clinical features may include mouth breathing and snoring due to nasal obstruction, pulsation of the tumor synchronous with pulse or respiration, and associated facial deformities. Rarely, the lesion may be discovered by the presence of CSF rhinorrhea or recurrent meningitis.[46,48,49]

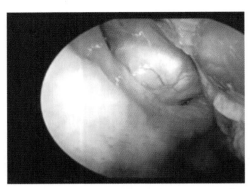

Figure 9.24 Meningoencephalocele on nasal endoscopy.

Differential diagnosis
Other midline masses such as glioma, dermoid, nasal polyp, hemangioma, and neoplastic lesion.

Workup
Imaging of a suspected meningoencephalocele should be performed before a biopsy is taken. Biopsy is not recommended due to the possibility of CSF leak. On endoscopy, meningoencephalocele may be seen as a smooth lobulated mass hanging down in the nasal cavity (Figure 9.24). Both CT and MRI are encouraged for complete radiologic evaluation of suspected meningoencephaloceles. Imaging can identify intracranial connections and the presence of herniated brain tissue. CT evaluation is recommended to delineate the bony defect and to help with surgical resection. Rarely the lesion is missed on a CT scan and the diagnosis is only made by MRI. MRI also helps pick up the presence of associated cranial anomalies as mentioned earlier.

Treatment
The treatment of meningoencephaloceles is solely surgical. The surgical approach depends on the location of the lesion and the size of the defect. Lesions may be removed using a craniotomy or endoscopic approach. Endoscopic transnasal approach is becoming increasingly more common. Currently, it is recommended for lesions with small skull base defects; however, in the hands of advanced endoscopic surgeon, larger lesions may be addressed. Key points in surgical resection include the identification of the skull base, bipolar resection of the neck of the meningoencephalocele sac, and multilayer closure. Prior to grafting, the skull base should be prepared by gentle resection of the mucosa around the skull base defect. Various grafting materials have been advocated including cartilage, bone, fat, fascia, and alloderm.[50–52]

References

1. Natvig K, Larsen TE. 1978. Mucocele of the paranasal sinuses. A retrospective clinical and histological study. *Journal of Laryngology* 92:1075–1082.
2. Yuca K, Bayram I, Kiroglu AF et al. 2006. Evaluation and treatment of antrochoanal polyps. *Journal of Otolaryngology* 35:420–423.
3. Ozdek A, Samim E, Bayiz U, Meral I, Safak MA, Oguz H. 2002. Antrochoanal polyps in children. *International Journal of Pediatric Otorhinolaryngology* 65:213–218.
4. Jang YJ, Rhee CK, Oh CH, Ryoo HG, Kim HG, Ha M. 2000. Arachidonic acid metabolites in antrochoanal polyp and nasal polyp associated with chronic paranasal sinusitis. *Acta Oto-Laryngologica* 120:531–534.
5. Yaman H, Yilmaz S, Karali E, Guclu E, Ozturk O. 2010. Evaluation and management of antrochoanal polyps. *Clinical and Experimental Otorhinolaryngology* 3:110–114.
6. Ozcan C, Zeren H, Talas DU, Kucukoglu M, Gorur K. 2005. Antrochoanal polyp: A transmission electron and light microscopic study. *European Archives of Oto-Rhino-Laryngology* 262:55–60.

7. Myatt HM, Cabrera M. 1996. Bilateral antrochonanal polyps in a child: A case report. *Journal of Laryngology* 110:272–274.
8. Basu SK, Bandyopadhyay SN, Bora H. 2001. Bilateral antrochoanal polyps. *Journal of Laryngology* 115:561–562.
9. Frosini P, Picarella G, De Campora E. 2009. Antrochoanal polyp: Analysis of 200 cases. *Acta otorhinolaryngologica Italica: Organo ufficiale della Societa italiana di otorinolaringologia e chirurgia cervico-facciale* 29:21–26.
10. Lee TJ, Huang SF. 2006. Endoscopic sinus surgery for antrochoanal polyps in children. *Otolaryngology—Head and Neck Surgery* 135:688–692.
11. Balikci HH, Ozkul MH, Uvacin O, Yasar H, Karakas M, Gurdal M. 2013. Antrochoanal polyposis: Analysis of 34 cases. *European Archives of Oto-Rhino-Laryngology* 270:1651–1654.
12. Lund VJ, Stammberger H, Nicolai P et al. 2010. European position paper on endoscopic management of tumours of the nose, paranasal sinuses and skull base. *Rhinology Supplement* 1–143.
13. Li JR, Qian J, Shan XZ, Wang L. 1998. Evaluation of the effectiveness of preoperative embolization in surgery for nasopharyngeal angiofibroma. *European Archives of Oto-Rhino-Laryngology* 255:430–432.
14. Mann WJ, Jecker P, Amedee RG. 2004. Juvenile angiofibromas: Changing surgical concept over the last 20 years. *Laryngoscope* 114:291–293.
15. McCombe A, Lund VJ, Howard DJ. 1990. Recurrence in juvenile angiofibroma. *Rhinology* 28:97–102.
16. Onerci M, Gumus K, Cil B, Eldem B. 2005. A rare complication of embolization in juvenile nasopharyngeal angiofibroma. *International Journal of Pediatric Otorhinolaryngology* 69:423–428.
17. Ramezani A, Haghighatkhah H, Moghadasi H, Taheri MS, Parsafar H. 2010. A case of central retinal artery occlusion following embolization procedure for juvenile nasopharyngeal angiofibroma. *Indian Journal of Ophthalmology* 58:419–421.
18. Douglas R, Wormald PJ. 2006. Endoscopic surgery for juvenile nasopharyngeal angiofibroma: Where are the limits? *Current Opinion in Otolaryngology and Head and Neck Surgery* 14:1–5.
19. Hackman T, Snyderman CH, Carrau R, Vescan A, Kassam A. 2009. Juvenile nasopharyngeal angiofibroma: The expanded endonasal approach. *American Journal of Rhinology and Allergy* 23:95–99.
20. Thakar A, Gupta G, Bhalla AS et al. 2011. Adjuvant therapy with flutamide for presurgical volume reduction in juvenile nasopharyngeal angiofibroma. *Head and Neck* 33:1747–1753.
21. Chakraborty S, Ghoshal S, Patil VM, Oinam AS, Sharma SC. 2010. Conformal radiotherapy in the treatment of advanced juvenile nasopharyngeal angiofibroma with intracranial extension: An institutional experience. *International Journal of Radiation Oncology, Biology, Physics* 80:1398–1404.
22. Baughman RP, Teirstein AS, Judson MA et al. 2001. Clinical characteristics of patients in a case control study of sarcoidosis. *American Journal of Respiratory and Critical Care Medicine* 164:1885–1889.
23. Reed J, deShazo RD, Houle TT, Stringer S, Wright L, Moak JS, 3rd. 2010. Clinical features of sarcoid rhinosinusitis. *American Journal of Medicine* 123:856–862.
24. Aloulah M, Manes RP, Ng YH et al. 2013. Sinonasal manifestations of sarcoidosis: A single institution experience with 38 cases. *International Forum of Allergy and Rhinology* 3:567–572.
25. deShazo RD, O'Brien MM, Justice WK, Pitcock J. 1999. Diagnostic criteria for sarcoidosis of the sinuses. *Journal of Allergy and Clinical Immunology* 103:789–795.
26. Baudin B. 2005. Angiotensin I-converting enzyme (ACE) for sarcoidosis diagnosis. *Pathologie Biologie* 53:183–188.

27. Nunes H, Bouvry D, Soler P, Valeyre D. 2007. Sarcoidosis. *Orphanet Journal of Rare Diseases* 2:46.
28. Fauci AS, Haynes BF, Katz P, Wolff SM. 1983. Wegener's granulomatosis: Prospective clinical and therapeutic experience with 85 patients for 21 years. *Annals of Internal Medicine* 98:76–85.
29. Rasmussen N. 2001. Management of the ear, nose, and throat manifestations of Wegener granulomatosis: An otorhinolaryngologist's perspective. *Current Opinion in Rheumatology* 13:3–11.
30. Gubbels SP, Barkhuizen A, Hwang PH. 2003. Head and neck manifestations of Wegener's granulomatosis. *Otolaryngologic Clinics of North America* 36:685–705.
31. Cannady SB, Batra PS, Koening C et al. 2009. Sinonasal Wegener granulomatosis: A single-institution experience with 120 cases. *Laryngoscope* 119:757–761.
32. Bullen CL, Liesegang TJ, McDonald TJ, DeRemee RA. 1983. Ocular complications of Wegener's granulomatosis. *Ophthalmology* 90:279–290.
33. Sproson EL, Jones NS, Al-Deiri M, Lanyon P. 2007. Lessons learnt in the management of Wegener's Granulomatosis: Long-term follow-up of 60 patients. *Rhinology* 45:63–67.
34. Barnes L. 2009. Surgical pathology of the head and neck. In: Barnes, L. (ed.), *Diseases of the Nasal Cavity, Paranasal Sinuses and Nasopharynx.* New York: Informa Healthcare, pp. 343–422.
35. Schneyer MS, Milam BM, Payne SC. 2011. Sites of attachment of Schneiderian papilloma: A retrospective analysis. *International Forum of Allergy and Rhinology* 1:324–328.
36. Jeon TY, Kim HJ, Chung SK et al. 2008. Sinonasal inverted papilloma: Value of convoluted cerebriform pattern on MR imaging. *American Journal of Neuroradiology* 29:1556–1560.
37. Ojiri H, Ujita M, Tada S, Fukuda K. 2000. Potentially distinctive features of sinonasal inverted papilloma on MR imaging. *American Journal of Roentgenology* 175:465–468.
38. Karkos PD, Fyrmpas G, Carrie SC, Swift AC. 2006. Endoscopic versus open surgical interventions for inverted nasal papilloma: A systematic review. *Clinical Otolaryngology* 31:499–503.
39. Busquets JM, Hwang PH. 2006. Endoscopic resection of sinonasal inverted papilloma: A meta-analysis. *Otolaryngology—Head and Neck Surgery* 134:476–482.
40. Sautter NB, Cannady SB, Citardi MJ, Roh HJ, Batra PS. 2007. Comparison of open versus endoscopic resection of inverted papilloma. *American Journal of Rhinology* 21:320–323.
41. Lawson W, Kaufman MR, Biller HF. 2003. Treatment outcomes in the management of inverted papilloma: An analysis of 160 cases. *Laryngoscope* 113:1548–1556.
42. Smith SC, Patel RM, Lucas DR, McHugh JB. 2013. Sinonasal lobular capillary hemangioma: A clinicopathologic study of 34 cases characterizing potential for local recurrence. *Head and Neck Pathology* 7:129–134.
43. Suwanwela C, Suwanwela N. 1972. A morphological classification of sincipital encephalomeningoceles. *Journal of Neurosurgery* 36:201–211.
44. Sakoda K, Ishikawa S, Uozumi T, Hirakawa K, Okazaki H, Harada Y. 1979. Sphenoethmoidal meningoencephalocele associated with agenesis of corpus callosum and median cleft lip and palate. Case report. *Journal of Neurosurgery* 51:397–401.
45. Cohen MM, Jr., Lemire RJ. 1982. Syndromes with cephaloceles. *Teratology* 25:161–172.
46. Dempsey PK, Harbaugh RE. 1988. Encephalomeningocele presenting with spontaneous cerebrospinal fluid rhinorrhea in an elderly man: Case report. *Neurosurgery* 23:637–640.
47. Copty M, Verret S, Langelier R, Contreras C. 1979. Intranasal meningoencephalocele with recurrent meningitis. *Surgical Neurology* 12:49–52.
48. Brunon J, Duthel R, Motuo-Fotso MJ, Huppert J. 1990. Spontaneous rhinorrhea disclosing intranasal meningoencephalocele and ependymoma of the 4th ventricle. *Neuro-Chirurgie* 36:383–387.

49. Hasegawa T, Sugeno N, Shiga Y et al. 2005. Transethmoidal intranasal meningoencephalocele in an adult with recurrent meningitis. *Journal of Clinical Neuroscience: Official Journal of the Neurosurgical Society of Australasia* 12:702–704.

50. Schlosser RJ, Bolger WE. 2004. Nasal cerebrospinal fluid leaks: Critical review and surgical considerations. *Laryngoscope* 114:255–265.

51. Lanza DC, O'Brien DA, Kennedy DW. 1996. Endoscopic repair of cerebrospinal fluid fistulae and encephaloceles. *Laryngoscope* 106:1119–1125.

52. Lorenz RR, Dean RL, Hurley DB, Chuang J, Citardi MJ. 2003. Endoscopic reconstruction of anterior and middle cranial fossa defects using acellular dermal allograft. *Laryngoscope* 113:496–501.

CHAPTER 10

Benign Skull Base Tumors

Monica Oberoi Patadia, Kevin Swong, and Anand V. Germanwala

- **Pituitary adenomas**
- **Benign fibro-osseous lesions**
- **Suggested reading**

Pituitary adenomas

Monica Oberoi Patadia, Kevin Swong, and Anand V. Germanwala

DEFINITION AND CLINICAL FEATURES

Pituitary adenomas represent approximately 15% of all intracranial tumors. These tumors usually cause symptoms by compression of the optic chiasm or functionally through overproduction of hormones; smaller nonfunctioning or nonsecreting adenomas may be found incidentally. Tumors less than 10 mm in diameter are described as microadenomas, while those 10 mm or larger are referred to as macroadenomas.

Nonfunctioning tumors are most common and usually present with a classic bitemporal visual field deficit from compression of the optic chiasm (Figure 10.1). Compression of other adjacent structures can occasionally create additional symptoms: headache due to compression of the dura, diplopia, oculomotor palsies, and rarely facial numbness from compression of the cavernous sinuses, and hypopituitarism from compression of the remnant pituitary gland. With functioning or secreting adenomas, symptoms on presentation are related to hormone secretion. While prolactin (PRL)-secreting tumors are the most common functioning pituitary tumor and lead to oligo-/amenorrhea and galactorrhea, adrenocorticotropin (ACTH)-secreting tumors cause Cushing's disease/hypercortisolism, growth hormone (GH)-secreting tumors cause acromegaly/gigantism, and thyroid-stimulating hormone (TSH)-secreting tumors cause hyperthyroidism. Pituitary apoplexy refers to the rare occurrence of pituitary infarction or hemorrhage within an existing adenoma and can often be a clinical emergency. It occurs in 2%–7% of tumors and can be the initial presentation of a patient with an

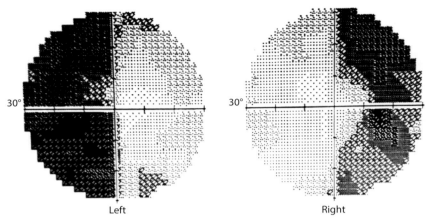

Figure 10.1 Humphrey visual field testing revealing a bitemporal homonymous hemianopsia. This finding is highly suggestive of compression of the optic chiasm.

unknown adenoma. Presenting symptoms are commonly acute headache, rapid vision deterioration, and, rarely, an altered level of consciousness. Patients may require immediate steroid and thyroid hormone replacement and urgent surgical resection of the adenoma with decompression of the visual pathways.

DIFFERENTIAL DIAGNOSIS

Other intracranial masses may present in this location with similar symptoms. They include Rathke's cleft cysts, craniopharyngiomas, meningiomas, infundibular granular cell tumors, chordomas, epidermoids, pituitary hyperplasia, arachnoid cysts, ectopic germinomas, and, rarely, metastatic tumors. Extracranial sphenoid lesions with similar findings include a mucocele or fungus ball. Granulomatous/infectious disorders include sarcoidosis and tuberculomas.

WORKUP

Magnetic resonance imaging (MRI) with and without gadolinium is the test of choice to help identify the presence of an adenoma and define its boundaries. It is important to determine if the mass has extended superiorly toward the suprasellar optic nerve or chiasm, laterally toward the cavernous sinus with encroachment on the internal carotid artery and/or sixth cranial nerve, inferiorly into the sphenoid sinus, and posteriorly toward the brainstem. Adenomas are avidly contrast enhancing (Figure 10.2). Compression of the visual apparatus and identification of the normal gland and infundibulum can also be visualized. A computerized tomography (CT) scan can also provide information on the presence of acute hemorrhage and the bony anatomy along the skull base and within the sinuses.

Workup ideally should involve a multidisciplinary team with evaluation by a neurosurgeon, endocrinologist, neuroophthalmologist, and otolaryngologist. Serum hormone levels for all six of the anterior pituitary hormones should be checked: ACTH, TSH, GH, PRL, follicle-stimulating hormone (FSH), and luteinizing hormone (LH) for women

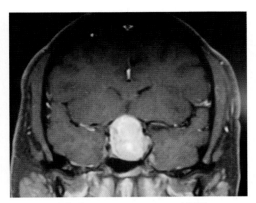

Figure 10.2 Preoperative coronal MRI T1 with gadolinium demonstrating a large contrast-enhancing mass within the sella with suprasellar extension and chiasmatic compression.

and testosterone for men. Additional information regarding the hypothalamic–pituitary–adrenal axis can be gained by checking serum levels of sodium (to assess for hypernatremia from vasopressin deficiency), free thyroxine, insulin-like growth factor-1, and cortisol. Formal visual acuity and field testing should also be performed.

TREATMENT

Treatment recommendations depend on several factors, including size, the presence of neurologic visual symptoms, and the functional status of the tumor. Small, incidental, nonfunctioning tumors are commonly observed with serial imaging on an annual basis. Intervention in these cases is usually offered when there is significant growth or the development of symptoms.

PRL-secreting tumors are usually first managed pharmacologically with dopamine receptor agonists such as bromocriptine

or cabergoline. GH-secreting adenomas may be initially treated with somatostatin analogs, while ACTH-secreting adenomas may be treated with medications that lower the adrenal gland's production of cortisol; however, medical therapy is not as effective in these cases and many patients undergo a multidisciplinary treatment with surgery and/or radiation therapy/radiosurgery.

Symptomatic and large adenomas, or non-PRL-secreting functioning tumors, are usually treated with surgery. Surgical interventions for adenomas are most commonly performed through transsphenoidal approaches (microscopic sublabial or endoscopic endonasal). Craniotomy for resection is reserved for very large tumors that require significant additional exposure. The endoscopic endonasal transsphenoidal approach for resection of adenomas with four-handed technique can be performed by an otolaryngologist and neurosurgeon and is gaining increasing popularity (Figures 10.3 through 10.9). This team approach combines otolaryngology expertise for

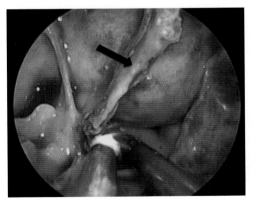

Figure 10.3 Intraoperative endoscopic endonasal photo demonstrating drilling of an intersphenoidal septum (black arrow).

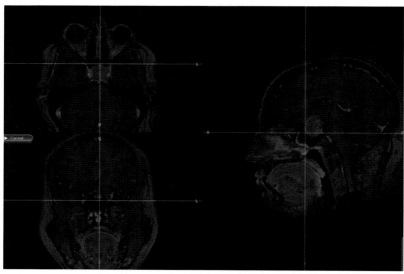

Figure 10.4 Intraoperative stereotactic navigation system that is used during the approach and resection to verify landmarks. A midline location along the floor of the sella is verified prior to dural opening.

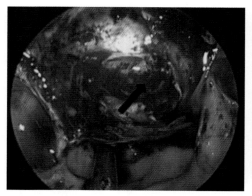

Figure 10.5 Intraoperative endoscopic endonasal photo demonstrating expression of the adenoma after dural opening (black arrow).

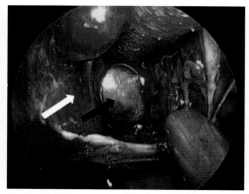

Figure 10.6 Intraoperative endoscopic endonasal photo demonstrating the medial right cavernous wall (white arrow), identification of the diaphragma during adenoma resection (black arrow), and suction removing left-sided residual adenoma.

access and closure and neurosurgical expertise for adenoma resection. Surgery is also offered to patients with adenomas that are medically refractory or who are unable to tolerate the side effects of medical therapy.

With surgically unresectable tumors, nonsurgical candidates, or in patients

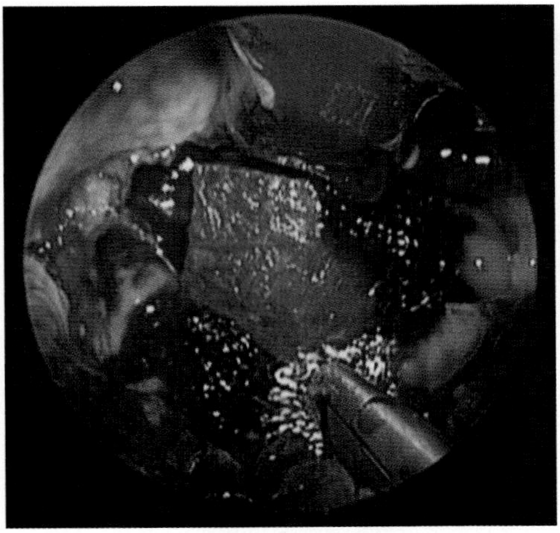

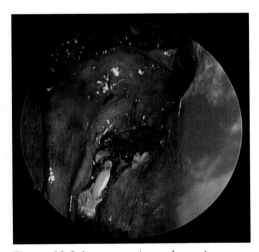

Figure 10.7 Intraoperative endoscopic endonasal photo demonstrating dural reconstruction with onlay collagen allograft.

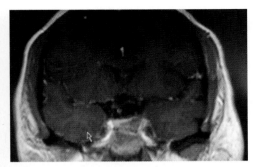

Figure 10.9 Postoperative coronal MRI T1 with gadolinium of the patient in Figure 10.2 demonstrating gross total resection of the large adenoma, decompression of the optic apparatus, and visualization of the infundibulum. The patient had an immediate full resolution of her preoperative bitemporal visual field deficit.

Figure 10.8 Intraoperative endoscopic endonasal photo demonstrating placement of a right-sided Hadad nasoseptal flap over the dural repair.

with recurrent or residual disease who do not want to undergo additional surgery, radiation therapy/radiosurgery may be considered.

Benign fibro-osseous lesions

Monica Oberoi Patadia

DEFINITION AND CLINICAL FEATURES

There is a wide spectrum of benign bone containing lesions within the paranasal sinuses and head and neck. All of these lesions share the common denominator of normal bone that is replaced by fibroblasts with a variable level of mineralized collagen matrix. Fibrous dysplasia has the least amount of bone present and osteomas result in the greatest amount of bone present.

Due to the varied histomorphologic patterns of stroma and bone in these lesions, there has been controversy and confusion concerning classification of these lesions. There are many entities and some may indeed have overlapping microscopic or clinical features. The most common entities affecting the paranasal sinuses are described later.

Fibrous dysplasia

Fibrous dysplasia results from an excess production of immature bone. Osseous

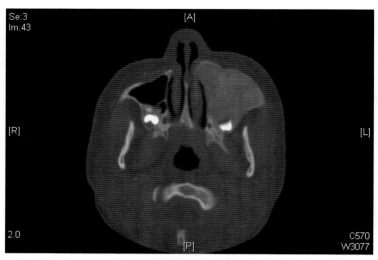

Figure 10.10 Axial CT scan revealing extensive ground glass appearance of the left maxillary sinus. This is highly suggestive of fibrous dysplasia. The dysplasia resulted in facial asymmetry with enlargement of the left cheek and superior and anterior displacement of the orbit.

proliferation of the maxilla is most common, followed by the mandible. This disease most commonly affects adolescents, usually in the late first and early second decades. Asymmetric and painless osseous expansion is often present (see Figure 10.10). This lesion can also cause significant pain or result in loss of vision if the bone growth results in obstruction of neural foramina. Growth often stops when the bones stop growing; however, growth can resume when a patient is pregnant.

Bone involvement can involve a solitary bone (monostotic) or many bones (polyostotic). The monostotic variant is more common at approximately 70%. In less than 5% of cases, patients with polyostotic bone may also present with precocious puberty or other endocrine dysfunction and café-au-lait spots. In these cases, McCune–Albright syndrome should be considered. McCune–Albright syndrome is thought to be due to a mutation in the gene encoding the G protein alpha-subunit (Gs-alpha) that couples cAMP to hormone receptors. Mazabraud syndrome is an extremely rare combination of fibrous dysplasia with soft tissue myxomas. Cherubism, also known as familial fibrous dysplasia, is another benign dysplastic bone disease that is limited to the maxilla and mandible. It was once considered a variant of fibrous dysplasia; however, it is no longer included in the classification of fibro-osseous lesions.

Ossifying fibroma

These lesions are present in the slightly older population compared to fibrous dysplasia. They can occur in the mandible and maxilla (most common), but also in the orbit, paranasal sinuses, and anterior skull base. Older terminology including cementifying fibroma and cemento-ossifying fibroma may be used for lesions noted in the mandible. Findings can be incidental or due to symptomatic swelling.

Osteomas

Osteomas are slow-growing, dense, well-delineated, radiopaque lesions (see Figure 10.11). They are usually present within the frontal sinus (80%) or ethmoid sinuses (15%). Osteomas are often found due to

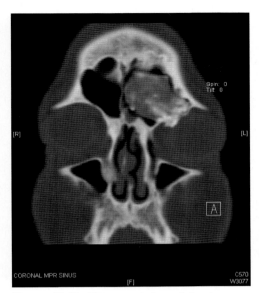

Figure 10.11 CT coronal view of the sinus revealing a large fibro-osseous lesion, consistent with an osteoma. This osteoma involves the frontal sinus and erodes the superior aspect of the orbital roof on the left side. Patient presented with headaches and diplopia.

sinonasal obstruction resulting in sinusitis or rarely mucocele formation. Direct mass effect of adjacent structures can also be noted. They are often found as an incidental finding in up to 3% of sinus imaging scans or present with facial pain or craniofacial deformity. Three possible mechanisms for pain are suggested including local effect, referred pain via the trigeminal nerve, and a prostaglandin E-2–mediated mechanism.

Sinonasal osteomas are solitary; however, a finding of multiple osteomas should raise the possibility of familial adenomatous polyposis (Gardner syndrome).

DIFFERENTIAL DIAGNOSIS

Fibrous dysplasia, osteomas, osteoblastoma, ossifying fibroma, Gardner syndrome, juvenile (aggressive) ossifying fibroma, McCune–Albright, osteoradionecrosis, osteosarcoma, Paget's disease, osteomyelitis, familial fibrous dysplasia (cherubism), hyperparathyroidism

WORKUP

The definitive diagnosis of any fibro-osseous lesion requires a complete history with correlation with radiographic findings, as well as histopathology. On history, the age of the patient, sex of the patient, race of the patient, location of the lesion, and the progression of growth should all be considered.

Fibrous dysplasia

Fibrous dysplasia often has the typical ground glass appearance on CT imaging, as noted in Figure 10.10. There are no discrete margins noted on imaging. The affected bone blends subtly into the normal appearing bone, which is critical to its diagnosis. Histologically, there is an expanded intramedullary space that contains immature spindle fibroblast cells. Malignant transformation to an aggressive osteosarcoma would be very rare. Serial CTs and monitoring for any loss of vision should be done.

Ossifying fibroma

The radiographic findings of ossifying fibroma can range anywhere from radiolucent to radiopaque, depending on the maturity of the lesion. On histology, an outer border of cellular fibrous tissue is noted. Within this there is an avascular fibrous tissue that can range from acellular to highly cellular collagen.

Osteoma findings

The CT findings include a very well-circumscribed mass with varying densities ranging from dense cortical bone to a less dense ground-glass appearance. The osteomas are often found within a sinus but can also have an exophytic growth pattern. Histologically, osteomas can be divided into ivory, mature, or mixed types. Distinguishing an osteoma from an osteoblastoma can be challenging.

TREATMENT
Fibrous dysplasia

Surgery should be considered for any disfiguring fibrous dysplasia or neurologic deficits due to foraminal compression (i.e., visual loss). Bisphosphonates can be considered for patients with pain due to fibrous dysplasia. Sculpting procedures may be considered for esthetic indications.

Ossifying fibroma

In contrast to fibrous dysplasia, ossifying fibromas should be completely resected as the growth rate is not predictable. Usually, the lesions are well demarcated, and hence, a narrow margin may be used.

Aggressive behavior or recurrence may require wider margins.

Osteomas

Surgical intervention is required only if lesions are symptomatic due to pain or obstruction of the sinus outflow tracts or impingement on surrounding structures. Depending on the location and size, an endoscopic or open or combined approach may be used.

Suggested reading

Eversole R, Su L, ElMofty S. 2008. Benign fibro-osseous lesions of the craniofacial complex: A review. *Head and Neck Pathology* 2(3): 177–202.

Kennedy DW, Hwang PH. 2012. Pathology of the sinonasal region and anterio and central skull base. *Rhinology: Diseases of the Nose, Sinuses, and Skull Base*. New York: Thieme.

Malignant Skull Base Tumors

Caitlin McLean and Pete S. Batra

- Introduction
- Squamous cell carcinoma
- Adenoid cystic carcinoma
- Adenocarcinoma
- Mucosal melanoma
- Esthesioneuroblastoma
- Sinonasal undifferentiated carcinoma
- Chondrosarcoma
- Nasopharyngeal carcinoma
- Chordoma
- Hemangiopericytoma
- Osteosarcoma
- Financial disclosures
- References

Introduction

Malignant neoplasms of the sinonasal tract are uncommon tumors of the head and neck region accounting for approximately 5% of upper respiratory tract malignancies. Presenting symptoms are often similar to those associated with paranasal sinus inflammatory disease, and thus, early diagnosis requires a high index of clinical suspicion. Key distinguishing features, including the relative age of the patient (<50 years old for inflammatory disease vs. >50 years old for sinonasal malignancy), insidious onset of unilateral symptoms, and lack of prior history of sinus disease, should raise concern for underlying malignancy. This is further compounded by the advanced stage at presentation given the nonspecific nature of the presenting symptomatology.[1]

Sinonasal malignancies are generally divided into two main groups: epithelial origin (SCC, adenocarcinoma [AC], and adenoid cystic carcinoma [ACC]) and nonepithelial origin (mucosal melanoma, esthesioneuroblastoma, and chondrosarcoma). Accurate histopathologic confirmation and tumor staging is critical for optimal treatment planning. Computed tomography (CT) and magnetic resonance (MR) imaging are required for evaluation of sinonasal malignancy and play complementary roles to delineate the extent of local disease and identify tumor extension relative to the orbit and skull base. Positron emission tomography (PET)/CT assessment is imperative for accurate staging and is commonly utilized to identify regional and distant disease. The combination of full-body CT and focal radioactive glucose uptake by cells can also provide standard uptake value information for posttreatment surveillance.

No standardized protocols are available for management of sinonasal malignancy. Typically, the generalized treatment strategy consists of multimodality therapy.

Surgical resection, with intraoperative frozen section control, forms the mainstay for treatment of sinonasal malignancy. Open craniofacial resection has served as the workhorse for tumor extirpation for more than 60 years; newer techniques rely on the utility of minimally invasive endoscopic techniques for tumor removal. Minimally invasive endoscopic resection (MIER) has been successfully employed with acceptable oncologic outcomes and low complication rate. Postoperative radiation therapy is also a mainstay for treatment, with chemotherapy being reserved for aggressive high-grade malignancies.[2]

While the general presentation, diagnostic workup, and treatment of sinonasal malignancies are similar for each specific histology, the following subsections elaborate on the various malignant subtypes, defining key features of each.

Squamous cell carcinoma

DEFINITIONS AND CLINICAL FEATURES
Squamous cell carcinoma (SCC) represents the most common malignant neoplasm of the sinonasal tract, accounting for ~80% of sinonasal carcinomas. SCC most frequently arises in the maxillary sinus (60%–70%), followed by the ethmoid sinus (20%–30%), and the frontal and sphenoid sinuses (~1%). The majority of SCCs are keratinizing and nonkeratinizing lesions, with the undifferentiated type occurring less frequently and having a more rapid growth pattern. The basaloid variant also has a more aggressive biologic behavior.

Males have a higher incidence, and SEER (Surveillance, Epidemiology, and End Result) incidence data suggest that although most cases occur among whites, paranasal sinus SCC is more likely to affect African-Americans and other non-white populations. Peak incidence occurs during the seventh decade of life. SCC has been associated with environmental and occupational exposure to wood dust, metal industry products (nickel and chromate), industrial fumes, and textile dust. Additional risk factors include high levels of asbestos, formaldehyde, and cigarette smoke.[3] More recently, human papilloma virus (HPV) has been associated with malignant transformation of inverted papilloma into SCC. Similar to HPV-related SCC of the oropharynx, HPV-positive sinonasal tumors have a better treatment outcome, although the role of HPV as a primary carcinogen in the sinonasal tract is unclear.[4] The incidence of sinonasal SCC has shown a statistically significant decline over three decades, perhaps related to reduced exposures and increased awareness.[3]

DIFFERENTIAL DIAGNOSIS
Other epithelial lesions, including AC and ACC, should be included.

WORKUP/INVESTIGATIONS
CT and MR imaging is required to determine the extent of disease (Figure 11.1a through c). PET imaging is required to rule out nodal or distant disease.

TREATMENT
Complete tumor extirpation with negative margins followed by adjuvant chemoradiation is the cornerstone of treatment. If complete resection is not technically feasible, induction chemotherapy followed by chemoradiation or definitive chemoradiation may be employed with reasonable success rate (Figure 11.2). Salvage surgery may be required for residual disease after concurrent chemoradiation. Cervical lymph node metastasis at the time of diagnosis is reported to occur in 3%–33% of patients. Elective treatment of the neck should be considered, as failure with N0 disease ranges from 9% to 33%.[5] The SEER 5-year survival rate for local disease is 85.71%. The 5-year survival with regional and distant metastases decreases to 47.80% and 39.98%, respectively. Mean overall 20-year survival remains 29.37% despite decreased incidence of SCC.[6,7]

Adenoid cystic carcinoma

DEFINITIONS AND CLINICAL FEATURES
ACC is a malignant epithelial tumor arising from minor salivary glands of the upper respiratory tract. It is the most common minor salivary gland malignant histology, representing 10% of all salivary gland tumors. The sinonasal tract is a common site for this tumor, accounting for 10%–25% of all head and neck ACC, making it the second most common malignancy of the nose and paranasal sinuses. The maxillary sinus is the most frequently involved site (47%–80%), followed by the nasal cavity (22%–30%), ethmoid sinus (11%), and sphenoid sinus (5%) (Figure 11.3).[8]

Histologically, ACC is divided into three major growth patterns: cribriform (well-differentiated and described as having a "Swiss cheese" appearance), tubular, and solid (less differentiated), although most tumors have mixtures of cytoarchitectural patterns. The histopathology confers prognostic significance, as the tubular and cribriform types tend to have a more favorable prognosis, while the solid form has the worst prognosis.[9] Thorotrast exposure, a radioactive substance (thorium dioxide), has been previously reported as an etiology for ACC.[10]

ACCs have historically had a female predominance, with a majority reported in whites. Age of onset is between 40 and 60 years, with most presenting in patients 55 years and older. ACCs are known for their prolonged history, slow progression, and late diagnosis, with high propensity for recurrence. Local invasion coincides with late presentation, most commonly with tumor spread to the orbit, less frequently to the skull base. It has a tendency for recurrence, submucosal spread, and

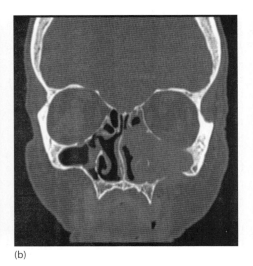

(a)

(b)

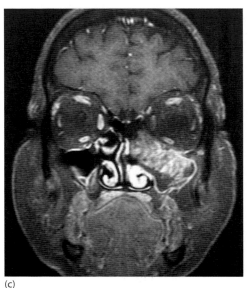

(c)

Figure 11.1 (a) Endoscopic view demonstrates exophytic friable mass filling the left middle meatus. (b) Coronal bone window CT scan demonstrates a left maxillary sinus mass with erosion of the maxilla and orbital floor. (c) Coronal T1-weighted MRI with gadolinium illustrates a heterogeneously enhancing maxillary sinus mass with extension to the left middle meatus.

neurotropism with metastases throughout major and minor nerves. This high propensity for perineural invasion can result in increased incidence of pain and neuropathies.[8,11]

DIFFERENTIAL DIAGNOSIS

ACC is considered in the differential diagnosis of most sinonasal malignancies, particularly poorly differentiated carcinoma, olfactory neuroblastoma, and pleomorphic adenoma.

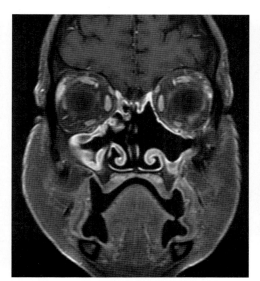

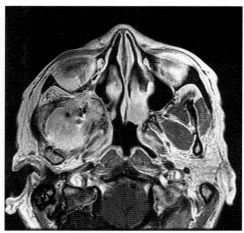

Figure 11.4 Corresponding axial T1-weighted MRI with gadolinium in the previous patient demonstrates the soft tissue mass involving the left posterior nasal cavity. A second larger soft-tissue mass is noted in the previous maxillectomy region with involvement of the pterygomaxillary fossa and infratemporal fossa.

Figure 11.2 Coronal T1-weighted MRI with gadolinium 3 years post definitive chemoradiation demonstrates complete resolution of the mass. Both maxillary sinuses show mild peripheral mucosal enhancement.

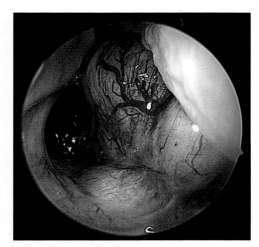

Figure 11.3 Endoscopic exam demonstrates a lobulated mass with multiple dilated vessels involving the left posterior nasal cavity with extension into the sphenopalatine region.

WORKUP/INVESTIGATIONS

Careful workup should include high-resolution CT and MR imaging to define the extent of local disease and PET imaging to rule out regional and distant metastasis (Figure 11.4). Propensity for perineural spread necessitates that trigeminal nerve branches be carefully evaluated on the MRI.

TREATMENT

The most common treatment modality is surgery followed by postoperative radiotherapy (Figure 11.5). Single modality radiotherapy is indicated to treat unresectable T4 tumors, reduce tumor burden prior to surgical resection, improve probability of achieving local control, and provide palliative therapy.[12] Additionally, the effective use of gamma knife radiosurgery has been shown for unresectable ACC, and may provide local control.[13] Occasionally, chemotherapy is used pre- or postoperatively to reduce tumor burden. Five-year disease-specific

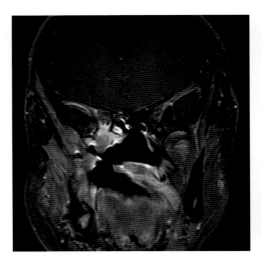

Figure 11.5 The patient underwent combined open and endoscopic resection of both masses followed by neutron beam radiation therapy. Coronal T1-weighted MRI with gadolinium illustrates resolution of the left nasal cavity mass. Small residual enhancing mass is noted in the right pterygomaxillary fossa, which has remained stable on imaging for 2 years.

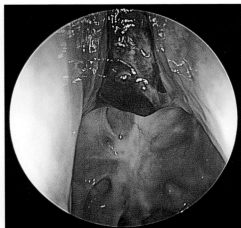

Figure 11.6 Endoscopic exam demonstrates an exophytic, friable mass involving the right superior nasal cavity. Biopsy confirmed diagnosis of recurrent nonintestinal adenocarcinoma.

survival has been reported in 50%–86% and up to 100% in patients without distant disease. Despite the relentless course of ACC, patients often survive for long periods with recurrent and/or metastatic disease. Five-year local recurrence and distant metastasis rates are 30% and 25%, respectively.[8,11]

Adenocarcinoma

DEFINITIONS AND CLINICAL FEATURES

AC represents the third most common malignant sinonasal histology. The most common site for AC is the ethmoid sinuses (5%–30%), followed by nasal cavity (27%) and maxillary sinus (20%) (Figure 11.6). It is usually considered an occupational pathology, and the most notable exposure is wood dust, which has been identified as an important risk factor in the European literature. The large-particle dust from particular hardwoods, such as ebony, oak, and beech, is believed to provide a 900-fold risk of development of AC.[14] Additional etiologic factors include formaldehyde, nickel, or chrome exposure and leather tannins.

AC of the sinonasal tract is classified into intestinal and nonintestinal subtypes. Intestinal type (IT) can be further subclassified (papillary, colonic, solid, mucinous, or mixed) and is generally more aggressive with local recurrence rate in 50%, lymphatic spread in 10%, and distant metastasis in 20% of patients. Hardwood dust exposure typically gives rise to ITAC, and in woodworkers, ITAC is most often found in the olfactory cleft and appears as a polyp-like mass.[15] Non-intestinal type (non-ITAC) is classified as low or high grade and most commonly occurs in the ethmoid and maxillary sinuses, respectively. Current evidence points to histologic subtypes and anatomic features as important predictors of survival.[16]

The mean age at diagnosis is 60–65 years, although it may present in the fifth to sixth decades in wood dust–related exposures. There is a male predominance, which likely reflects occupational factors. Prolonged exposure time (mean 28 years) conveys increased risk, with delayed latency to presentation by ~40 years. Exposures appear to be more common in Europe where such work is more prevalent.[17]

DIFFERENTIAL DIAGNOSIS

AC should be considered in the differential diagnosis of most sinonasal malignancies. Primary sinonasal ITAC should be diagnosed after ruling out metastasis from GI tract and lung primary.[18] Additionally, benign pathology, such as hamartoma, should be considered.

WORKUP/INVESTIGATION

This lesion requires both CT scan and MRI to determine its precise extension (Figure 11.7a and b). Immunohistochemistry (IHC) of low-grade non-ITAC shows cytokeratin 7 positivity with no myoepithelial or basal cells. Additionally, colonoscopy may be indicated if the microscopic appearance of the sinonasal carcinoma resembles that of colorectal carcinoma.[18,19]

TREATMENT

Although there is no standardized treatment for AC, surgical excision followed by radiotherapy is the mainstay treatment approach (Figure 11.8). Tumor resection can often be achieved by an endoscopic approach, though open craniofacial resection may be warranted for more advanced disease, especially with disease that extends laterally over the orbit. Overall, AC is associated with a relatively favorable prognosis, despite a local failure rate approaching 30%. The overall survival is 60% at 5 years. Of the ITAC, papillary subtype has a more favorable prognosis (80% 5-year disease free survival) compared to mucinous and solid subtypes. Low-grade non-ITAC are generally more localized at presentation and carry a favorable prognosis (80% disease free survival at 5 years), while

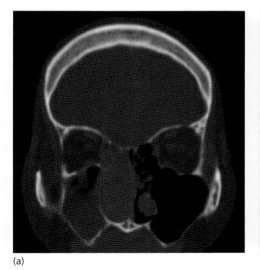
(a)

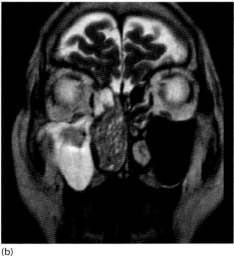
(b)

Figure 11.7 (a) Coronal bone window CT demonstrates a right nasal cavity soft tissue mass with opacification of the adjacent maxillary and ethmoid sinuses. The septum is bowed to the contralateral side. No skull base erosion is noted. (b) Coronal T2-weighted MRI demonstrates the hypointense mass with mild enhancement after contrast administration. High signal in the adjacent paranasal sinuses from postobstructive secretions is noted.

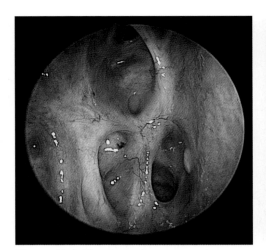

Figure 11.8 The previous patient underwent endoscopic resection of the mass followed by radiation therapy. Endoscopic exam at 3.5 years demonstrates healed surgical cavity without evidence of recurrence.

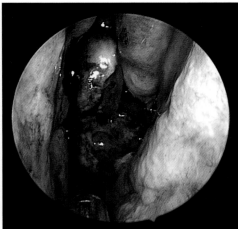

Figure 11.9 Endoscopic exam shows a pigmented, friable mass involving the left sphenoethmoid recess with extension into the posterior nasal cavity.

high-grade tumors have a very poor prognosis with a 3-year survival of ~20%. Advanced stage tumors, sphenoid sinus extension, skull base invasion, and high-grade histology portend a poorer prognosis.[16]

Mucosal melanoma

DEFINITIONS AND FEATURES

Primary mucosal melanoma of the sinonasal region is rare, accounting for 0.3%–2% of all melanomas, and only about 4% of head and neck melanomas. The sinonasal tract represents the most common site of mucosal melanoma, with the majority of tumors involving the nasal cavity (65.5%), followed by the septum, or combination of the nasal cavity and sinuses. Caucasians represent the majority of patients (90.8%), with most cases occurring between the fifth to eighth decades, with a mean age at diagnosis of 71.2 years. There is no gender predilection. Additionally, no risk factors are known for this condition. Clinical presentation varies with tumor location and includes epistaxis,

mass lesion, and/or obstructive nasal symptoms. The endoscopic view of malignant mucosal melanoma may demonstrate a pigmented, polypoid mass in the nasal and paranasal sinus regions (Figure 11.9).[20]

DIFFERENTIAL DIAGNOSIS

Sinonasal undifferentiated carcinoma (SNUC), poorly differentiated carcinoma, AC, lymphoma, rhabdomyosarcoma, angiosarcoma, neuroendocrine carcinoma, olfactory neuroblastoma, and plasmacytoma should be considered.

WORKUP/INVESTIGATIONS

Histologically, most sinonasal mucosal melanomas are comprised of large, epithelioid cells with abundant eosinophilic cytoplasm and round nuclei showing eosinophilic nucleoli, or spindle cells. Approximately one-third of tumors have undifferentiated, small, round, blue cells that may be mistaken for lymphoma. IHC profile of sinonasal malignant mucosal melanoma is identical to that of cutaneous lesions. Markers include S-100 protein, tyrosinase, HMB-45, melan A,

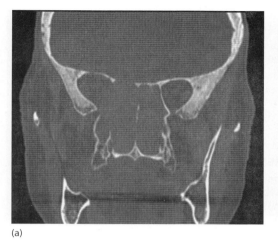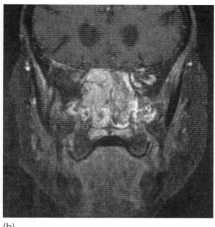

(a)   (b)

Figure 11.10 (a) Coronal bone window CT scan demonstrates soft tissue mass involving bilateral posterior ethmoid sinuses with nasal cavity extension. Erosion of the right orbital apex and ethmoid roof is noted. (b) Coronal T1-weighted MRI with gadolinium shows a moderately enhancing mass involving bilateral ethmoid sinuses. No orbital or intracranial extension is noted.

and microphthalmia transcription factor (MITF). Positivity for a series of markers is needed to make the accurate diagnosis. In addition to routine CT and MR evaluation (Figure 11.10a and b), PET imaging is mandatory to establish the presence of regional and distant metastases.[21]

TREATMENT

Optimal management of mucosal melanoma remains a significant dilemma. The primary treatment modality is complete surgical resection, although wide margins can be difficult to achieve due to restrictions of the paranasal sinus confines adjacent to critical structures (Figure 11.11). Primary neck dissection is not routinely recommended as regional lymph node metastasis is generally low and has not been shown to impact survival. Endoscopic or open surgery accompanied by radiation and/ or chemotherapy is frequently employed. Hypofractionated radiotherapy is the preferred regimen, while chemotherapy is currently only used for disseminated disease and surgical failures. Recurrences are

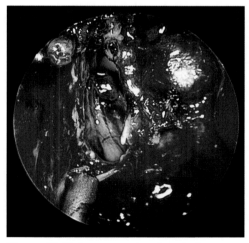

Figure 11.11 Intraoperative view during endoscopic anterior skull base resection of sinonasal mucosal melanoma demonstrates tumor extension to the left olfactory bulb.

common with many patients succumbing to disseminated disease. There is a high risk of local recurrence (37%–54%) with an average time from surgery to recurrence of 5–20 months. Distant metastasis occurs in

51.5% of patients. Local failure predicts distant metastasis in 73.1% of patients, with an average of 12 months to development of distant disease. Nodal and distant metastases can occur late. Overall survival is worse than cutaneous melanomas with only 20% 5-year survival rate.[22]

Esthesioneuroblastoma

DEFINITIONS AND CLINICAL FEATURES
Esthesioneuroblastoma (ENB) or olfactory neuroblastoma is a rare sinonasal neuroectodermal malignancy accounting for 2%–3% of intranasal neoplasms. It is thought to arise from olfactory epithelium in the region of the cribriform plate. It can occur in children and adults, reported to occur from 3 to 90 years of age, with a bimodal peak in the second and sixth decades of life. There is no gender predilection.

Histologically, ENB typically presents as a lobulated tumor surrounded by sustentacular cells with rosettes, pseudo-rosettes, calcifications, and fibrillary stroma in some areas. A histologic grading system based on growth, architecture, mitotic activity, necrosis, nuclear polymorphism, rosette formation, and fibrillary matrix has been reported by Hyams and classifies four different grades from well-differentiated (Grade I) to undifferentiated (Grade IV). Hematoxylin and eosin stain demonstrates a small round blue cell tumor. The tumor presents clinically as a discrete sinonasal mass. It can vary in size from a small nodule to a large friable mass, which may cause local destruction and extend beyond the confines of the sinonasal tract into the orbit or brain. It may have an engorged red appearance because of the richly vascularized tumor matrix, or could exhibit surface ulceration and granulation tissue, particularly in higher-grade tumors (Figure 11.12).[23]

Several classification schemes have been proposed to stage ENB. Kadish staging, the most common staging system, was first described in 1976. Group A tumors are

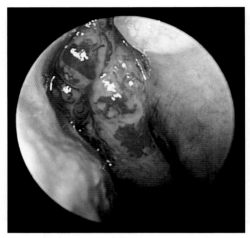

Figure 11.12 Endoscopic view of right nasal cavity demonstrates a large exophytic mass with multiple dilated vessels on the surface. Biopsy confirmed diagnosis of high-grade esthesioneuroblastoma.

confined to the nasal cavity, group B involve the paranasal sinuses, and group C extend beyond the sinonasal cavity. This system was modified to add stage D, which includes cervical or distant metastasis.[24] Dulguerov and Calcaterra described a third system in 1992, based on the TNM classification system, to take into account lymph node involvement and distant metastases.[25]

DIFFERENTIAL DIAGNOSIS
Sinonasal-undifferentiated carcinoma (SNUC), nasopharyngeal carcinoma (NPC), sinonasal neuroendocrine carcinomas, Ewing sarcoma, rhabdomyosarcoma (alveolar type), lymphoma, mucosal melanoma, ectopic pituitary adenoma, and paraganglioma should be considered.[23]

WORKUP/INVESTIGATIONS
ENB has a distinctive immunoprofile that includes keratin negativity, neuroendocrine marker positivity (neuron specific enolase and synaptophysin), and S100-positive sustentacular cells, which surround and support nests of tumor. High-resolution

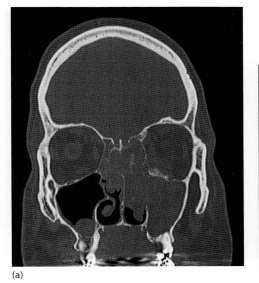

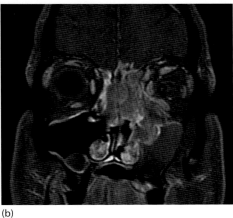

(a)   (b)

Figure 11.13 (a) Coronal bone window CT illustrates left sinonasal mass destruction of left ethmoid air cells and superior septum. The lesion extends to the contralateral ethmoid region. Subtle erosion of the left cribriform plate is noted. (b) Coronal T1-weighted MRI with gadolinium demonstrates enhancing mass involving the bilateral ethmoid and left maxillary sinuses. The mass extends through the skull base with involvement of the left olfactory bulb. Extensive dural enhancement is noted.

CT should be carefully reviewed for erosion of the lamina papyracea, cribriform plate, and ethmoid roof. T1-weighted MR images will show decreased signal intensity of tumor compared to brain parenchyma. On T2-weighted images, tumor may be iso- or hyperintense relative to the brain. Intratumoral calcifications and cysts along the intracranial margin are highly suggestive for ENB (Figure 11.13a and b).

TREATMENT

There is no consensus regarding optimal treatment. The most frequently used regimen is a combined approach with radiotherapy given before or after surgical resection. Early-stage lesions (Kadish A or T1) may not require adjuvant radiotherapy if clear surgical margins are obtained. The classic craniofacial resection is being gradually replaced by expanded endoscopic approaches in select cases, without adverse impact on 5-year control rate (Figure 11.14). The impact of chemotherapy remains unknown, but it may be added as a radiosensitizer to reduce tumor growth and to manage potential micrometastasis for Kadish B or C lesions. Concurrent chemoradiation may be used before surgery to avoid delay in therapy and to reduce tumor size prior to surgery. In contrast to other sinonasal malignancies, treatment of N0 neck should be considered given 15% risk of regional recurrence. There is potential benefit to neck dissection or radiotherapy aimed at lowering the risk of regional recurrence. Survival rates can be >80% for early-stage tumors. The 5-year disease-specific survival rate is reported as 52%–90%.[26] Local recurrence rates vary widely by 16%–40% and distant metastasis by 0%–60%, which

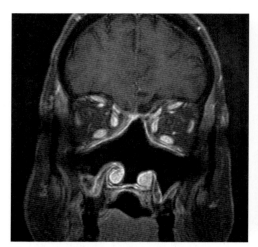

Figure 11.14 This patient underwent endoscopic anterior skull base resection followed by concurrent chemoradiation. T1-weighted MRI with gadolinium at 2 years shows resolution of the mass with minimal signal enhancement consistent with mild ongoing inflammation in the surgical bed.

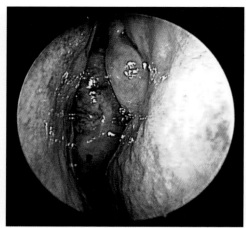

Figure 11.15 Endoscopic view of left nasal cavity demonstrates an exophytic mass filling the olfactory region with lateral displacement of the middle turbinate. Biopsy confirmed diagnosis of SNUC.

could reflect inclusion of different histologic grades of ENB and/or misdiagnosed tumors such as SNUC.[27]

Sinonasal undifferentiated carcinoma

DEFINITIONS AND CLINICAL FEATURES

SNUC is a rare, highly aggressive carcinoma of uncertain histogenesis, thought to be part of the spectrum of neuroendocrine malignancies that includes ENB, neuroendocrine carcinoma, and small cell carcinoma. The age range affected is broad, from 30 to 90 years old, with the sixth decade as the median age at presentation. There is a male predominance (2–3:1). Patients typically present with multiple complaints including nasal and orbital (diplopia, vision change) symptoms, facial pain, and cranial nerve involvement, which characteristically develop over a relatively short duration of time. SNUC typically presents as a rapidly enlarging mass involving multiple sinonasal sites, often

with extrasinus extension (Figure 11.15). Clinically positive regional nodes are present at diagnosis in 10%–30% of patients. Distant metastases often involve the lungs and bone and can be seen at initial presentation. SNUC may rarely seed the cerebrospinal fluid and result in spinal metastasis, also known as "drop metastases."

DIFFERENTIAL DIAGNOSIS

ENB, small cell carcinoma, and classic neuroendocrine carcinoma should be considered.

WORKUP/INVESTIGATIONS

Histologic diagnosis requires clinical correlation between light microscopic and IHC studies. SNUCs are consistently immunoreactive with epithelial markers, including pankeratins (diffuse, intense staining) and simple keratins (i.e., CK 7, CK 8, CK 9). Radiographic imaging shows a large sinonasal mass typically with invasive growth pattern extending beyond bony confines with orbital and/or skull base involvement (Figure 11.16a and b).

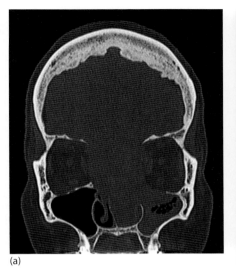
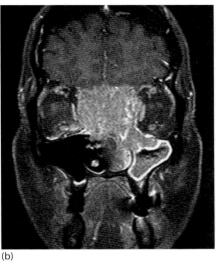

(a)   (b)

Figure 11.16 (a) Coronal CT scan shows an extensive, destructive mass involving bilateral ethmoid sinuses. Complete erosion of bilateral lamina papyracea and skull base is evident. (b) Coronal T1-weighted MRI with contrast shows an enhancing ethmoid mass abutting bilateral frontal lobes and orbits.

TREATMENT

It is generally accepted that multimodality therapy including surgery, radiation, and chemotherapy provides the best oncologic outcomes (Figure 11.17). A meta-analysis review of 30 studies involving 167 cases demonstrated that surgery represented the best single modality treatment, but patients who underwent surgical resection with the addition of radiation and/or chemotherapy had a 260% increased chance of survival compared to surgery alone.[28] Moreover, aggressive trimodality therapy including surgery and postoperative chemoradiation has yielded significantly improved locoregional control and overall survival compared to surgery alone or nonsurgical treatment.[29] Additionally, the use of neoadjuvant chemotherapy and/or radiation therapy prior to definitive surgery has been proposed by some investigators to improve the therapeutic ratio. A review of SNUC treatments and outcomes suggests that preoperative radiation therapy may allow reduced treatment volumes with more accurate targeting and

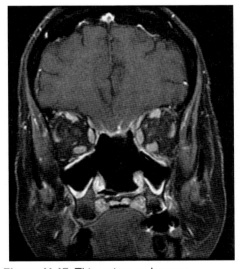

Figure 11.17 This patient underwent induction chemotherapy followed by gross total endoscopic resection of the mass. Coronal T1-weigthed MRI with gadolinium 1 year after completion of concurrent chemoradiation demonstrates interval resection of mass with minimal inflammatory signal in the surgical cavity.

delivery of radiation therapy, and decrease toxicity to normal tissues.[30] However, despite aggressive treatment regimens, the prognosis of patients suffering from SNUC remains poor. Recently, morphoproteomics has been described to help define the biology of SNUC tumors and provide targets for the employed agents.[31]

Chondrosarcoma

DEFINITIONS AND CLINICAL FEATURES

Chondrosarcomas are slow-growing malignant tumors that generally arise from hyaline cartilage. Sinonasal chondrosarcomas are relatively rare and constitute 10%–20% of malignant primary bone tumors, of which approximately 5%–10% originate in the head and neck. Given the tendency for hyaline cartilage differentiation, there is increased occurrence in the maxilla and skull base, theoretically due to its initial cartilaginous composition and subsequent ossification.

Chondrosarcomas represent a heterogeneous group of lesions with variable clinical presentation and morphologic features. A unique feature is its ability to arise in either bone or soft tissue with a 2:1 predilection for the skeleton.[32] A recent review shows a slight female predominance of 1.27:1 with a peak age of onset between 30 and 60 years.[33] Nasal obstruction is the most frequently reported presenting symptom (50.3%). They cause local destruction, and due to their indolent growth and late presentation, multiple sites may be affected at the time of diagnosis.

DIFFERENTIAL DIAGNOSIS

Chondroma, aggressive osteoblastoma, and osteochondroma should be considered.

WORKUP/INVESTIGATIONS

Accurate histologic characterization is essential; there are three histologic grades of chondrosarcoma, which vary by cellularity, nuclear size, and mitotic rate. Grade I has small, densely staining nuclei. Grade II and III chondrosarcomas are distinguished by mitotic rate, with low (<2 mitoses per 10 high power field [HPF]) and high mitoses (≥2 mitoses per 10 HPF), respectively. Historically, plain skull radiographs were used with calcification demonstrated in ~60% of cases. CT characteristics include hyperdense mass with clumps of calcification, foci of bone destruction, and moderate contrast enhancement. MR features include iso-/hypointense on T1-weighted images with pronounced contrast enhancement and high signal intensity on T2 sequences, possibly isointense to CSF (Figure 11.18a and b).[34,35]

TREATMENT

Aggressive surgical resection is the mainstay of treatment for chondrosarcomas (Figure 11.19). In selected patients, complete resection can be achieved using a transnasal endoscopic approach.[36] Adjuvant radiotherapy is shown to have survival benefit in some studies and may decrease local recurrence.[33] A variety of factors influence the addition of radiotherapy, including tumor size (5 cm threshold indicated in some studies), margin status, aggressive tumor type (mesenchymal), and skull base or neurovascular involvement.[37,38] For small tumors, proton beam radiation therapy as a single modality treatment has been reported with some success.[39,40] Although local recurrence is common, regional and distant metastases are rare, and long-term prognosis is good with complete surgical excision. Survival rate has been reported from 44% to 87%.

Nasopharyngeal carcinoma

DEFINITIONS AND CLINICAL FEATURES

NPC is an upper airway tract malignancy originating from interactions between epithelial and B-cells in the nasopharynx.

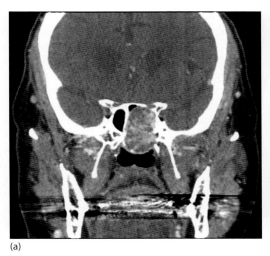
(a)

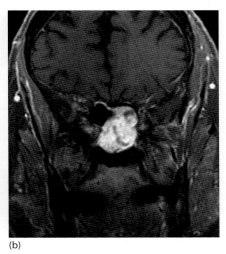
(b)

Figure 11.18 (a) Coronal soft tissue CT scan with contrast demonstrates a moderately enhancing mass involving the left sphenoid region. The lesion abuts the left optic nerve and erodes the floor of the sphenoid sinus. Biopsy confirmed diagnosis of low-grade chondrosarcoma. (b) Coronal T1-weighted MRI with contrast shows the hyperintense mass. No intracranial or orbital extension is noted.

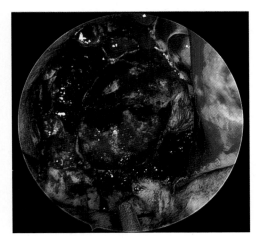

Figure 11.19 This patient underwent uneventful endoscopic resection of the mass after an extended sphenoid approach with a posterior septectomy. Endoscopy demonstrates the immediate intraoperative view of the sphenoclival region.

It accounts for ~1% of all childhood malignancies. Almost all adult nasopharyngeal cancers are carcinomas, whereas only 35%–50% of nasopharyngeal malignancies are carcinomas in children. NPC has a bimodal age distribution with a small peak in late childhood and a second peak occurs at 50–60 years. There is a 2:1 male/female predominance.

Three subtypes of NPC are recognized in the World Health Organization (WHO) classification: (1) squamous cell carcinoma, (2) nonkeratinizing carcinoma, and (3) undifferentiated carcinoma. Endemic areas include Southern China, Southeast Asia, Middle East, North Africa, Alaska, and Greenland. In these areas, there is a strong correlation between Epstein–Barr virus (EBV) latency and NPC. Most patients have poorly or undifferentiated carcinoma (WHO type 2 or 3) and present with locally advanced stage disease. NPC is rare in the United States and Western Europe, and the frequency of SCC (WHO type 1) is

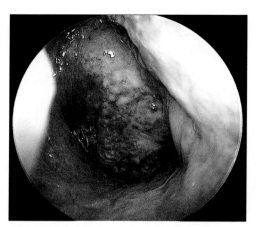

Figure 11.20 Endoscopic view of the right nasopharynx demonstrates a submucosal mass filling the right fossa of Rosenmuller.

about 25%, which is markedly higher than in endemic areas. Nodal involvement and bilateral nodal disease are more frequently observed with NPC than with other head and neck cancers. Additionally, it differs from nonnasopharyngeal head and neck SCC in its increased radio- and chemosensitivity and a greater propensity for distant metastases.

The tumor may appear as a submucosal bulge in the lateral nasopharynx or may form a large exophytic tumor mass (Figure 11.20). Enlargement and extension of the tumor in the nasopharynx may result in symptoms of nasal obstruction, changes in hearing secondary to direct extension or eustachian tube dysfunction, and cranial nerve palsies due to tumor extension into the skull base. NPC with spread to the regional lymph nodes may also initially come to medical attention as a primary neck mass before the nasopharyngeal site of origin is established.

DIFFERENTIAL DIAGNOSIS
Nasal polyps, non-Hodgkin's lymphoma, and rhabdomyosarcoma should be considered.

WORKUP/INVESTIGATIONS
Blood work should be performed for EBV titers, immunoglobulin A, and immunoglobulin G antibodies to the viral capsid antigen, early antigen, and nuclear antigen. Titers may correlate with tumor burden and decrease with treatment. Additionally, pretreatment and postradiotherapy plasma EBV-DNA levels may be a helpful marker for risk assessment, initial treatment response, and time of relapse, outcome, and survival.[41,42] Biopsy of the lesion shows cells that generally stain with p63 and high-molecular-weight keratins; however, the extent of staining may be variable. EBV can be shown by in situ hybridization in nearly 100% of cases, although this is lower in non-Asian populations. CT or MRI is recommended to define the disease in the nasopharynx and to detect lymph node metastases (Figure 11.21a and b).

TREATMENT
Radiation therapy is the primary treatment modality. Intensity-modulated radiotherapy (IMRT) techniques are recommended with locoregional control rates exceeding 90%. Prophylactic neck irradiation is recommended and usually covers the entire neck lymph node drainage region. Radiotherapy alone is adequate for treating stage I NPC; however, the treatment for stage II and locally advanced NPC (stages III–IVb) is concurrent cisplatin-based chemoradiotherapy. Concurrent cisplatin, 5-fluorouracil, and radiotherapy have been shown to improve survival.[43,44] Sequential chemoradiotherapy with gemcitabine and cisplatin has been shown to improve survival in locoregionally advanced NPC.[45] Induction chemotherapy appears to be better tolerated, and induction-concurrent sequences show substantially improved compliance, but may not significantly improve prognosis in overall and recurrence-free survival.[46] IMRT and appropriate chemotherapeutic agents have resulted in marked improvement in the outcome of NPC. Nonetheless, about 10% of patients still develop recurrent disease in the

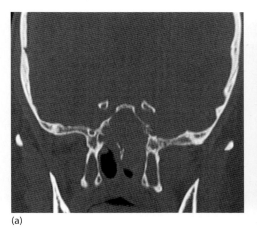 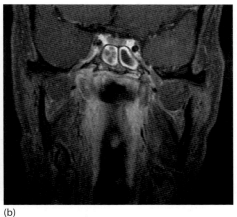

(a)   (b)

Figure 11.21 (a) Coronal bone window CT illustrates a soft tissue mass in the left nasopharynx with erosion of the sphenoid floor and extension into bilateral sphenoid sinuses. (b) Coronal T1-weighted MRI with contrast demonstrates an enhancing mass in bilateral nasopharynx, which is more prominent on the right. Abnormal enhancement in the right cavernous sinus is noted.

neck or at the primary site. The best salvage treatment for locally recurrent NPC remains to be determined, and the options include brachytherapy, external RT, stereotactic radiosurgery, nasopharyngectomy, and microwave coagulation therapy, either alone or in different combinations. The role of chemotherapy alone is primarily reserved for palliation in patients not suitable for radical radiation therapy or salvage nasopharyngectomy. The role of targeted therapy and EBV-specific immunotherapy is currently under investigation. The 5-year local control and overall survival rates are as high as 91% and 90%, respectively, for stage I NPC using conventional RT or IMRT. However, the treatment outcomes for locoregionally advanced NPC remain unsatisfactory and the 5-year overall survival rates are reported at 53%–80% and 28%–61% in NPC stages III and IV, respectively.[47]

Chordoma

DEFINITIONS AND CLINICAL FEATURES
Chordomas represent a rare clinical entity with an incidence of 0.08 per 100,000.[48] Chordomas are thought to arise from embryonic notochord remnants. They are most commonly located in the sacrococcygeal region or clivus, though the tumor can occur anywhere along the spine. Rarely, they occur in the cervical spine and can present as a paravertebral or parapharyngeal mass. Slightly over one-third of chordomas originate in the clivus where they present as midline, typically extradural masses, within the bone (Figure 11.22a through c). There are three histologic patterns: classic or conventional, chondroid, and dedifferentiated. Classic chordomas are most frequently encountered. Necrosis appears to be an important feature that portends a more aggressive course. Chondroid chordomas tend to be less aggressive than conventional chordomas, while dedifferentiated chordomas are more aggressive, faster growing, and more likely to metastasize. Dedifferentiated chordomas are often fatal within a year of diagnosis.

Chordomas can arise at any age, though most frequently occur between 30 and 50 years of age with a slight male predominance. They are slow growing with a propensity for locally aggressive behavior and

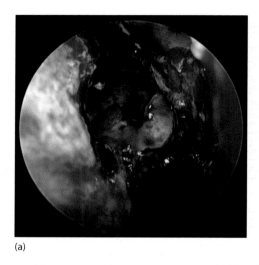

(a)

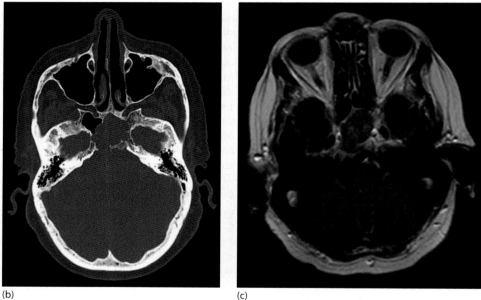

(b)   (c)

Figure 11.22 (a) Endoscopic view shows a gray to green submucosal mass partly filling the left sphenoid sinus. Biopsy confirmed the diagnosis of chordoma. (b) Axial bone window CT scan demonstrates a mass involving the left sphenoclival region. Erosion of bone over both paraclival carotid arteries is noted. (c) Axial T1-weighted MRI with gadolinium demonstrates a hypointense mass involving the sphenoclival region. The lesions abuts both paraclival carotids and extends to the posterior fossa.

rare metastasis, usually after recurrence. Cranial nerve involvement, particularly cranial nerve VI, is often seen at presentation.[49]

DIFFERENTIAL DIAGNOSIS

Chondrosarcoma, chordoid meningiomas, metastatic mucinous adenocarcinomas, and developmental lesion like ecchordosis physaliphora are in the differential.[50]

WORKUP/INVESTIGATIONS

Microscopic exam shows vacuolated cells that have been termed "physaliphorous cells" from the Greek meaning "bearer of bubbles."[49] By IHC, chordomas are positive for cytokeratin, epithelial membrane antigen, S-100 protein, and vimentin. Some are also positive for carcinoembryonic antigen (CEA).

TREATMENT

Optimal treatment is gross total resection via endoscopic endonasal approach when possible (Figure 11.23a and b). If the tumor location or extension is too lateral or inferior for effective endoscopic resection, an open or combined endoscopic/open approach should be utilized. Postoperative radiation therapy is typically indicated because of high likelihood for recurrence despite complete surgical resection. Recurrences tend to be local and late recurrences are relatively common.[50]

Hemangiopericytoma

Sinonasal-type hemangiopericytoma is an uncommon upper aerodigestive tract tumor of uncertain cellular differentiation. It comprises less than 1% of all vascular tumors and 15%–25% of these tumors are found in the head and neck.

Sinonasal hemangiopericytomas have no gender predilection and typically present in the third to fifth decade of life. Clinically, these tumors most often present with epistaxis and/or nasal obstruction. Endoscopic examination usually reveals a rubbery mass that is vascular and variable in color. Benign and malignant forms have been reported, with variable prognosis. Malignant sinonasal hemangiopericytomas are less common

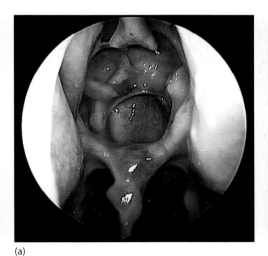
(a)

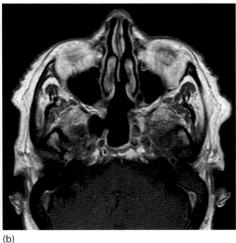
(b)

Figure 11.23 (a) Endoscopic exam at 1 year postendoscopic resection and postoperative radiation therapy demonstrates a completely healed sphenoclival region. (b) Axial T1-weighted MRI with contrast illustrates no evidence of recurrence at 2 years.

and can metastasize, most frequently to the lung, and also to the brain, bone, and liver. This tumor has also been reported to cause a paraneoplastic syndrome, called osteogenic osteomalacia. The tumor is relatively radioresistant and surgery is the mainstay of treatment. Most lesions can be resected completely via the endoscopic route. Adjuvant radiotherapy has proven beneficial if complete surgical resection is not feasible. However, recurrence remains a challenge in managing this tumor, with rates reported between 9% and 51%.[51]

Osteosarcoma

Osteosarcoma is a rare bone tumor arising in the long bones, with 6%–13% of cases occurring in the head and neck region. Osteosarcomas account for 0.5%–1% of sinonasal neoplasms. Most cases of sinonasal osteosarcoma are metastatic tumors or high-grade primary osteosarcomas. Well-differentiated osteosarcomas are low-grade malignant tumors and can de-differentiate to high-grade osteosarcomas and exhibit more aggressive biological behavior. Reports of long bone osteosarcomas indicate an average age of onset in the teenage years, whereas the mean age of onset of head and neck osteosarcomas is between 26 and 40 years of age. Craniofacial osteosarcomas may arise either de novo or postradiation and exhibit variable imaging features depending on the extent of bone destruction, soft tissue extension, and matrix composition. Surgery with adequate margins remains the mainstay of treatment, although the benefits of preoperative or adjuvant therapy are disputed. Factors affecting prognosis include adequacy of surgical resection and tumor grade. Hematogenous metastases occur less frequently in high-grade sinonasal osteosarcoma than in osteosarcomas of long bones, although metastasis to the lungs, lymph nodes, and other bones has been reported. Progressive local disease is the most common cause of death in patients with osteosarcomas of the head and neck. The overall 5-year survival rate has been reported as 55%, despite the preponderance of high-grade tumors.[52]

Financial disclosures

Batra: Research grants (ARS, Medtronic), consultant (Medtronic), SAB (Merck).
    McLean: None.

References

1. Haerle SK, Gullane PJ, Witterick IJ, Zweifel C, Gentili F. 2013. Sinonasal carcinomas: Epidemiology, pathology, and management. *Neurosurgery Clinics of North America* 24:39–49.
2. Harvey RJ, Dalgorf DM. 2013. Chapter 10: Sinonasal malignancies. *American Journal of Rhinology and Allergy* 27(Suppl. 1):S35–S38.
3. Ansa B, Goodman M, Ward K et al. 2013. Paranasal sinus squamous cell carcinoma incidence and survival based on Surveillance, Epidemiology, and End Results data, 1973 to 2009. *Cancer* 119:2602–2610.
4. Syrjanen K, Syrjanen S. 2013. Detection of human papillomavirus in sinonasal carcinoma: Systematic review and meta-analysis. *Human Pathology* 44:983–991.
5. Guan X, Wang X, Liu Y, Hu C, Zhu G. 2013. Lymph node metastasis in sinonasal squamous cell carcinoma treated with IMRT/3D-CRT. *Oral Oncology* 49:60–65.
6. Hanna EY, Cardenas AD, DeMonte F et al. 2011. Induction chemotherapy for advanced squamous cell carcinoma of the paranasal sinuses. *Archives of Otolaryngology—Head and Neck Surgery* 137:78–81.
7. Sanghvi S, Khan MN, Patel NR, Yeldandi S, Baredes S, Eloy JA. 2014. Epidemiology of sinonasal squamous cell carcinoma: A comprehensive analysis of 4,994 patients. *Laryngoscope* 124:76–83.

8. Husain Q, Kanumuri VV, Svider PF et al. 2013. Sinonasal adenoid cystic carcinoma: Systematic review of survival and treatment strategies. *Otolaryngology: Head and Neck Surgery* 148:29–39.

9. Moskaluk CA. 2013. Adenoid cystic carcinoma: Clinical and molecular features. *Head and Neck Pathology* 7:17–22.

10. Adelglass JM, Samara M, Cantor JO, Rankow RM, Blitzer A, Luken MG. 1980. Thorotrast-induced multiple carcinomatosis of the frontal sinus. *Bulletin of the New York Academy of Medicine* 56:453–457.

11. Sanghvi S, Patel NR, Patel CR, Kalyoussef E, Baredes S, Eloy JA. 2013. Sinonasal adenoid cystic carcinoma: Comprehensive analysis of incidence and survival from 1973 to 2009. *Laryngoscope* 123:1592–1597.

12. Vikram B, Strong EW, Shah JP, Spiro RH. 1984. Radiation therapy in adenoid-cystic carcinoma. *International Journal of Radiation Oncology, Biology, Physics* 10:221–223.

13. Mori Y, Kobayashi T, Kida Y, Oda K, Shibamoto Y, Yoshida J. 2005. Stereotactic radiosurgery as a salvage treatment for recurrent skull base adenoid cystic carcinoma. *Stereotactic and Functional Neurosurgery* 83:202–207.

14. Nylander LA, Dement JM. 1993. Carcinogenic effects of wood dust: Review and discussion. *American Journal of Industrial Medicine* 24:619–647.

15. Jankowski R, Georgel T, Vignaud JM et al. 2007. Endoscopic surgery reveals that woodworkers' adenocarcinomas originate in the olfactory cleft. *Rhinology* 45:308–314.

16. Lund VJ, Chisholm EJ, Takes RP et al. 2012. Evidence for treatment strategies in sinonasal adenocarcinoma. *Head and Neck* 34:1168–1178.

17. Choussy O, Ferron C, Vedrine PO et al. 2008. Adenocarcinoma of Ethmoid: A GETTEC retrospective multicenter study of 418 cases. *Laryngoscope* 118:437–443.

18. Leivo I. 2007. Update on sinonasal adenocarcinoma: Classification and advances in immunophenotype and molecular genetic make-up. *Head and Neck Pathology* 1:38–43.

19. Franchi A, Massi D, Palomba A, Biancalani M, Santucci M. 2004. CDX-2, cytokeratin 7 and cytokeratin 20 immunohistochemical expression in the differential diagnosis of primary adenocarcinomas of the sinonasal tract. *Virchows Archiv* 445:63–67.

20. Gal TJ, Silver N, Huang B. 2011. Demographics and treatment trends in sinonasal mucosal melanoma. *Laryngoscope* 121:2026–2033.

21. Clifton N, Harrison L, Bradley PJ, Jones NS. 2011. Malignant melanoma of nasal cavity and paranasal sinuses: Report of 24 patients and literature review. *Journal of Laryngology and Otology* 125:479–485.

22. Dauer EH, Lewis JE, Rohlinger AL, Weaver AL, Olsen KD. 2008. Sinonasal melanoma: A clinicopathologic review of 61 cases. *Otolaryngology: Head and Neck Surgery* 138:347–352.

23. Faragalla H, Weinreb I. 2009. Olfactory neuroblastoma: A review and update. *Advances in Anatomic Pathology* 16:322–331.

24. Foote RL, Morita A, Ebersold MJ et al. 1993. Esthesioneuroblastoma: The role of adjuvant radiation therapy. *International Journal of Radiation Oncology, Biology, Physics* 27:835–842.

25. Dulguerov P, Calcaterra T. 1992. Esthesioneuroblastoma: The UCLA experience 1970–1990. *Laryngoscope* 102:843–849.

26. Devaiah AK, Andreoli MT. 2009. Treatment of esthesioneuroblastoma: A 16-year meta-analysis of 361 patients. *Laryngoscope* 119:1412–1416.

27. Malouf GG, Casiraghi O, Deutsch E, Guigay J, Temam S, Bourhis J. 2013. Low- and high-grade esthesioneuroblastomas display a distinct natural history and outcome. *European Journal of Cancer* 49:1324–1334.

28. Reiersen DA, Pahilan ME, Devaiah AK. 2012. Meta-analysis of treatment outcomes for sinonasal undifferentiated carcinoma. *Otolaryngology: Head and Neck Surgery* 147:7–14.

29. Yoshida E, Aouad R, Fragoso R et al. 2013. Improved clinical outcomes with multi-modality therapy for sinonasal undifferentiated carcinoma of the head and neck. *American Journal of Otolaryngology* 34:658–663.

30. Mendenhall WM, Mendenhall CM, Riggs CE, Jr., Villaret DB, Mendenhall NP. 2006. Sinonasal undifferentiated carcinoma. *American Journal of Clinical Oncology* 29:27–31.

31. Ansari M, Guo S, Fakhri S et al. 2013. Sinonasal undifferentiated carcinoma (SNUC): Morphoproteomic-guided treatment paradigm with clinical efficacy. *Annals of Clinical Laboratory Science* 43:45–53.

32. Lightenstein L, Bernstein D. 1959. Unusual benign and malignant chondroid tumors of bone. A survey of some mesenchymal cartilage tumors and malignant chondroblastic tumors, including a few multicentric ones, as well as many atypical benign chondroblastomas and chondromyxoid fibromas. *Cancer* 12:1142–1157.

33. Khan MN, Husain Q, Kanumuri VV et al. 2013. Management of sinonasal chondrosarcoma: A systematic review of 161 patients. *International Forum of Allergy and Rhinology* 3:670–677.

34. Connor SE, Umaria N, Chavda SV. 2001. Imaging of giant tumours involving the anterior skull base. *British Journal of Radiology* 74:662–667.

35. Korten AG, ter Berg HJ, Spincemaille GH, van der Laan RT, Van de Wel AM. 1998. Intracranial chondrosarcoma: Review of the literature and report of 15 cases. *Journal of Neurology, Neurosurgery, and Psychiatry* 65:88–92.

36. Kharrat S, Sahtout S, Tababi S et al. 2010. Chondrosarcoma of sinonasal cavity: A case report and brief literature review. *La Tunisie médicale* 88:122–124.

37. Knott PD, Gannon FH, Thompson LD. 2003. Mesenchymal chondrosarcoma of the sinonasal tract: A clinicopathological study of 13 cases with a review of the literature. *Laryngoscope* 113:783–790.

38. Mark RJ, Tran LM, Sercarz J, Fu YS, Calcaterra TC, Parker RG. 1993. Chondrosarcoma of the head and neck. The UCLA experience, 1955–1988. *American Journal of Clinical Oncology* 16:232–237.

39. Mokhtari S, Mirafsharieh A. 2012. Clear cell chondrosarcoma of the head and neck. *Head and Neck Oncology* 4:13.

40. Weber DC, Rutz HP, Pedroni ES et al. 2005. Results of spot-scanning proton radiation therapy for chordoma and chondrosarcoma of the skull base: The Paul Scherrer Institut experience. *International Journal of Radiation Oncology, Biology, Physics* 63:401–409.

41. Gastpar H, Wilmes E, Wolf H. 1981. Epidemiologic, etiologic and immunologic aspects of nasopharyngeal carcinoma [NPC]. *Journal of Medicine* 12:257–284.

42. Henle G, Henle W. 1976. Epstein-Barr virus-specific IgA serum antibodies as an outstanding feature of nasopharyngeal carcinoma. *International Journal of Cancer* 17:1–7.

43. Al-Sarraf M, LeBlanc M, Giri PG et al. 1998. Chemoradiotherapy versus radiotherapy in patients with advanced nasopharyngeal cancer: Phase III randomized Intergroup study 0099. *Journal of Clinical Oncology* 16:1310–1317.

44. Chan AT, Teo PM, Leung TW, Johnson PJ. 1998. The role of chemotherapy in the management of nasopharyngeal carcinoma. *Cancer* 82:1003–1012.

45. Gu MF, Liu LZ, He LJ et al. 2013. Sequential chemoradiotherapy with gemcitabine and cisplatin for locoregionally advanced nasopharyngeal carcinoma. *International Journal of Cancer* 132:215–223.

46. Liang ZG, Zhu XD, Tan AH et al. 2013. Induction chemotherapy followed by concurrent chemoradiotherapy versus concurrent chemoradiotherapy with or without adjuvant chemotherapy for locoregionally advanced nasopharyngeal carcinoma: Meta-analysis of 1,096 patients from 11 randomized controlled trials. *Asian Pacific Journal of Cancer Prevention* 14:515–521.

47. Zhang L, Chen QY, Liu H, Tang LQ, Mai HQ. 2013. Emerging treatment options for nasopharyngeal carcinoma. *Drug, Design, Development and Therapy* 7:37–52.

48. Safwat A, Nielsen OS, Jurik AG et al. 1997. A retrospective clinicopathological study of 37 patients with chordoma: A danish national series. *Sarcoma* 1:161–165.

49. Barnes L, Kapadia SB. 1994. The biology and pathology of selected skull base tumors. *Journal of Neuro-Oncology* 20:213–240.

50. Fernandez-Miranda JC, Gardner PA, Snyderman CH et al. 2014. Clival chordomas: A pathological, surgical, and radiotherapeutic review. *Head and Neck* 36:892–906.

51. Dahodwala MQ, Husain Q, Kanumuri VV, Choudhry OJ, Liu JK, Eloy JA. 2013. Management of sinonasal hemangiopericytomas: A systematic review. *International Forum of Allergy and Rhinology* 3:581–587.

52. Ha PK, Eisele DW, Frassica FJ et al. 1999. Osteosarcoma of the head and neck: A review of the Johns Hopkins experience. *Laryngoscope* 109:964–969.

SECTION 3

LARYNGOLOGY

Common Problems of the True Vocal Folds

Glendon M. Gardner and Michael S. Benninger

- **Normal examination**
- **Nodule**
- **Cyst**
- **Polyp**
- **Granuloma: Contact ulcer**
- **Granulation tissue**
- **Recurrent respiratory papilloma**
- **Polypoid corditis, polypoid degeneration, Reinke's edema**
- **Sulcus vocalis**
- **Laryngopharyngeal reflux disease**
- **Laryngocele**
- **Vocal fold paralysis**
- **Squamous cell carcinoma**
- **Leukoplakia**
- **Infectious laryngitis**
- **Vocal fold hemorrhage and vascular ectasias**

Normal examination

Examination of the larynx begins with listening to the patient's voice while they give you their history. Voice is not something we can quantify like hearing. We have yet to create the easily measurable voicegram like the audiogram. Yet, most of us know a "normal" voice when we hear it, and an abnormal voice when we hear that. A normal speaking voice does not draw attention to itself, unless it is an unusually beautiful or powerful voice, although some "normal" voices are simply unpleasant to listen to. For most normal voices, the listener does not think about the quality of the voice; rather they listen to what is being said.

The larynx can be viewed in several different ways. Indirect laryngoscopy with a mirror is the simplest method and is successful in approximately 2/3 of patients. This is often adequate to rule out many pathologies. The mirror exam also provides a better appreciation of color of the larynx, since no video or lens is involved, which could distort color. For those patients in whom indirect laryngoscopy is not possible, due to an overly sensitive gag reflex, difficult anatomy, the patient's inability to do the task, or certain anatomy cannot be adequately seen (anterior commissure), flexible fiber-optic laryngoscopes are used. This allows a clear view of all regions of the larynx, with the possible exception of the subglottis. Also, motion of the vocal folds can be best assessed with the flexible scope, since it allows the patient to sniff to maximally stimulate the posterior cricoarytenoid muscles, something not possible, or at least very difficult, with transoral examination with a mirror or rigid scope. The transoral route, which involves grasping the extended tongue, can cause the appearance of excessive tension, which may be induced by the exam and not how the person typically phonates, leading to a misdiagnosis of muscle tension dysphonia.

The larynx is composed of three large singular cartilages, thyroid, cricoid, and epiglottic; a pair of arytenoid cartilages; and pairs of smaller cartilages, corniculate and cuneiform. The three main cartilages are connected by ligaments as well as muscles, named for their attachments and positions: cricothyroid muscles, lateral cricoarytenoid muscles, posterior cricoarytenoid muscles, and thyroarytenoid muscles (also known as the vocalis muscle). The larynx is lined with mucosa draped over the muscles and ligaments. Motor and sensory innervation is supplied by the recurrent laryngeal nerve and the internal and external branches of the superior laryngeal nerve, which are branches of the vagus nerve.

The laryngoscopist will see several structures, including the epiglottis, aryepiglottic folds, false vocal folds, the entrance to the ventricles, mucosa overlying the corniculate and arytenoid cartilages and the true vocal folds (Figures 12.1 and 12.2). The anterior 2/3 of the true vocal folds extend from the anterior commissure, which is attached to the thyroid cartilage, to the vocal processes of the mobile arytenoid cartilages. This portion of the true vocal folds is referred to as the musculomembranous portion. This is the portion that vibrates and is responsible for the sound of the voice. The posterior 1/3 is posterior to the vocal processes and extends to the inner surface of the cricoid cartilage. Although this portion of the

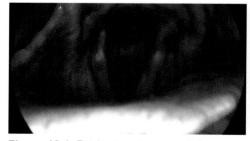

Figure 12.1 Epiglottis at bottom of picture, right aryepiglottic fold upper left.

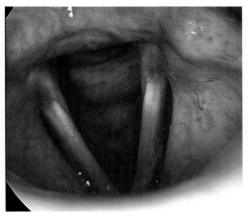

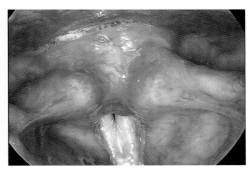

Figure 12.3 Normal closure during phonation. Normal pyriform sinuses with no pooling.

Figure 12.2 Normal vocal folds in fully abducted position.

glottis is typically referred to as the posterior commissure, it is not a true commissure and should be called the posterior larynx. The glottis is the tissue at the level of the true vocal folds. The supraglottis is above the ventricles and includes the false vocal folds, the epiglottis, and all the tissue connecting them. The subglottis starts 1 cm below the superior edge of the true vocal folds.

The basic parameters to observe when examining the larynx include relative symmetry of the two sides, the presence of lesions, color of tissue, the contours of the vocal folds (straight or concave), motion of the vocal folds, closure of the glottis during phonation, the size of the airway, and pooling of secretions in the pyriform sinuses. Obvious abnormalities in any of these categories will be apparent with indirect laryngoscopy or flexible laryngoscopy (Figure 12.3).

Videostroboscopy and high-speed videography are both techniques used to see vibrating vocal folds in slow motion. When vocal folds are vibrating at 100 Hz or greater, they appear fuzzy to the eye. Being able to slow this motion down allows us to see how well the vocal folds are vibrating. The mucosa of a normal true vocal fold slides over the vocal ligament when vibrating,

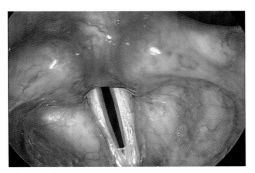

Figure 12.4 Normal mucosal waves, open phase of glottal cycle of vibration, as seen with videostroboscopy. Small amount of mucus at anterior commissure.

creating a wave, referred to as the "mucosal wave" (Figure 12.4). Loss of the wave indicates an abnormality of the mucosa or superficial layer of the lamina propria. Sometimes normal-appearing vocal folds do not vibrate normally, thereby explaining why the voice is not normal. These techniques also often reveal subtle lesions of the vocal folds not seen with the unaided eye. It also best demonstrates closure (Figure 12.3). Either technique can and should be done with either a rigid telescope or a distal chip (chip tip) flexible scope, depending on the patient's tolerance and anatomy. The telescopes with a 3-chip camera or the distal chip flexible scope provide the best detail.

Recording the exam enables the clinician to review the exam in slow motion and have more than one viewer, both increasing the sensitivity of the examination. The patient is also able to see the pathology (or lack thereof), which helps the patient understand the problem they have and appreciate what is necessary for treatment. Having an image is extremely valuable for follow-up examinations to determine if lesions, vocal motion, closure, excessive muscle tension, or a variety of other parameters have changed.

If the pathology is subglottic or tracheal, flexible endoscopy with topical anesthesia in the office is employed. After topically anesthetizing the nose, the larynx can be anesthetized several different ways. The simplest technique is using a laryngeal mirror to guide a curved cannula or sprayer transorally to drip or spray an anesthetic, such as tetracaine, on the glottis. A scope with a side port can also be used to spray the vocal folds directly, if the patient does not tolerate the transoral approach. Last, bilateral superior laryngeal nerve blocks can be performed with injection of lidocaine at the lateral aspect of the thyrohyoid membrane bilaterally. This last technique is rarely necessary. Once adequate anesthesia is achieved, the scope can be passed beyond the glottis, providing an excellent view of the subglottis and trachea. The exam should be recorded because, despite the anesthetic, patients often cough and tolerate the exam only briefly and being able to review the exam frame by frame afterward can be critical.

Experienced clinicians often know before they look at the larynx what they will see. A singer whose voice became a bit rough while performing and has a barely perceptible abnormality when they come to the office is likely to have a submucosal hemorrhage. A man who awoke from a thyroidectomy with a weak breathy voice will have a paralyzed vocal fold. The loud soccer mom with a moderately rough voice typically has vocal fold nodules. A 60-year-old woman smoker who sounds like a man has polypoid degeneration of the vocal folds. These pathologies will be presented in the following section.

Images obtained in the office or clinic will be oriented anterior down, while operative images will be oriented anterior up, reflecting how the clinician sees the larynx in these different settings.

This section will feature pathology that can be appreciated in still images. Some conditions, such as adductor spasmodic dysphonia and voice tremor, can only be diagnosed by observing the larynx in motion and will not be addressed in this section in detail.

Be aware that the definitions of a variety of benign lesions of the vocal folds have not been agreed upon by the community of laryngologists in the United States. In addition, many general otolaryngologists use several of the names interchangeably, mostly "nodule" and "polyp," but may, in fact, be describing a cyst or pseudocyst. The following definitions are those used most commonly among laryngologists. Also, pathologists often use the terms "nodule" and "polyp" for lesions that are grossly quite different, but may appear similar microscopically.

Nodule

DEFINITION
Nodules are bilateral relatively symmetric lesions in the midportion of the musculomembranous portion of the vocal folds, which is the area of greatest vibration.

CLINICAL FEATURES
Patients typically have a long history of phonotrauma (voice overuse or abuse). Screaming children, teachers, "soccer moms," sports coaches, and untrained singers are prone to nodule formation. Early in their development, they are soft raised areas of edema located in the epithelium and/or

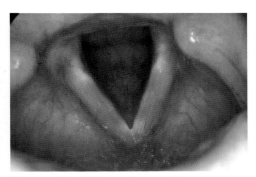

Figure 12.5 Subtle, soft prenodules in a female alto singer.

the subepithelium or superficial layer of the lamina propria. At this stage, they are often referred to as *pre*nodules to avoid the anxiety associated with a diagnosis of nodules for singers (Figures 12.5 and 12.6).

DIFFERENTIAL DIAGNOSIS

Soft nodules can be differentiated from cysts or pseudocysts with videostroboscopy or high-speed digital video because they "ride" the mucosal wave rather than disrupt or abolish it. There is absence of

the mucosal wave at a cyst. Mature fibrotic nodules are the end result of chronic phonotrauma. The lesions are thicker and harder as seen on videostroboscopy and when palpated in the operating room during direct microlaryngoscopy (Figures 12.7 through 12.11). The fibrosis is in the epithelium and/or immediately deep to the epithelium in the superficial layer of the lamina propria.

Often, a unilateral cyst or pseudocyst will cause swelling of the contralateral vocal fold and this may appear very similar to symmetric classic vocal fold nodules. The contralateral lesion is often referred to as a reactive nodule. It can be difficult to determine which is the primary lesion and which is reactive. The behavior of the mucosal wave can help with diagnosis. See the following text for the treatment considerations.

Classic nodules will be aligned with each other. The presence of unaligned "bamboo shoot" nodules, which have a transverse white line, raises the possibility of lupoid or rheumatic nodules, due to autoimmune disease (Figures 12.12 and 12.13). The mucosal wave is impaired at the site of the

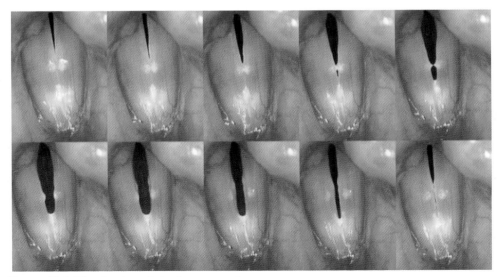

Figure 12.6 The glottic cycle in the same patient.

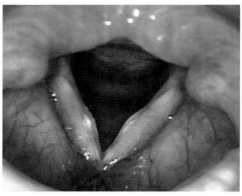

Figure 12.7 More mature nodules.

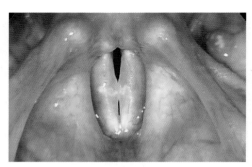

Figure 12.10 Incomplete closure.

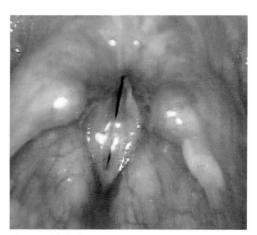

Figure 12.8 Same patient, nodules causing incomplete closure.

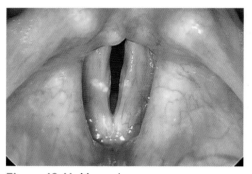

Figure 12.11 Mucosal waves.

lesion and the appearance can be mistaken for a submucosal cyst. An appropriate autoimmune workup should be carried out. Excision of a portion of the submucosal fibrous tissue may improve voice. The tissue, however, is not diagnostic of a particular disease.

TREATMENT

With vocal hygiene and voice therapy, soft *pre*nodules usually resolve.

While the voice may improve with voice therapy, the more mature nodules often do not resolve with therapy. If further improvement is desired, the nodules can be conservatively excised with microsurgical technique, taking care not to injure the underlying vocal ligament or surrounding normal tissue (Figures 12.14 through 12.18).

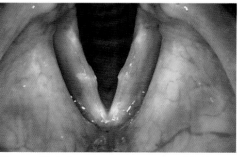

Figure 12.9 Prominent mature vocal fold nodules in a singer and athlete.

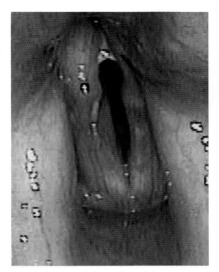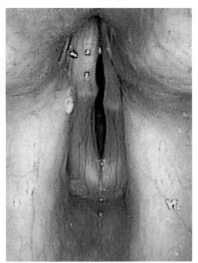

Figure 12.12 "Bamboo shoot" nodules impairing the mucosal wave.

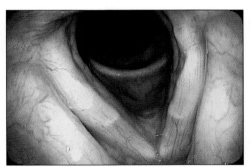

Figure 12.13 "Bamboo shoot" nodules, transverse white lines, not aligned from side to side.

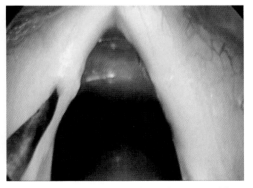

Figure 12.14 Incision made with microsickle knife at superior junction of the nodule and normal mucosa. Incision into superficial layer of lamina propria. Right true vocal fold nodule has already been removed.

Cyst

DEFINITION
A cyst has a well-defined membrane that contains liquid. Old "burned-out" cysts may have a similar appearance, but are a fibrotic mass, with no fluid within.

CLINICAL FEATURES
Patients may have a history of phonotrauma, similar to nodule patients or have no features in common with that population. Cysts may be congenital or acquired and are mucus filled. Acquired cysts are thought to occur when inflammation leads to plugging of the duct of a mucinous gland. This inflammation could be due to smoking, phonotrauma, or reflux. The mucus backs up slowly dilating the gland/duct, forming the mucus-filled cyst. The cyst is an ovoid structure that resides in the superficial layer of the lamina propria and tethers the

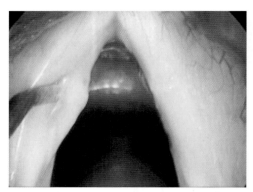

Figure 12.15 Elevation of lesion with 30° blunt tipped elevator.

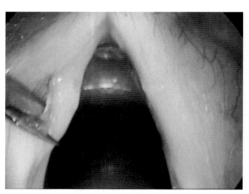

Figure 12.16 Posterior cut being made with upbiting microscissors.

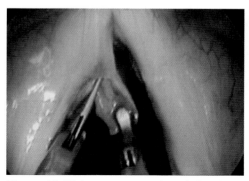

Figure 12.17 Lesion retracted medially while inferior and anterior incisions are made.

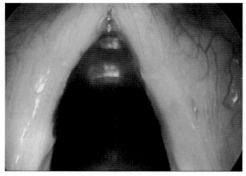

Figure 12.18 Final defect.

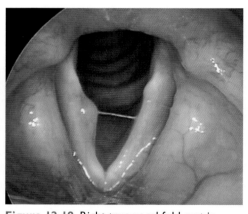

Figure 12.19 Right true vocal fold cyst in 66-year-old woman with 5 years of hoarseness.

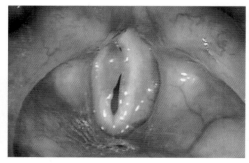

Figure 12.20 Closure.

overlying mucosa so that it is unable to slide over the vocal ligament or the cyst, interfering with propagation of the mucosal wave (Figures 12.19 through 12.22). A pseudocyst has a similar appearance but lacks a true

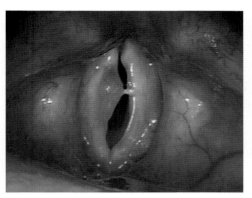

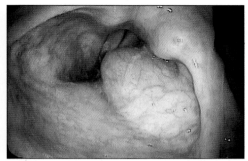

Figure 12.23 Left false vocal fold cyst.

Figure 12.21 Mucosal wave is abolished on the right.

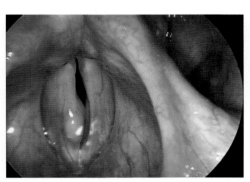

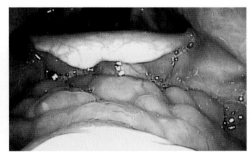

Figure 12.24 Epiglottic cyst, lingual surface, close-up.

Figure 12.22 Very large right true vocal fold cyst.

capsule. Cysts can also occur in many other locations in the larynx and pharynx, rarely causing symptoms and are usually incidental finding (Figures 12.23 through 12.28).

DIFFERENTIAL DIAGNOSIS

Cysts most closely resemble vocal fold nodules or sessile polyps. They are easily mistaken for classic nodules when there is a contralateral "reactive nodule." The lack of a mucosal wave differentiates between cysts and nodules. Voice therapy will often cause resolution of the reactive nodule, while the cyst remains.

TREATMENT

While voice therapy may result in an improved voice, it does not lead to

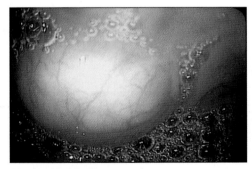

Figure 12.25 Close up of cyst.

resolution of the cyst. Cysts have been known to rupture either externally, which can result in a sulcus vocalis, or internally, but both are infrequent occurrences (Figures 12.29 through 12.31). If the cyst persists and the patient's voice remains poor, then excision of

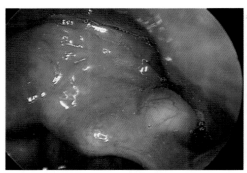

Figure 12.26 Left pyriform sinus cyst.

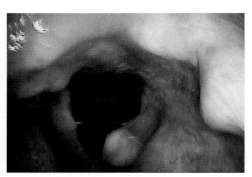

Figure 12.29 Left vocal fold cyst.

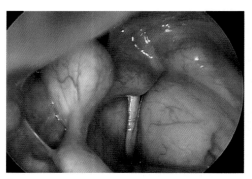

Figure 12.27 Right aryepiglottic fold cyst.

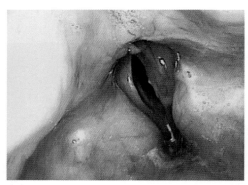

Figure 12.30 Same patient within weeks after spontaneous internal rupture of the cyst.

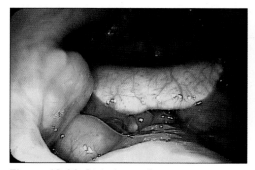

Figure 12.28 Right base of tongue cyst.

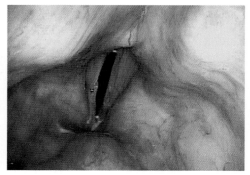

Figure 12.31 Same patient several months later with normal mucosal waves. No recurrence of cyst.

the cyst is recommended. This is one of the more technically difficult surgeries performed on the vocal folds, requiring magnification, the appropriate fine microlaryngeal instruments, very steady hands, and a delicate technique. The goal is to dissect out the cyst, preserving all of the normal overlying mucosa, not injuring the underlying vocal ligament and not rupturing the capsule of the cyst. If the cyst is removed unruptured, then there is no doubt that the entire cyst has been removed. If it ruptures, then some of the wall may remain and the cyst may reform in the future. Since the cyst arises from and is therefore attached to the epithelium, dissecting it free from the mucosa is very difficult, and this is the site where rupturing the cyst is most likely to occur. If the overlying mucosa is completely preserved, the recovery is usually very smooth and rapid with improvement in voice in the vast majority of cases. The mucosal wave may or may not be restored, however (Figures 12.22, 12.31 through 12.39).

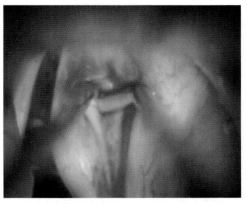

Figure 12.33 After an incision over the top of the cyst, a mucosal microflap is elevated over the medial aspect of the cyst.

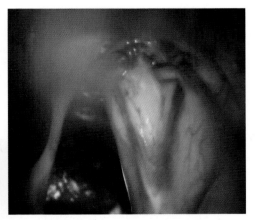

Figure 12.34 The cyst is elevated off the vocal ligament.

As mentioned in the "Nodules" section, there may be a reactive nodule opposite the cyst. If it is soft, it may resolve once the cyst has been excised. If it is firm, it should be excised at the same time as the cyst.

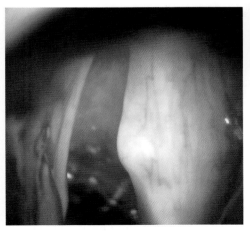

Figure 12.32 Intraoperative view.

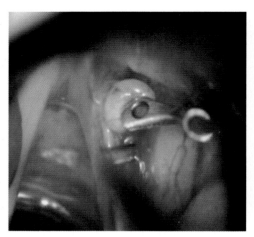

Figure 12.35 Cyst is being removed intact.

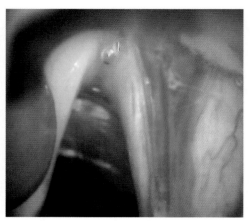

Figure 12.36 Intact microflap redraped at the end of the case.

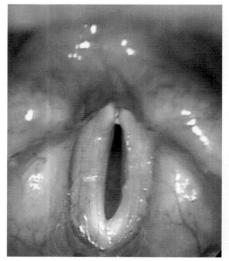

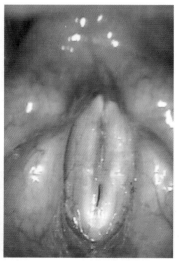

Figure 12.37 Eighteen months post excision. Mucosal wave still slightly blunted on the right. Tiny gap anteriorly.

Polyp

DEFINITION

Laryngeal polyps are not considered neoplasms (although some neoplasms may be polypoid in appearance). A polyp generally has a thin epithelium overlying an edematous or gelatinous matrix.

CLINICAL FEATURES

They can be long and pedunculated, sessile and broad based, single or multiple. The cause of the edema within the superficial layer of the lamina propria can be an episode of bleeding, smoking, hypothyroidism, chronic phonotrauma, perhaps laryngopharyngeal reflux. Polyps come in many

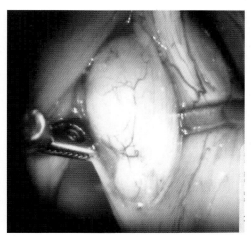

Figure 12.38 Intraoperative photo of cyst being dissected.

different shapes and sizes and can occur in several different locations in the larynx. The most common location is the musculomembranous true vocal fold. They have also been seen extending from the ventricle. The history may vary considerably from patient to patient, depending on the etiology (Figures 12.40 through 12.46).

DIFFERENTIAL DIAGNOSIS

Occasionally, a polyp emanating from the ventricle or false vocal fold may be mistaken for an internal laryngocele. If there is concern as to whether the mass is a polyp or a neoplasm, a biopsy must be done (Figures 12.47 and 12.48).

TREATMENT

If the likely etiology is smoking, cessation of smoking may result in some decrease in the size of the polyp(s). Voice therapy may also be helpful, if not to decrease the size of the polyp(s), to improve postoperative healing. With time, some polyps recede or fall off. Most polyps require excision to restore a normal voice, but the urgency and timing depend on the size and location of the polyp(s) and the patient's needs. Surgical excision is relatively easy, but care must still be taken to avoid trauma to the surrounding normal tissue and vocal ligament. They can be removed with cold instruments or lasers. Coagulation of the polyp with a fiber-optically delivered laser in the office may also provide an excellent result (Figures 12.49 and 12.50). The shape and

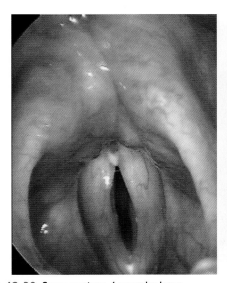
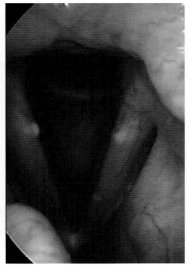

Figure 12.39 Same patient 4 months later.

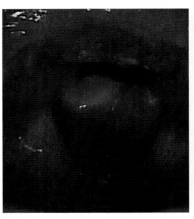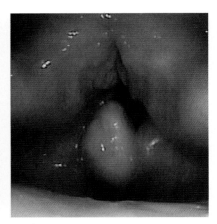

Figure 12.40 Severe polypoid degeneration in a smoker.

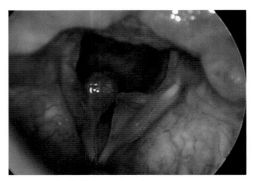

Figure 12.41 Bilateral polyps.

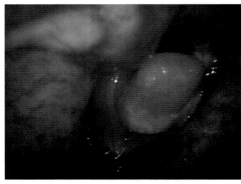

Figure 12.42 Large left vocal fold polyp.

location of the polyp, the surgical technique as well as how well the patient complies with postoperative rehabilitation will determine how well the patient heals and how good the postoperative voice is.

Granuloma: Contact ulcer

DEFINITION
The classic vocal fold granuloma is a smooth mass, often bilobed, arising from the vocal process of the arytenoid cartilage. There is usually no epithelium present. It is essentially an ulcer, composed of a mass of inflammatory cells. It is not a true "granuloma" as there are rarely multinucleated giant cells.

CLINICAL FEATURES
A vocal process ulcer or granuloma arises from trauma to the thin mucosa overlying the vocal process of the arytenoid cartilage. Endotracheal intubation, chronic throat clearing, laryngopharyngeal reflux, hard glottal onset, hard compression of the vocal processes due to an incompetent musculomembranous glottis, have all been listed as sources of that trauma (Figures 12.51 through 12.55). For intubation granulomas

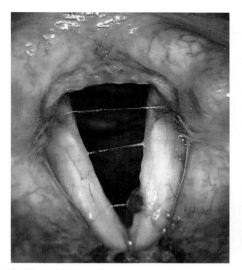
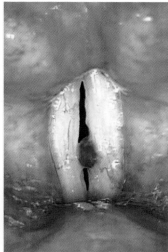

Figure 12.43 Left hemorrhagic or vascular polyp, incomplete closure.

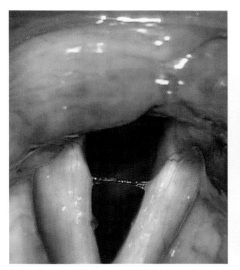
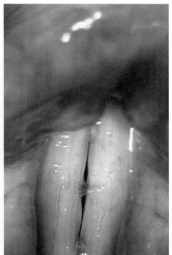

Figure 12.44 Tiny right true vocal fold vascular polyp.

or ulcers, the typical symptoms of globus sensation, throat clearing, pain (possibly with referred unilateral otalgia), and variable degrees of hoarseness may not appear for several weeks or months after the intubation. Very large granulomas may cause airway compromise.

DIFFERENTIAL DIAGNOSIS

Lesions that have been mistaken for granulomas include granular cell tumors, cysts, and polyps (Figures 12.56 through 12.58). A cancer is more likely to resemble an ulcer than an exophytic granuloma. A Teflon granuloma is a true granuloma (foreign

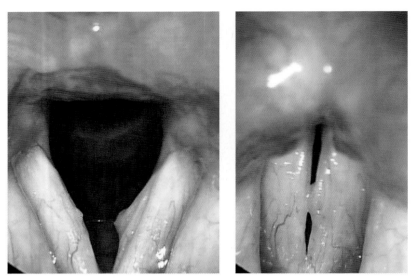

Figure 12.45 Left sessile vocal fold polyp, incomplete closure.

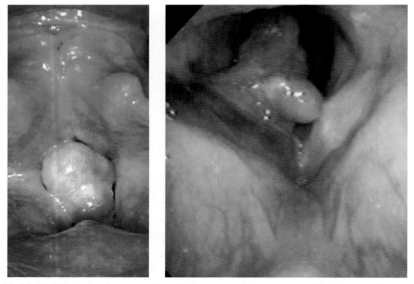

Figure 12.46 Multilobed polyp as well as likely recent right true vocal fold hemorrhage.

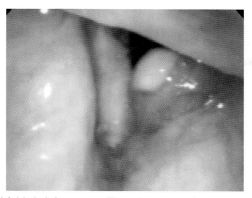

Figure 12.47 Left vocal fold rhabdomyoma. The white area is the result of an attempt at pulsed dye laser coagulation of what was thought to be a polyp emanating from the left ventricle. When it did not respond in a typical manner, it was biopsied, revealing the pathology and then excised in the operating room with the CO_2 laser. It arose from the superior aspect of the true vocal fold. The white area is *not* typical of this lesion, whereas the more lateral aspect is.

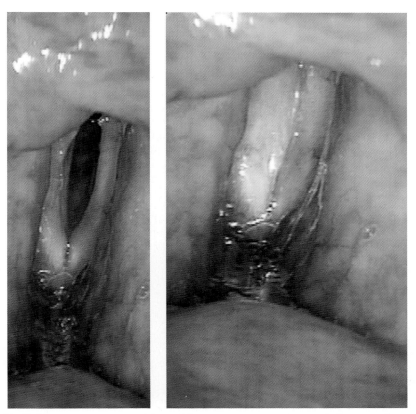

Figure 12.48 Three years post excision, with no recurrence and normal closure and mucosal waves.

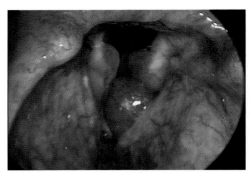

Figure 12.49 Multiple large polyps and polypoid corditis in a 60-year-old woman recent ex-smoker.

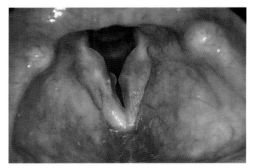

Figure 12.50 Same patient 1 month post pulsed dye laser coagulation of the polyps (no excision done).

body reaction) and has a variable appearance and is the result of injection of Teflon into the vocal fold to treat unilateral vocal fold paralysis. This substance is no longer used for this purpose (Figure 12.59).

WORKUP

If the lesion varies in appearance from the classic granuloma, if it grows, or if it does not respond to the antireflux and voice therapy discussed, or if the physician has any doubt regarding the diagnosis or the patient has significant anxiety, then it should be excised, or at least biopsied to confirm the diagnosis, keeping in mind that there is a high recurrence rate after excision. Ulcers and granulomas may develop in patients with an incompetent glottis, so glottic closure must be assessed. While calcified arytenoid cartilages have been associated with granulomas or ulcers, imaging is not routinely done (Figure 12.54).

TREATMENT

With intubation granulomas, the underlying cause has already been eliminated. With time and avoidance of throat clearing, the granuloma may resolve on its own either by shrinking or falling off. Most (but not all) laryngologists treat patients

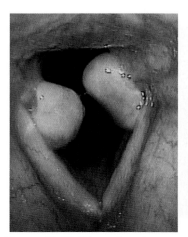
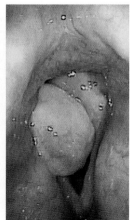
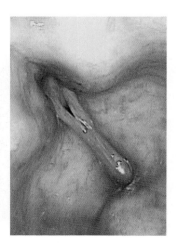

Figure 12.51 Bilateral intubation granulomas.

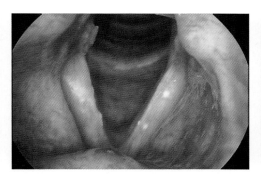

Figure 12.52 Right vocal fold ulcer in a professional singer.

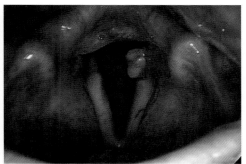

Figure 12.55 Patient with acid reflux and chronic throat clearing.

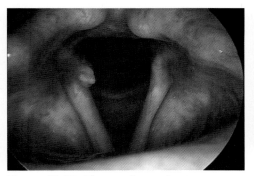

Figure 12.53 Chronic throat clearing.

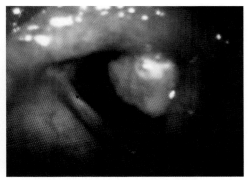

Figure 12.56 Granular cell tumor. Note different consistency of tissue and lack of bilobed appearance.

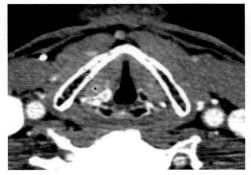

Figure 12.54 Calcified arytenoid cartilage on same side as granuloma.

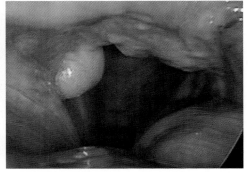

Figure 12.57 Right-sided lesion that appeared to be granuloma, but was a cyst.

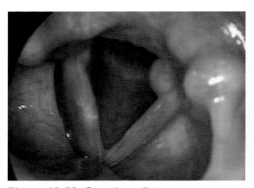

Figure 12.58 Granular cell tumor.

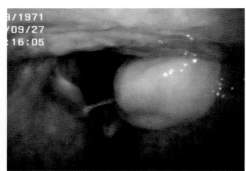

Figure 12.60 Left vocal process granuloma 5 months post 2 intubations.

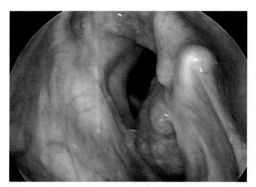

Figure 12.59 Teflon granuloma 29 years after injection.

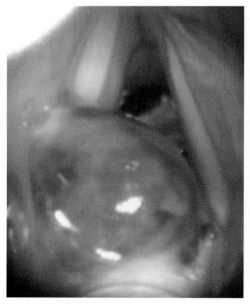

Figure 12.61 Large left vocal process granuloma, endoscopic view post intubation with laser proof endotracheal tube.

with granulomas with antacid medications. Voice therapy may be required to decrease throat clearing and/or hard glottal attack to decrease the trauma to the vocal processes. Simple excision of the granuloma often fails with at least a 50% recurrence rate. If the granuloma is excised, the base can be injected with steroids (Figures 12.60 through 12.64). Botox injections to the thyroarytenoid muscles help prevent forceful contact between the vocal processes postoperatively to prevent recurrence or have been employed as the sole therapy with great success. Use of botox will cause a period of weaker voice lasting days to weeks, depending on the dosage and the patient's response. On the other hand, if inability to achieve good closure of the musculomembranous vocal folds has caused someone to squeeze so hard that the vocal processes are injured, correcting the glottal incompetence

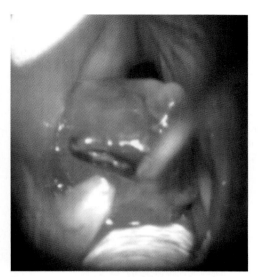

Figure 12.62 Right angle probe retracting the granuloma anteriorly demonstrating the stalk attachment of the mass to the vocal process.

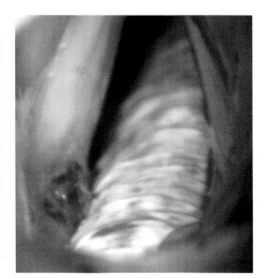

Figure 12.63 After excision with the CO_2 laser. Triamcinolone was then injected into the base of the wound. Patient treated with antacids postoperatively.

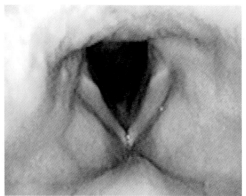

Figure 12.64 One year post excision.

by medializing the vocal folds is the key to resolution of the granuloma, or recurrence after excision.

Occasionally, the granuloma will be so large that it obstructs the airway and excision is mandatory. If the lesion recurs after it has been removed, the physician and patient are at least comfortable with the knowledge that it is only a granuloma and not something more serious. The author has treated several granulomas and ulcers over the years that recurred and due to minimal symptoms were finally left alone, only to finally resolve spontaneously. Some of these same patients have had recurrences years later on the contralateral side.

Granulation tissue

DEFINITION
Granulation tissue is a mass of inflammatory cells that can occur anywhere in the larynx where there is a wound.

CLINICAL FEATURES
Granulation tissue can occur in the midmusculomembranous vocal fold after an intubation injury or after excision of a T1 carcinoma. It often occurs due to irritation from foreign bodies such as laryngeal stents,

tracheal T-tubes, tracheal stents, suture material, and tracheotomy tubes. Tracheal granulation tissue above the tracheotomy tube is a common reason why patients fail capping trials (Figures 12.65 through 12.72).

DIFFERENTIAL DIAGNOSIS

If the patient has a history of carcinoma, one must consider that the abnormal tissue may be a recurrence. With presence of foreign bodies, especially in patients with no history of carcinoma, the likelihood of a neoplasm is extremely low. The author has seen at least

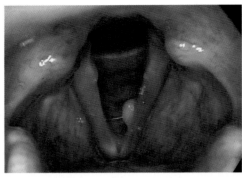

Figure 12.67 Granuloma left midvocal fold. No inciting etiology. Excised twice.

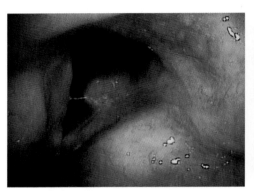

Figure 12.65 Granuloma which formed within 4 weeks of left partial cordectomy for TI SCC. Excised due to significant deterioration of voice and to rule out rapid recurrence.

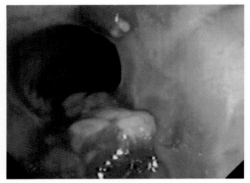

Figure 12.68 Granulation tissue at anterior rib graft site in subglottis 2 months postoperative.

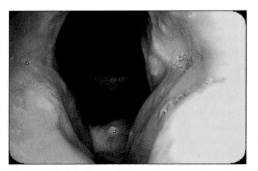

Figure 12.66 Granulation tissue at anterior inferior aspect of right partial cordectomy site for TI SCC. Biopsied to confirm diagnosis.

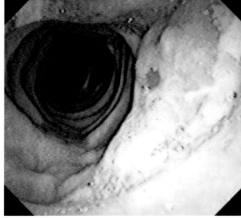

Figure 12.69 Granulation tissue at left distal end of tracheal stent.

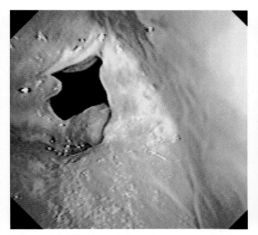

Figure 12.70 Granulation tissue at tracheal anastomosis post tracheal resection.

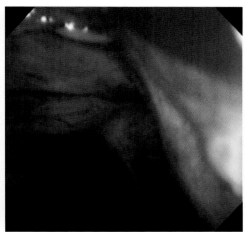

Figure 12.72 Flap of granulation tissue seen through the tracheotomy stoma with the tube removed in the same patient.

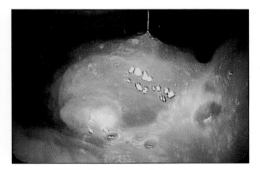

Figure 12.71 Flap of granulation tissue immediately superior to tracheotomy tube, obstructing airway. Anterior tracheal wall is down in picture.

one case of an angiosarcoma that appeared to be typical granulation tissue around a tracheotomy tube. Biopsy revealed the true diagnosis.

TREATMENT

Many laryngologists treat patients with antireflux measures and medications to help prevent granulation tissue formation, especially after laryngeal and tracheal reconstructions. The granulation tissue will usually resolve with time and removal of the foreign body. Injection with steroids can be helpful. Excision may be necessary to maintain the voice or airway and is often done to facilitate decannulation of tracheotomy patients. Excision can be done with cold instruments, microdebriders, coblation, electrocautery, or lasers depending on the location of the tissue, the instruments available, and the surgeon's experience.

Recurrent respiratory papilloma

DEFINITION

Papillomata in the larynx are benign neoplasms caused by the human papilloma virus (HPV), typically the lower-risk types 6 and 11. They can grow anywhere in the respiratory tract, but, within the upper respiratory tract, occur mostly on the true vocal folds.

CLINICAL FEATURES

The virus is contracted during birth or later in life, likely through sexual contact, although the mode of transmission has not been perfectly delineated. The virus may

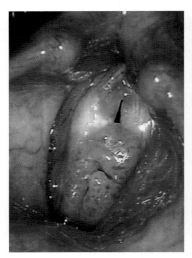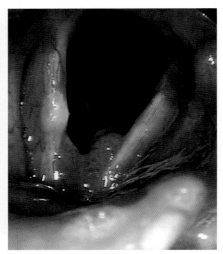

Figure 12.73 Typical glottic papilloma with characteristic vessels.

remain dormant for years and the papillomata start growing with an alteration in the immune system or hormonal balance. The disease will usually be more complicated or aggressive when it presents at age less than 5 years.

Voice is affected first and if left untreated, airway may be impaired. Laryngoscopy reveals the lesions. The characteristic feature that differentiates the papilloma from other laryngeal lesions is the presence of spiral vessels in the core of the lesions that look like red dots (Figures 12.73 through 12.76). There is a low (less than 5%) likelihood that squamous papilloma of the larynx will degenerate to a squamous cell carcinoma (SCC) over the patient's lifetime, but specimens should always be sent for pathology. Various grades of dysplasia may be seen within the papilloma and may vary over time (Figure 12.77). It is not a given that if mild or moderate dysplasia is seen on one occasion, then the degree of dysplasia will worsen over time.

DIFFERENTIAL DIAGNOSIS

Other lesions that sometimes have a similar appearance are papillomatous dysplastic lesions and SCCs.

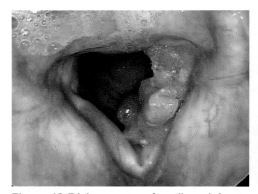

Figure 12.74 Large mass of papilloma left true vocal fold. Anterior commissure and right true vocal fold are not involved.

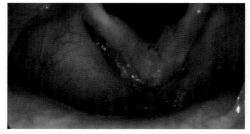

Figure 12.75 Less bulky, but more diffuse involvement of glottis with small anterior web.

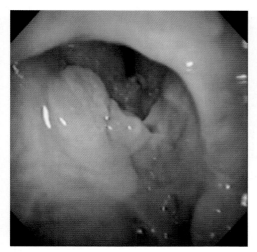

Figure 12.76 Severe case with near obstruction of the larynx.

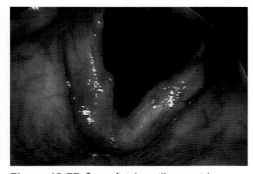

Figure 12.77 Superficial papilloma with severe dysplasia.

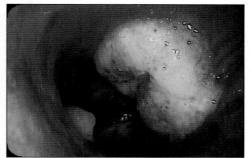

Figure 12.78 Papilloma in distal trachea.

TREATMENT

Treatment consists primarily of excising lesions carefully to maintain the voice and/or the airway while avoiding trauma to the surrounding and underlying tissue. Excision can be performed with cold microinstruments, microdebriders, CO_2 laser, pulsed KTP, pulsed dye laser, and coblation wands. At the anterior commissure, opposing raw surfaces must be avoided to prevent formation of a web. If the anterior commissure is involved bilaterally, staged surgeries may be necessary. Radiation therapy should *not* be used for completely benign papilloma. Various medications have been investigated over the years. Local injections of cidofovir and bevacizumab seem to be effective without systemic side effects, while other drugs, including interferon, are also effective but cause significant side effects. None of the medications consistently cause resolution of the disease. It is likely that the relatively new HPV vaccine will dramatically decrease the incidence of this disease.

WORKUP

Bronchoscopy should be performed at the same time as laryngoscopy to look for distal spread of the disease. If papillomas are found in the distal trachea or bronchi, imaging should be obtained to rule out involvement of the pulmonary parenchyma (Figure 12.78). Lung involvement is a very bad prognostic sign. Tissue should be obtained to rule out malignancy.

Polypoid corditis, polypoid degeneration, Reinke's edema

DEFINITION

Polypoid corditis is also known as polypoid degeneration or Reinke's edema. There is severe edema of the superficial layer of the lamina propria. The overlying mucosa can be thin, normal, or have areas of leukoplakia. The edema involves only the

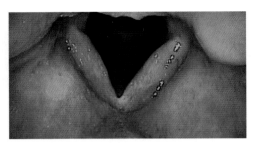

Figure 12.79 A 44-year-old woman with 25 pack-year smoking history with mild-to-moderate Reinke's edema.

musculomembranous portion of the vocal fold, ending at the vocal process of the arytenoid (Figures 12.79 through 12.82).

CLINICAL FEATURES

Primarily the voice is affected, but in severe cases, breathing can also be impaired. Smoking is the primary cause of this condition, and it is much more common in women. The typical patient is a woman in her 50s or 60s, smoker since her teens, who is often mistaken for a man over the phone. Fortunately, cancer rarely coexists with this condition, despite the mutual risk factor.

DIFFERENTIAL DIAGNOSIS

The clinician should always look for a coexistent neoplasm, although that occurs rarely. Otherwise, few lesions appear similar to classic polypoid corditis.

WORKUP

If there are other symptoms or signs of hypothyroidism, the appropriate laboratory tests should be obtained, starting with a directed thyroid-stimulating hormone level.

TREATMENT

The patient must quit smoking if there is any hope for improvement. After many months of abstaining, there may be some decrease

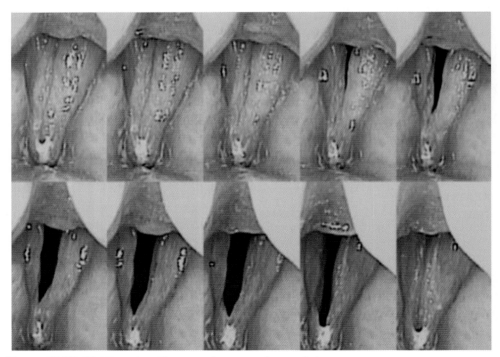

Figure 12.80 Glottic cycle with mucosal waves and normal closure.

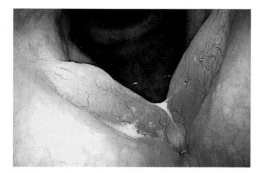

Figure 12.81 A 53-year-old woman with 30 pack-year smoking history with moderate Reinke's edema.

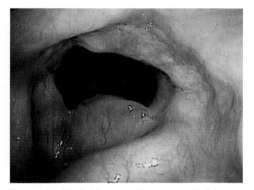

Figure 12.82 A 65-year-old woman with 30 pack-year smoking history with more severe edema.

in the edema and improvement in voice. If further improvement is desired, excision of the redundant tissue with redraping of the mucosal microflap will result in a better voice, although a truly normal voice is not to be expected. Care must be taken not to remove too much of the gelatinous matrix creating vocal folds that are too thin with incomplete closure. Also, mucosa must remain anteriorly and medially on at least one vocal fold to avoid development of an anterior glottic web (Figures 12.83 through 12.87). Many laryngologists will not offer the patient surgery if they have not quit smoking for several months, since smoking will almost certainly cause a recurrence of the condition. If there is concern for a neoplasm, the suspicious tissue should be excised even if the patient has continued to smoke.

Sulcus vocalis

DEFINITION
This is a fairly uncommon condition in which the mucosa along the medial edge of the vocal fold is scarred down to the vocal ligament, creating a groove, which eliminates the mucosal wave. The resulting sulcus

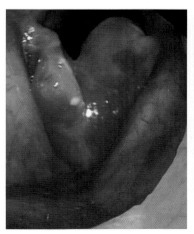

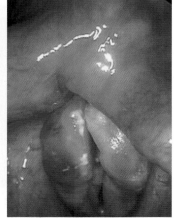

Figure 12.83 A 60-year-old woman with 40 pack-year smoking history and several year history of gradually worsening dysphonia.

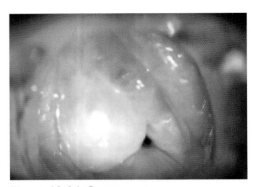

Figure 12.84 Operative view.

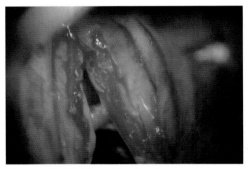

Figure 12.85 Most of redundant mucosa excised leaving intact mucosa along medial edge up to anterior commissure and *not* removing the entire gelatinous matrix.

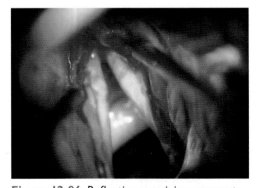

Figure 12.86 Reflecting remaining mucosa to demonstrate anterior commissure. Avoiding opposing raw surfaces prevents anterior glottic web. Minimal mucosal defect.

is usually in the midportion of the musculomembranous vocal fold, not extending beyond the vocal process of the arytenoid cartilage (as opposed to "pseudosulcus" seen in patients with laryngopharyngeal reflux) (Figures 12.88 and 12.89).

CLINICAL FEATURES

The cause of sulcus vocalis could be chronic phonotrauma or a vocal fold cyst that ruptures medially, leaving a deep groove attached to the vocal ligament laterally. Often, the sulcus can be seen when the vocal folds are abducted, or with stroboscopy or high-speed video during phonation when the mucosal wave is abolished. Sometimes, however, the sulcus is not confirmed until the vocal fold is palpated during direct microlaryngoscopy and is sometimes surprisingly deep (Figures 12.90 through 12.92). Closure is often incomplete with a midglottal gap.

DIFFERENTIAL DIAGNOSIS

A mucosal bridge may appear similar to a sulcus vocalis and is probably a variant of the same process.

TREATMENT

As with most cases of dysphonia, voice therapy should be done first. Surgery for sulcus vocalis is much more difficult than for other glottic pathologies. If there is glottal incompetence, then medializing the vocal folds and improving closure may improve the voice adequately. Surgery that directly addresses the sulcus involves raising a microflap of mucosa that includes a small portion of the vocal ligament to avoid buttonholing the flap. This is a difficult task to achieve. Sometimes just raising and redraping the flap is adequate for restoring the mucosal wave. Others, including Paolo Pontes and Charles Ford, slice the mucosa vertically to break up the scar along the medial edge of the vocal fold. Sulcus vocalis and other cases of vocal fold scarring are some of the most difficult conditions to treat.

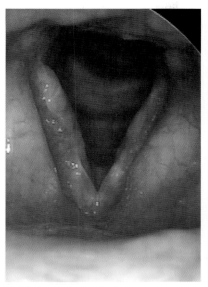 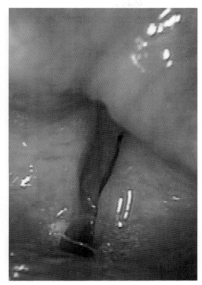

Figure 12.87 Several months later.

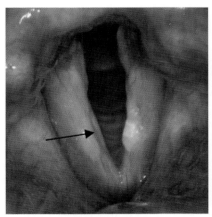 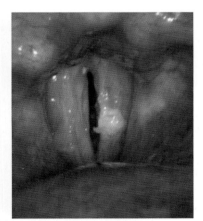

Figure 12.88 Right sulcus vocalis (arrow). Also thickening of the vocal processes and very thick adherent mucus.

Laryngopharyngeal reflux disease

DEFINITION

This is one of the more controversial topics in laryngology. Laryngopharyngeal reflux (LPR) refers to the reflux of gastric contents up to the level of the larynx. This causes inflammation within the larynx and a variety of symptoms. Not all people who reflux up to the larynx will experience the classic symptoms of gastroesophageal reflux disease (GERD), heartburn, and acid indigestion. This has made many patients and clinicians question whether the symptoms attributed to LPR are actually caused by it.

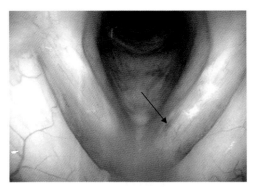

Figure 12.89 Left sulcus vocalis (arrow) as well as pseudosulcus.

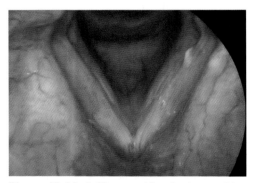

Figure 12.90 A 58-year-old male singer with bilateral sulci.

CLINICAL FEATURES

The symptoms most commonly attributed to LPR include globus sensation, urge to clear the throat, hoarseness (especially in the AM), mild chronic sore throat, chronic cough, mild dysphagia, and episodes of laryngospasm, especially at night. LPR has been purported to cause characteristic findings within the endolarynx that include thickening and inflammation of the posterior commissure, edema of the undersurface of the true vocal folds, causing the appearance of a sulcus between the true vocal fold edge and the edematous tissue, referred to as a "pseudosulcus." This sulcus extends posterior to the vocal process (unlike the true sulcus vocalis that stops anterior to the vocal process). Crowding of the ventricles and generalized erythema of the larynx is also often attributed to LPR. The components of the reflux finding score include subglottic edema, ventricular obliteration, erythema/hyperemia (of the arytenoids or diffusely), vocal fold edema, diffuse laryngeal edema, posterior commissure hypertrophy, granuloma/granulation, thick endolaryngeal mucus (Figures 12.93 through 12.101).

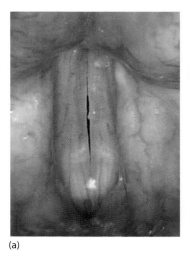

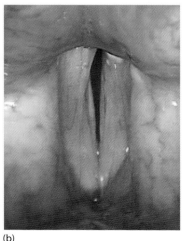

(a)   (b)

Figure 12.91 Incomplete closure (a) and impaired mucosal waves (b).

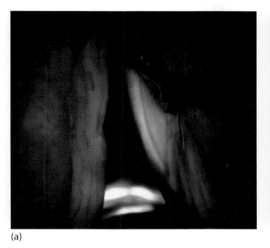

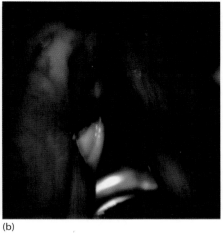

(a)

(b)

Figure 12.92 Intraoperative view of same patient showing depth of the sulci, which cannot be appreciated with in-office endoscopy. (a) shows the right true vocal fold sulcus and (b) shows the left true vocal fold sulcus.

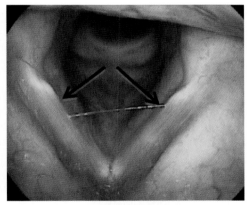

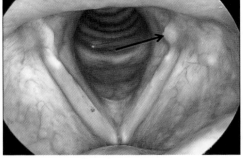

Figure 12.94 A 60-year-old male with classic reflux symptoms as well as chronic throat clearing and hoarseness. Has edema of undersurface of the vocal folds, pseudosulcus formation, and a left vocal process granuloma (arrow).

Figure 12.93 "Pseudosulcus" formation (arrows) due to edema of the undersurface of the true vocal folds. Note that the sulcus extends inferior and posterior to the vocal process of the arytenoid cartilage, unlike a true sulcus vocalis that stops anterior to the vocal process.

DIFFERENTIAL DIAGNOSIS AND WORKUP

If a patient has the classic symptoms of GERD, then it is usually safe to assume they have GERD. If they only have the symptoms associated with LPR and not GERD, then diagnostic testing (pH probe or impedance probe) is necessary to prove whether they do. Alarm symptoms, such as dysphagia and weight loss, are indications for further evaluation of the esophagus, including a swallow study and/or esophagoscopy, to rule out an esophageal neoplasm. Irritable larynx syndrome refers to hypersensitivity of the larynx of unknown etiology and

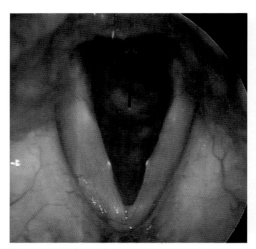

Figure 12.95 A 31-year-old untrained singer with early nodules as well as moderate thickening of the posterior commissure (arrow) and left vocal process.

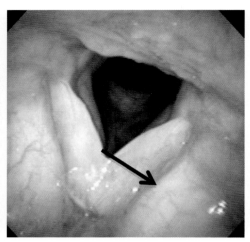

Figure 12.97 A 66-year-old woman never-smoker with severe thickening of posterior commissure, moderate edema of true vocal folds and pseudosulcus formation, and crowding of ventricles (arrow).

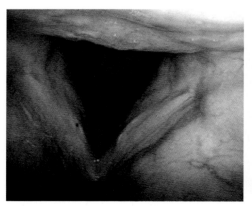

Figure 12.96 A 46-year-old woman with chronic hoarseness with severe thickening of the posterior commissure and edema of the undersurface of the true vocal folds.

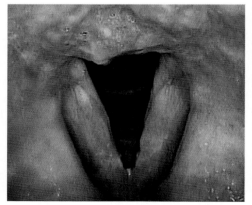

Figure 12.98 A 60-year-old male smoker with GERD and chronic hoarseness. Findings due to both his smoking and reflux. Severe posterior commissure thickening.

can also present with the same symptoms, although some believe it is caused by LPR.

TREATMENT

Many clinicians will treat patients for reflux for 2 months with proton pump inhibitors and behavior modifications and if they improve, there is a good chance that the diagnosis is correct. If not, either the diagnosis is not correct or the patient requires the formal testing. After treatment, the symptoms will usually resolve, but the physical exam findings may not change significantly or rapidly. Severe cases of classic

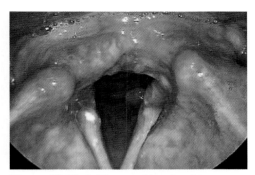

Figure 12.99 A 57-year-old male with hoarseness. Note severe inflammation of posterior larynx.

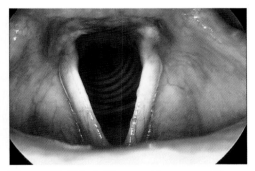

Figure 12.100 A 60-year-old woman with chronic sore throat and hoarseness. Note inflammation of posterior larynx, including subglottis.

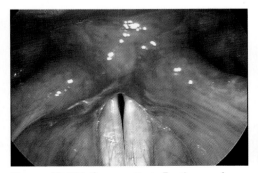

Figure 12.101 Same patient. Erythema of mucosa overlying the corniculate and arytenoid cartilages.

GERD may be treated with a gastric fundoplication with good results, but LPR does not respond as well to that surgery.

Laryngocele

DEFINITION

A laryngocele or saccular cyst is an air- or fluid-filled sac that arises from the saccule and/or ventricle. It can remain internal, in the false vocal fold or aryepiglottic fold medial to the thyroid cartilage lamina; can be external, extending through the thyrohyoid membrane; or mixed internal and external.

CLINICAL FEATURES

A very large internal laryngocele will cause bulging of the false vocal fold and can cause airway obstruction or can rest on the true vocal fold, impairing vibration and causing dysphonia (Figures 12.102 through 12.107). External laryngoceles may become infected, causing airway obstruction or other sequelae associated with neck abscesses. An external bulge in the neck at the thyrohyoid membrane that enlarges by blowing against closed lips or a modified Valsalva maneuver is almost diagnostic of an external or mixed laryngocele (Figures 12.108 through 12.116). Woodwind and brass musicians are at higher risk of developing laryngoceles due to the high pressures generated while playing.

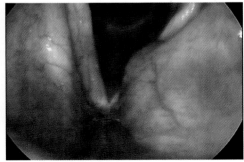

Figure 12.102 Left internal laryngocele.

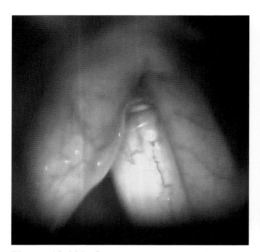

Figure 12.103 Operative view through microscope with bulging left false vocal fold.

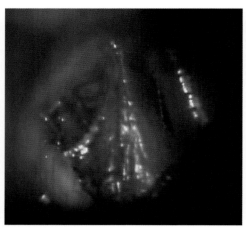

Figure 12.105 After excision with ventricle open, view of the superior aspect of the left true vocal fold.

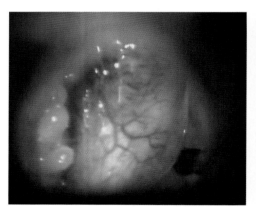

Figure 12.104 Incision made with CO_2 laser superior to laryngocele.

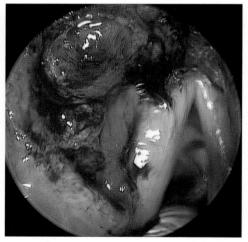

Figure 12.106 Telescopic view post resection showing defect.

DIFFERENTIAL DIAGNOSIS

Solid tumors must be ruled out. Also, a neoplasm may be present in the ventricle, causing an obstruction that led to retention of secretions in the saccule, in the case of cystic laryngoceles.

WORKUP

Imaging, usually with a CT scan, will delineate the lesion and rule out characteristics that would cause concern for a neoplasm such as solid components and erosion of cartilage (Figure 12.111).

TREATMENT

If a laryngocele is symptomatic, it should be excised or marsupialized. This can be done endoscopically for internal laryngoceles, usually with a CO_2 laser (Figures 12.103 through 12.106). Excision of an

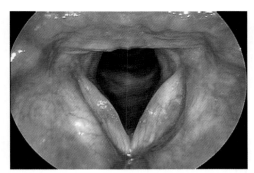

Figure 12.107 Same patient several months post endoscopic excision of left internal laryngocele.

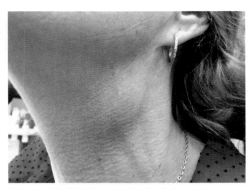

Figure 12.110 External bulge left neck in thyrohyoid region.

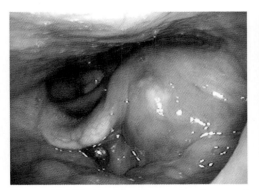

Figure 12.108 Combined internal and external laryngocele with swelling of left lateral glossoepiglottic fold. Endoscopic marsupialization had been performed previously.

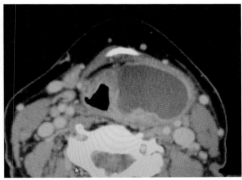

Figure 12.111 Axial CT of same patient at level of supraglottis.

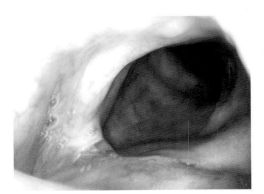

Figure 12.109 View of the glottis, same patient. Left false vocal fold bulging.

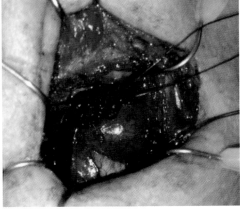

Figure 12.112 Exposure of external laryngocele.

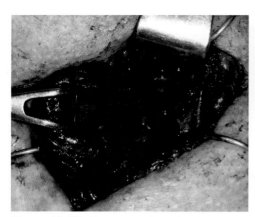

Figure 12.113 Dissecting through thyrohyoid membrane to remove remaining internal component.

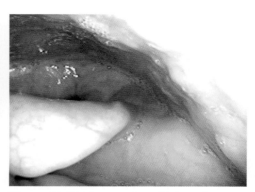

Figure 12.115 Same patient 12 days after open excision of left combined internal and external laryngocele via external approach only. Left lateral glossoepiglottic fold mildly edematous.

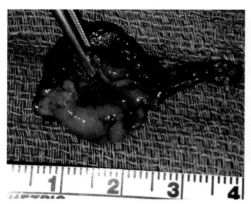

Figure 12.114 Laryngocele specimen.

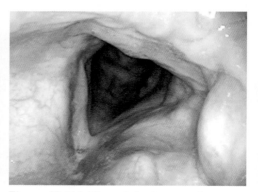

Figure 12.116 View of glottis, same time.

external or combined laryngocele requires an external approach, taking care to avoid trauma to the internal branch of the superior laryngeal nerve (Figures 12.112 through 12.114).

Vocal fold paralysis

DEFINITION
Unilateral and bilateral vocal fold paralyses are caused by vagus, superior laryngeal, and/or recurrent laryngeal nerve dysfunction.

CLINICAL FEATURES
These various nerves can be injured by tumors, infections, other inflammatory conditions, and most commonly by surgeons. The most common etiology is still thyroid or parathyroid surgery. A patient with unilateral vocal fold paralysis complains of voice changes, usually a weak or breathy voice due to an incompetent glottis with incomplete closure. Aspiration of thin liquids is also a common complaint (Figures 12.117 through 12.119). Patients with bilateral vocal fold paralysis have obstruction of the airway, as both vocal folds sit

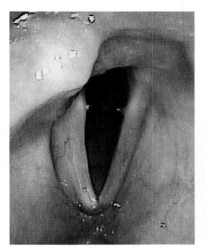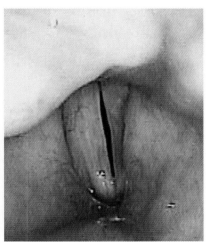

Figure 12.117 A 68-year-old woman 9 months post right parathyroidectomy with immobile bowed right vocal fold and incomplete closure.

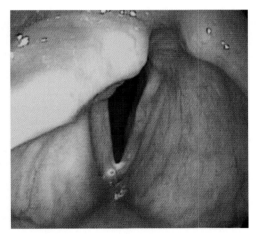

Figure 12.118 Eighteen months post right medialization laryngoplasty with silastic implant. Right vocal fold straight.

close together in the paramedian positions (Figures 12.120 and 12.121).

DIFFERENTIAL DIAGNOSIS

A vocal fold that is fixed in position by scar tissue, a dislocated arytenoid cartilage, or a tumor interfering with the cricoarytenoid joint will cause one or both vocal folds to not move, similar to paralysis (SCC or chondrosarcoma of the posterior cricoid cartilage).

WORKUP

The cause of the paralysis must be determined as it may be due to an undiagnosed malignancy in the neck or chest (Figures 12.122 and 12.123). If the history and physical examination do not reveal the cause, imaging of the length of the nerves of interest should be done. Laryngeal electromyography (LEMG) is the only test that can truly determine that a vocal fold is paralyzed, but the results often do not change the plan and LEMG is not necessary in all cases of suspected vocal fold paralysis. Palpation of the arytenoid will also reveal whether it is fixed or passively mobile, the latter indicating a paralysis.

TREATMENT

The goal of treating the paralysis is improving closure. Fortunately, many patients will have spontaneous recovery of the function of the vocal fold while others will slowly accommodate with the immobile vocal fold

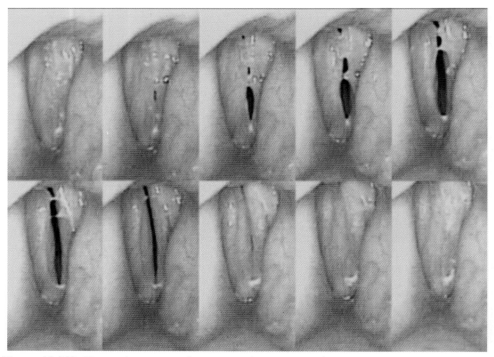

Figure 12.119 Closure is now complete, mucosal waves normal.

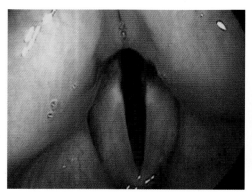

Figure 12.120 Bilateral vocal fold immobility post thyroidectomy. Airway limited, but adequate.

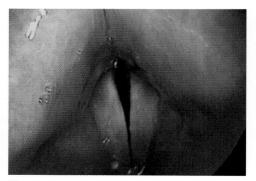

Figure 12.121 Closure with phonation.

moving into a position where the mobile vocal fold can achieve complete closure, or the mobile vocal fold crossing the midline. In these cases, the voice may be normal or near-normal and require no surgical intervention. Voice therapy may also help the patient's voice by improving their technique and maximizing vocal efficiency, although it does not affect recovery of the function of the nerve(s).

In those cases in which closure is not achieved spontaneously, the immobile

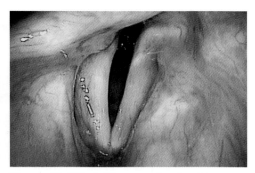

Figure 12.122 A 75-year-old male with 5-month hx of dysphonia with right vocal fold immobility.

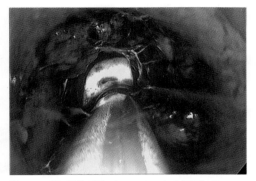

Figure 12.123 Workup revealed SCC of trachea located 2.5 cm below glottis.

vocal fold can be medialized by injecting a substance into the deep tissues of the vocal fold (vocal fold injection or injection medialization) or approaching the vocal fold through the thyroid cartilage and placing an implant that holds the vocal fold in place (medialization laryngoplasty with implant) (Figures 12.117 through 12.120). Reinnervation has also been successful in achieving these goals, although normal motion of the vocal fold is not restored.

Bilateral vocal fold paralysis presents a different problem. Because both vocal folds sit in the paramedian position, the airway is restricted and patients may have inspiratory stridor. Because most patients and many clinicians will refer to stridor as "wheezing," many of these patients are treated for asthma when they do not have that disease. The voice is also affected, but this problem is of secondary concern. If the airway obstruction is significant enough, it can be quickly remedied with a tracheotomy or a suture lateralization of one of the vocal folds. If one of the vocal folds recovers mobility, the tracheotomy or the suture is removed. If bilateral immobility is permanent, and the patient desires/needs a better airway, this can be achieved with an airway-enlarging procedure such as an arytenoidectomy, a cordotomy, or a partial cordectomy (Figures 12.124 through 12.127). These destructive procedures, however, will sacrifice some voice quality. Reinnervation of the posterior cricoarytenoid muscle has been shown to improve the airway as well, without removing any vocal fold tissue.

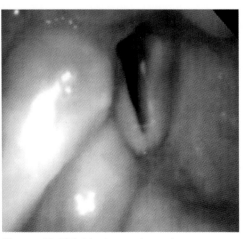

Figure 12.124 Maximum airway in woman with right vocal fold paralysis, left vocal fold paresis post three thyroid surgeries with dyspnea and inspiratory stridor.

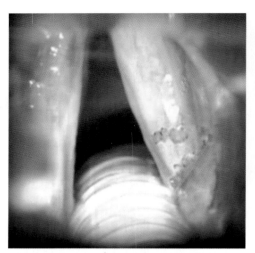

Figure 12.125 Right partial cordectomy incision outlined.

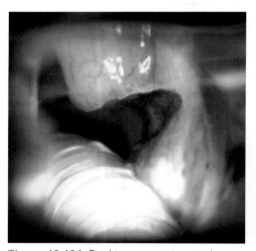

Figure 12.126 Final intraoperative result.

Squamous cell carcinoma

DEFINITION

SCC is a malignant epithelial neoplasm and is the most common malignant lesion of the larynx. "Precancerous" lesions include various grades of dysplasia and carcinoma in situ. The invasive lesions are staged from

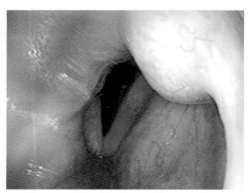

Figure 12.127 Improved airway 2 years postoperatively. (More typical result.)

T1 to T4 depending mostly on location and extension to other sites and structures and the mobility of the vocal fold(s).

CLINICAL FEATURES

The malignant lesions may be ulcerated, exophytic, papillomatous, or smooth (Figures 12.128, 12.131, 12.134 through 12.136, 12.138, 12.139, 12.142, 12.143). The primary risk factor for SCC is smoking followed

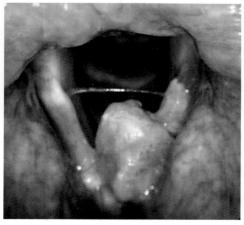

Figure 12.128 A 80-year-old male never smoker with T1a left vocal fold papillary SCC. Treated with radiation therapy. No evidence of disease at 5 years.

by alcohol use. The human papilloma virus is also emerging as a cause of development of SCC in the larynx.

SCC can involve any site in the larynx with the true vocal folds being the most common. Fortunately, voice changes early in the development of the tumor usually leads to diagnosis at an early stage. Supraglottic and hypopharyngeal lesions, however, often present much later with pain, dysphagia, hemoptysis, and development of metastatic neck lymphadenopathy being the initial symptoms and signs of cancer.

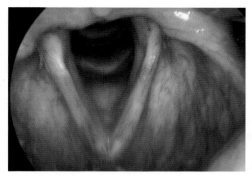

Figure 12.129 Same patient 4.5 years after treatment.

DIFFERENTIAL DIAGNOSIS
There are few other lesions that appear similar to SCC. Lymphoma may present in the larynx with similar symptoms and findings. Metastases to (as opposed to from) the larynx are rare. Renal cell carcinoma is one possibility.

WORKUP
Biopsy is imperative and can be done in the clinic with topical anesthesia or in the OR under general anesthesia, depending on the location, the patient's tolerance, and the surgeon's experience. Imaging of the larynx and neck is usually carried out with CT scan with contrast to evaluate the extent of the lesion and possible neck metastases (Figure 12.137).

TREATMENT
For dysplastic lesions and carcinoma in situ of the glottis, endoscopic excision with narrow margins is usually curative with a good voice result. This can be done with cold microinstruments or the CO_2 laser (see section on Leukoplakia). Small T1 lesions are also usually curable with endoscopic excision with the voice result dependent on the extent of normal tissue resected (Figures 12.131 through 12.133). Larger glottic lesions may be treated with endoscopic or open surgery alone or combined with radiation and chemotherapy (Figures 12.128 through 12.130). The same holds true for supraglottic and hypopharyngeal lesions (Figures 12.140 and 12.141). With these latter locations, metastases to the neck are much more common than with glottic lesions and therefore, the necks must also be treated, either surgically or with radiation therapy. The ultimate oncologic surgery for laryngeal carcinoma is the total laryngectomy, which is necessary in very large lesions and those that have failed radiation and chemotherapy (Figures 12.135 and 12.136).

Leukoplakia

DEFINITION
Leukoplakia literally a "white patch" refers to lesions often seen throughout the upper aerodigestive tract, both benign and malignant.

CLINICAL FEATURES
Although the true diagnosis can be known only through pathologic analysis, the patient's history and especially risk factors may suggest the diagnosis prior to biopsy. For smokers and alcohol drinkers, a patch

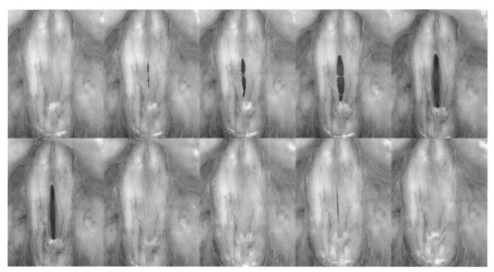

Figure 12.130 Same patient showing mucosal waves.

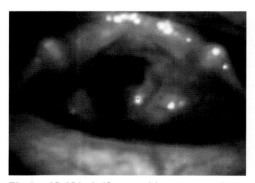

Figure 12.131 A 62-year-old woman smoker with T1 SCC left vocal fold.

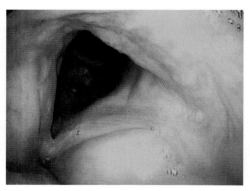

Figure 12.132 Same patient 4 years after CO_2 laser excision of tumor.

of leukoplakia should be considered to be at least dysplastic until proven otherwise. Patients on steroid inhalers may have very angry–appearing white lesions that interfere with the mucosal wave that resolve completely when treated for candida. Some lesions will resolve completely with no apparent intervention. Dysplastic white lesions have also been seen in patients with absolutely no risk factors (Figures 12.144 through 12.152).

DIFFERENTIAL DIAGNOSIS
Candida, parakeratosis, hyperkeratosis, dysplasia (varying degrees), carcinoma in situ, invasive SCC.

WORKUP
Biopsy done in clinic or operating room.

TREATMENT
Areas of leukoplakia that do not resolve over time should be excised. Elevation of

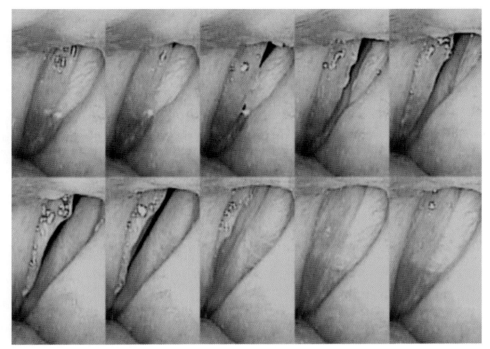

Figure 12.133 Same patient showing mucosal waves.

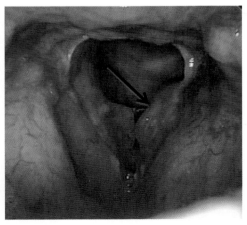

Figure 12.134 A 64-year-old male smoker with 4 months of hoarseness. T1 SCC of left true vocal fold (arrow) excised.

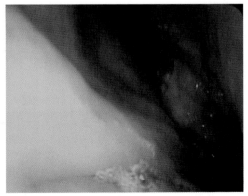

Figure 12.135 Same patient with recurrent T3 left transglottic SCC after failing endoscopic excision, then combined chemotherapy and radiation therapy.

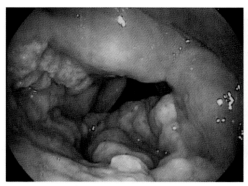

Figure 12.136 A 61-year-old male with 45 pack-year smoking history with T3 supraglottic SCC.

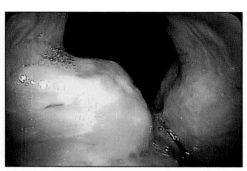

Figure 12.139 Closer view of same patient showing lesions of supraglottis.

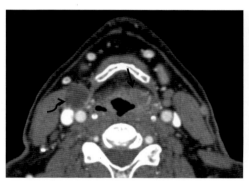

Figure 12.137 Axial CT at level of supraglottis demonstrating tumor on the left (straight arrow) and enlarged node on the right (curved arrow).

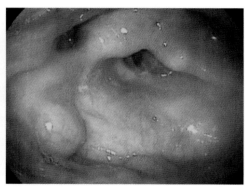

Figure 12.140 Same patient 1 year after endoscopic CO_2 laser supraglottic laryngectomy.

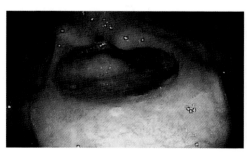

Figure 12.138 A 60-year-old female with 60 pack-year smoking history with T2 SCC of the supraglottis.

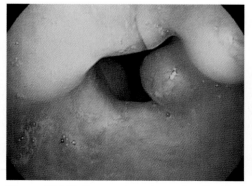

Figure 12.141 Same patient closer view. Residual left false vocal fold is edematous/polypoid.

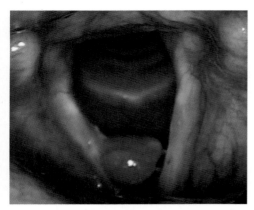

Figure 12.142 TI spindle cell carcinoma right anterior true vocal fold in a 60-year-old male occasional smoker.

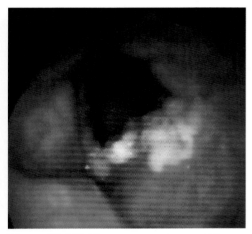

Figure 12.143 Verrucous carcinoma of the left true and false vocal folds.

a microflap that includes the entire lesion with very narrow margins in the superficial layer of the lamina propria will provide the pathologist with enough tissue and likely cure the patient (Figures 12.145 through 12.148, 12.153 through 12.156). There are, however, many cases of recurrence of dysplastic and hyperkeratotic lesions after complete excision, even in the absence of smoking. Thin areas of leukoplakia can also be removed in the office with topical anesthesia and lasers such as the pulsed

KTP or pulsed dye laser, thus saving the patient a general anesthetic.

Infectious laryngitis

DEFINITION
Inflammation of the larynx caused by an infectious agent.

CLINICAL FEATURES
The most common infectious laryngitis is what is simply referred to as "acute laryngitis" and is caused by cold and flu viruses. In addition to a rough hoarse voice, the patient experiences sore throat, odynophagia, and often cough and fever. The larynx is diffusely erythematous and edematous. It lasts only a few days. Candida laryngitis occurs in patients who are immunosuppressed, on antibiotics, systemic steroids, or steroid inhalers. While a whitish exudate is usually present on the glottis and supraglottis, it sometimes appears to be part of the tissue (leukoplakia) rather than on the tissue's surface. There are also etiologies common in the developing world that are rarely seen in the United States. *Bordetella pertussis*, *Corynebacterium diphtheriae*, and *Haemophilus influenzae* type B are important pathogens, usually affecting children, especially where vaccinations are not routine. The human papilloma virus may cause the development of papillomas, which are discussed in another section. Herpes simplex virus will appear as blisters, although that stage may be missed and only the inflammation be seen by the clinician. *Staphylococcus aureus* has also been identified as a laryngeal pathogen recently (Figures 12.157 through 12.163).

DIFFERENTIAL DIAGNOSIS
Some neoplastic lesions can appear the same as laryngitis caused by some of the less well-known infectious agents, such as histoplasmosis (Figure 12.164).

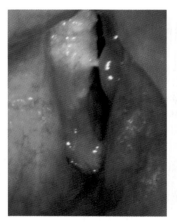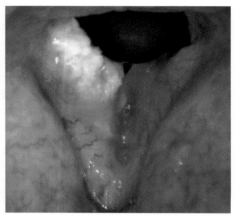

Figure 12.144 A 69-year-old female smoker with a history of excision of mild-to-moderate dysplasia from the right true vocal fold 18 months earlier, continued to smoke, and presented with new lesion.

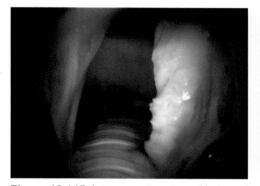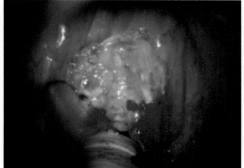

Figure 12.145 Intraoperative view of lesion of right true vocal fold.

Figure 12.146 Lesion reflected medially as CO_2 laser is used to incise tissue.

WORKUP

If the laryngitis persists beyond 2 weeks, it should be assumed to not be typical viral caused acute laryngitis. If the inflammation does not resolve with medical treatment for a presumed specific agent (e.g., fluconazole for candida), then cultures and/or biopsies should be obtained to guide therapy and rule out a neoplasm.

TREATMENT

Viral acute laryngitis is treated with supportive symptomatic measures (anti-inflammatories, antitussive, mucolytics, analgesics) and much water, until resolved. Candida laryngitis responds within days to fluconazole, usually given for a 2-week period. Other less common pathogens require specific medical therapy once they have been identified (Figure 12.165).

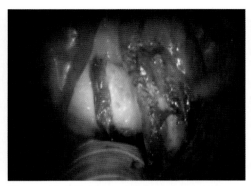

Figure 12.147 Mucosal defect post excision with vocal ligament visible, but intact in depth of wound.

Vocal fold hemorrhage and vascular ectasias

DEFINITION
The true vocal fold is not a particularly vascular structure, but submucosal hemorrhages may still occur. A vascular ectasia is a distended vessel, presumably with a somewhat weakened wall.

DIFFERENTIAL DIAGNOSIS
The appearance of an acute hemorrhage is very typical, not likely to mistaken for any other lesion.

CLINICAL FEATURES
Hemorrhage of the vocal fold is most likely to happen to people who are singing, shouting, straining, and on anticoagulants (Figures 12.166, 12.168, and 12.173). Women who are menstruating are also at risk. The most significant risk factor, however, is the presence of a vascular anomaly, referred to as a varix or a vascular ectasia (Figures 12.168 through 12.171).

Patients with an acute vocal fold hemorrhage will report a sudden or rapid change in voice, often while singing or shouting or straining and occasionally report pain. The dysphonia may be severe and obvious or may be a subtle control and range issue for a singer.

WORKUP
Examination of the larynx with almost any technique will reveal evidence of the

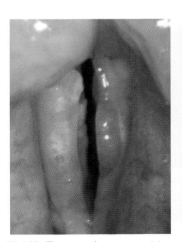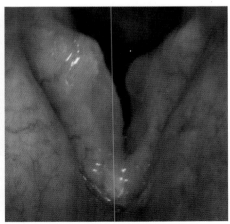

Figure 12.148 Ten months post excision of lesion, which was also mild-to-moderate dysplasia.

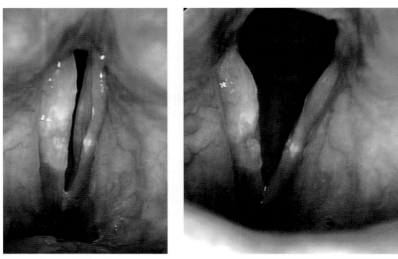

Figure 12.149 A 50-year-old ex-smoker woman (20 pack-year) with right vocal fold "leukoplakia" post excision of polyps bilaterally 13 years earlier. No mucosal wave. Had chronic cough, possibly due to pertussis. Treated with Advair.

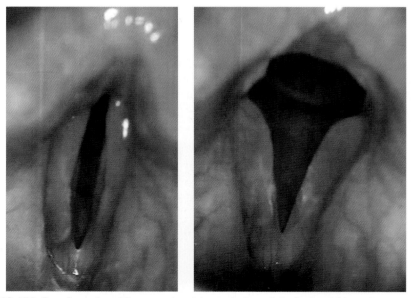

Figure 12.150 Post 2 weeks of fluconazole with resolution of the leukoplakia and restoration of the mucosal wave.

hemorrhage with varying amounts of submucosal blood. While underlying vascular ectasias are a common cause of hemorrhage, the lesion may be obscured by the surrounding blood on initial presentation. Follow-up examinations should be done, looking for a vascular lesion (Figures 12.168 through 12.171).

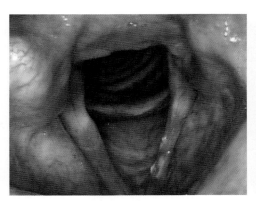

Figure 12.151 A 75-year-old male with 30 pack-year smoking history. No voice complaints. Incidental finding of left true vocal fold leukoplakia.

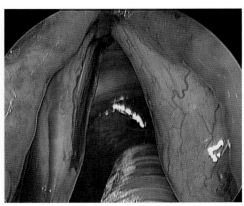

Figure 12.154 After excision of the lesion with 1–2 mm margin done with microsurgical instruments. Vocal ligament visible, but intact in base of wound.

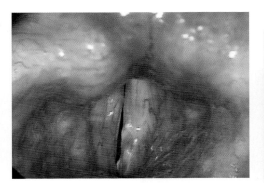

Figure 12.152 No mucosal wave on left.

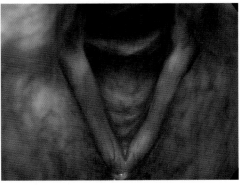

Figure 12.155 Fifteen months post excision of lesion, which was carcinoma in situ.

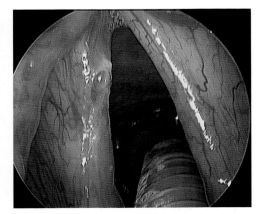

Figure 12.153 Intraoperative view showing leukoplakia left true vocal fold.

TREATMENT

Treatment is voice rest and avoidance of anticoagulants. Voice rest may be complete silence for a week or not singing and using a soft voice for several weeks, depending on the patient's needs. A singer who has an upcoming performance should be silent until cleared to start speaking and singing again, while a truck driver, who may not talk much during his typical day, could probably simply use a soft voice and avoid straining (Figures 12.166 through 12.175).

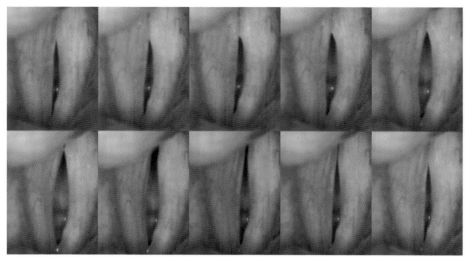

Figure 12.156 Incomplete closure and lack of left-sided mucosal wave.

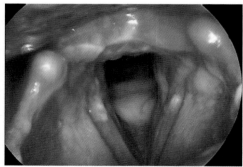

Figure 12.157 A 48-year-old male with several days of sore throat and raspy voice diffuse erythema of entire larynx with pus/mucus in subglottis is consistent with acute viral laryngitis.

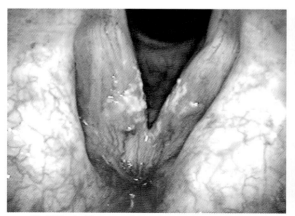
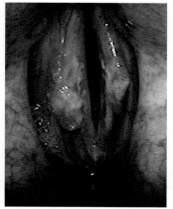

Figure 12.158 A 48-year-old male smoker with COPD on Advair for 5 months with hoarseness.

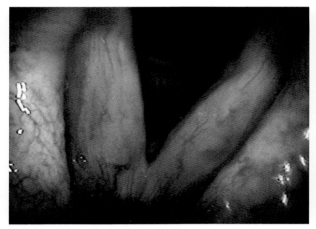
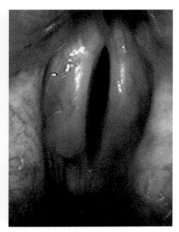

Figure 12.159 Same patient post 14 days of fluconazole with improvement in voice.

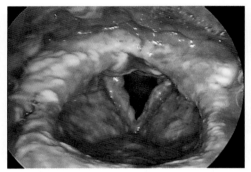

Figure 12.160 Severe, diffuse candida in a 47-year-old woman smoker with immunodeficiency.

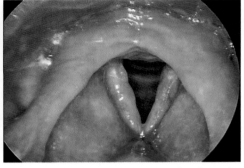

Figure 12.161 One month later after 2 weeks of fluconazole.

The patient should follow up within 1–2 weeks and when the blood has reabsorbed, they can return to normal voice use. The patient must be educated in vocal hygiene and avoidance of phonotrauma to avoid a recurrence. Also, at follow-up, an underlying vascular ectasia may become evident. If present, the risk of another hemorrhage is much higher. The patient should be counseled as to what to expect if there is another bleed and to immediately decrease voice use and return to see the clinician.

Surgery to coagulate or excise a vascular ectasia is indicated in patients who have had several recurrent hemorrhages. Most laryngologists use a laser to coagulate the vessel. Very low power must be used to avoid trauma to the surrounding normal tissue and resultant scar and stiffness (Figures 12.168 through 12.172). Hemorrhages may lead to formation of a hemorrhagic polyp if the blood is not able to reabsorb, which may occur with repeated trauma (voice use, straining) and bleeding (Figure 12.176).

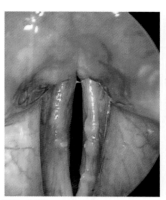
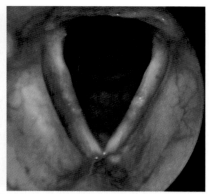

Figure 12.162 A 76-year-old ex-smoker on inhaled steroids and antibiotics referred with concerns regarding glottic leukoplakia.

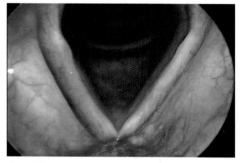

Figure 12.163 Post 2 weeks of fluconazole.

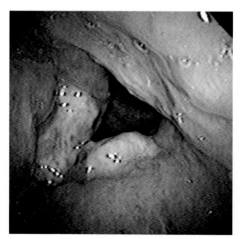

Figure 12.164 A 68-year-old woman smoker with 4-month history of hoarseness since neck surgery. No immunosuppression. Excision of the abnormal tissue revealed histoplasmosis.

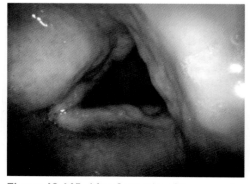

Figure 12.165 After 3 months of itraconazole.

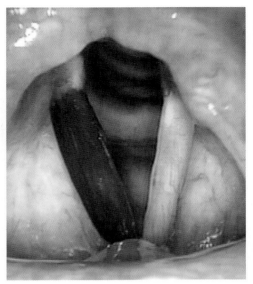 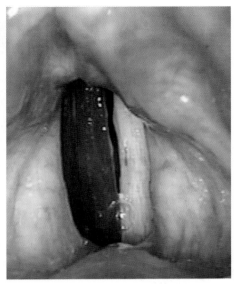

Figure 12.166 A 74-year-old woman with sudden-onset hoarseness 1 month earlier. Obvious right true vocal fold hemorrhage. No inciting event. No mucosal wave on right.

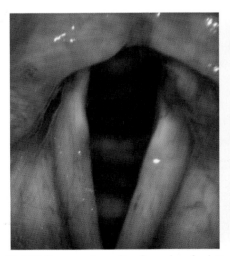 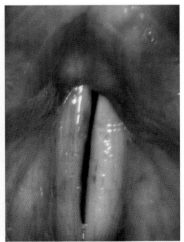

Figure 12.167 Same patient after 3 weeks of relative voice rest. No obvious underlying vascular ectasia. Mucosal wave restored.

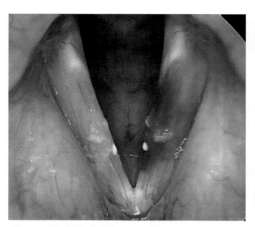

Figure 12.168 A 35-year-old professional soprano with pitch control problems at upper range. This is their second hemorrhage.

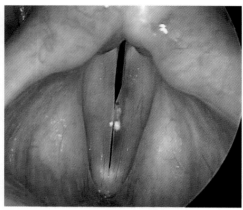

Figure 12.170 One week later with further improvement. Underlying vascular lesion is evident.

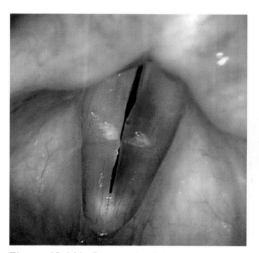

Figure 12.169 One week of absolute voice rest later with decreased submucosal blood.

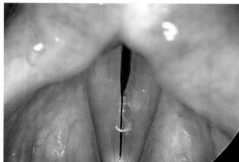

Figure 12.171 Another week of relative rest. Blood is reabsorbed, left vocal fold has residual edema and is stiff and vascular lesion remains.

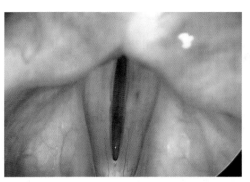

Figure 12.172 Two weeks after pulsed dye laser coagulation and excision of left vocal fold vascular ectasia. Mucosal wave is intact.

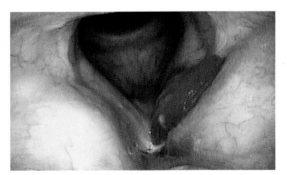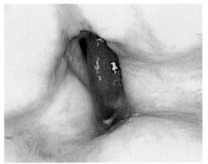

Figure 12.173 Sudden onset of hoarseness with sneeze 1 day prior to the exam in a 43-year-old workman smoker.

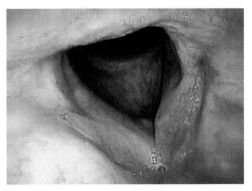

Figure 12.174 After 5 days of relative voice rest and avoidance of heavy lifting or straining.

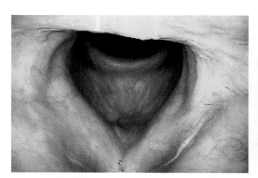

Figure 12.175 One month later, completely resolved, no underlying lesion.

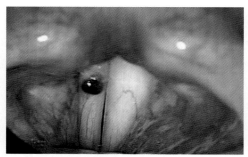

Figure 12.176 A 17-year-old female singer. Two months post coughing episode and change in voice. Hemorrhagic polyp superior surface of the right true vocal fold.

Laryngeal and Tracheal Stenosis

Glendon M. Gardner and Michael S. Benninger

- **Laryngeal and tracheal stenosis**
- **Sarcoidosis**
- **Cicatricial pemphigoid**

Laryngeal and tracheal stenosis

DEFINITION

We divide laryngeal stenosis into anterior and posterior glottic stenosis, supraglottic stenosis and subglottic stenosis. Anterior glottic stenosis consists most commonly of a web between the vocal folds (Figures 13.1 through 13.9). Posterior glottic stenosis is scarring of the posterior aspect of the glottis usually resulting in immobility of both vocal folds and narrowing of the airway (Figures 13.10 through 13.12). Supraglottic stenosis involves the epiglottis and/or the false vocal folds (Figure 13.13). Subglottic stenosis is at the level of the cricoid cartilage (Figures 13.14 through 13.21). Tracheal stenosis includes narrowing of the tracheal airway due to scarring within the lumen of an otherwise normal trachea or collapse of the wall of the trachea due to loss

of integrity and rigidity or external compression (Figures 13.22 and 13.23).

CLINICAL FEATURES

Patients with stenosis of the larynx and/or trachea complain of dyspnea and often have inspiratory stridor. Voice is often also affected but is of secondary concern. The etiology of most cases of laryngeal and tracheal stenosis is iatrogenic trauma.

Anterior glottic stenosis may be congenital and present at birth, but in adults is usually the result of laryngeal surgery in which tissue has been removed from both vocal folds anteriorly. External trauma with injury to the cartilaginous framework and the endolaryngeal mucosa can also result in anterior glottic stenosis. The voice is usually affected.

Posterior glottic stenosis is usually due to long-term intubation and results in immobile vocal folds and a very narrow

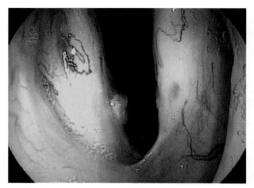

Figure 13.1 Small anterior glottic web (and a small right true vocal fold lesion) in a 52-year-old woman who had undergone excision and radiation therapy for a T1 squamous cell carcinoma of the right true vocal fold 18 years earlier.

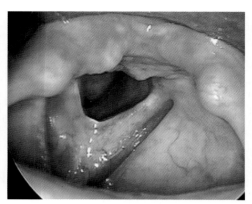

Figure 13.3 Anterior glottic web in 33-year-old woman who had been intubated several times. Had had lysis of the anterior web at least once. Patient is on liver transplant list and airway is small enough to interfere with intubation and postoperative airway management.

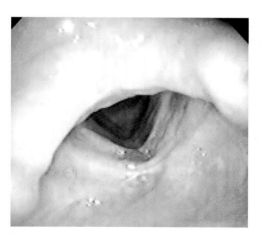

Figure 13.2 Anterior glottic and supraglottic webs in a 46-year-old woman who underwent three laryngeal surgeries at age 3.

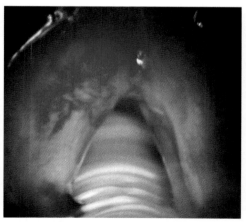

Figure 13.4 Intraoperative image prior to lysis of the anterior web with the CO_2 laser. Laser proof tube in airway.

airway, similar to bilateral vocal fold paralysis described earlier.

Supraglottic stenosis can be due to caustic ingestion, a variety of connective tissue and inflammatory disorders (pemphigoid, sarcoidosis), treatment of supraglottic carcinoma (radiation therapy, supraglottic laryngectomy), or external trauma.

Subglottic stenosis is usually due to long-term, frequent, or traumatic endotracheal intubation or that combined with a cricothyroidotomy or very high tracheotomy. There are also many cases of idiopathic subglottic stenosis, which almost always occur in women of childbearing age. Other diseases such as Wegener's granulomatosis, relapsing

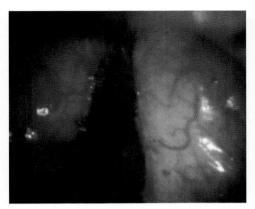

Figure 13.5 After lysis, prior to placement of stent.

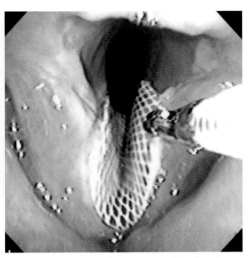

Figure 13.7 Stent being removed in the clinic 2 weeks after lysis of the web in the operating room with application of mitomycin and placement of the stent.

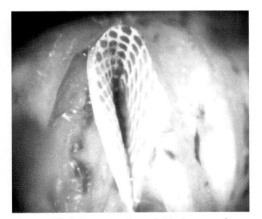

Figure 13.6 Stent in place, folded piece of silastic sheeting secure with one 2-0 prolene suture passed from externally through the cricothyroid membrane through the inferior aspect of the stent and then through the superior aspect above the level of the glottis, secured externally over a button.

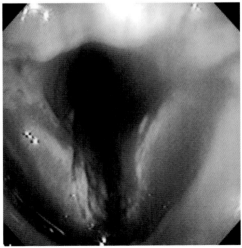

Figure 13.8 Glottis immediately after stent removal. Long-term follow-up is not available for this patient. Some degree of reformation of the web is expected.

polychondritis, and carcinoma may also be responsible.

Tracheal stenosis, like subglottic stenosis, is usually due to prolonged endotracheal intubation, often followed by tracheotomy. While the patient still has the tracheotomy tube in place, capping trials may fail, leading to endoscopy and discovery of the stenosis. Or, the patient may be decannulated after successful capping trials and then, within a month or two, develop stridor and dyspnea.

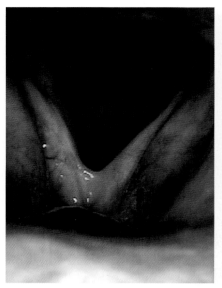
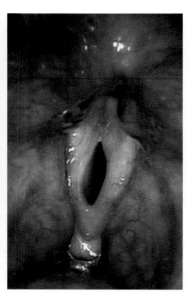

Figure 13.9 A 73-year-old male post excision of recurrent respiratory papillomatosis with resultant anterior glottic web. Only a small portion of the glottis is vibrating.

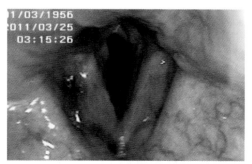

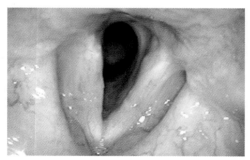

Figure 13.10 Type 2 posterior glottic stenosis in a 55-year-old woman with history of prolonged intubation, tracheotomy.

Figure 13.11 Mild residual stenosis 2 years post incision of the scar.

DIFFERENTIAL DIAGNOSIS

Rarely would anterior glottic stenosis be due to anything other than trauma of some sort. Posterior glottic stenosis should be differentiated from bilateral vocal fold paralysis, the latter requiring a workup for the etiology of the paralysis. A tumor of the cricoid cartilage (chondrosarcoma) can cause narrowing posteriorly, fixed vocal folds, or subglottic stenosis. Supraglottic stenosis may be due to rare conditions such as cicatricial pemphigoid, which appears similar to scar tissue. Glottic and subglottic stenosis can be due to any number of inflammatory conditions including Wegener's granulomatosis, relapsing polychondritis, sarcoidosis, amyloidosis, chondromas or chondrosarcomas, and carcinoma. The potential diagnoses are similar for tracheal stenosis. External compression of the trachea must also be considered.

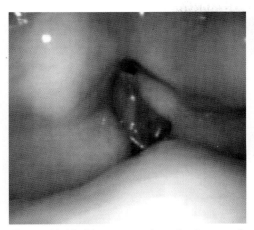

Figure 13.12 Almost complete glottic stenosis after intubation after CVA. Tracheotomy.

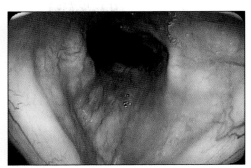

Figure 13.14 A 39-year-old woman with 1-year history of progressively worsening dyspnea and stridor. Vocal folds in foreground with stenosis of subglottis and proximal trachea seen in distance.

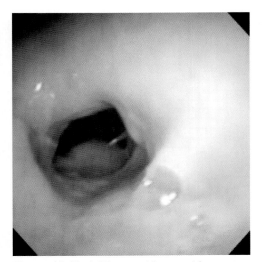

Figure 13.13 A 33-year-old man with cicatricial pemphigoid causing supraglottic stenosis beyond the turban-shaped epiglottis. Bulge in center of view is the right false vocal fold. The true vocal folds are normal, but not seen well in this image.

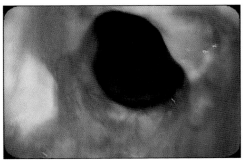

Figure 13.15 Closer view of stenosis. Patient underwent biopsy, incisions, and dilation of the stenosis with application of mitomycin. Workup revealed Wegener's granulomatosis.

WORKUP

Prior to any surgical intervention, a CT scan of the larynx and trachea should be done to evaluate the outer contours of the larynx and trachea to determine if endoscopic surgery is safe or likely to be successful and if there are any neoplastic lesions causing the airway obstruction (Figures 13.24 and 13.25). This is also an easy way to measure the extent of stenosis and, in the case of tracheal stenosis, how much of the trachea may need to be resected. Biopsies of any abnormal tissue are necessary to rule out causes of stenosis other than scarring, such as those listed earlier (Figures 13.26 and 13.27). Bronchoscopy of the remainder of the airway may also reveal other abnormalities such as tracheomalacia, bronchomalacia, and tracheo-esophageal fistulas (Figures 13.28 through 13.30).

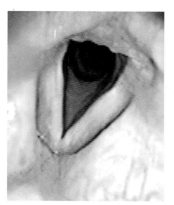

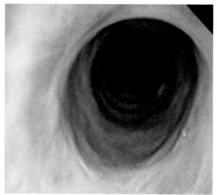

Figure 13.16 Nine months post only surgical intervention and now with medical treatment. Closer view of patent airway on right.

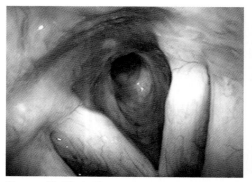

Figure 13.17 A 50-year-old woman with idiopathic subglottic stenosis.

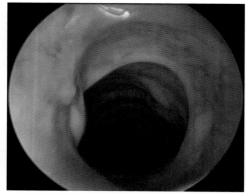

Figure 13.19 Close-up of stenosis.

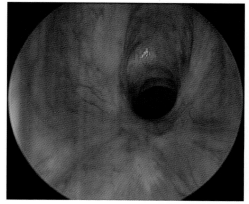

Figure 13.18 Intraoperative view prior to incisions and dilation. Direct microlaryngoscopy done with jet ventilation and CO_2 laser.

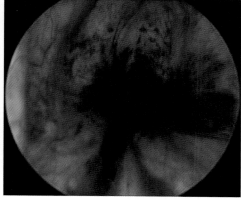

Figure 13.20 After incisions, before dilation.

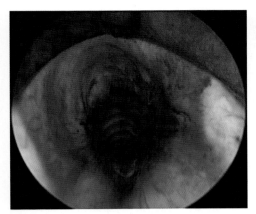

Figure 13.21 After dilation with balloon.

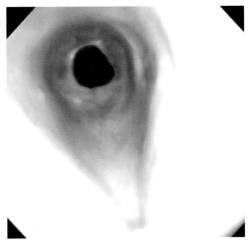

Figure 13.23 Four weeks post tracheal resection. View of anastomosis. Carina seen in distance.

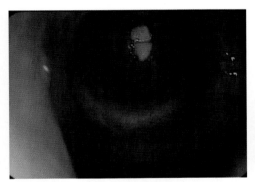

Figure 13.22 Multiple intubations and tracheotomy for chronic lung disease. Stenosis at tracheotomy site seen with tip of scope at glottis.

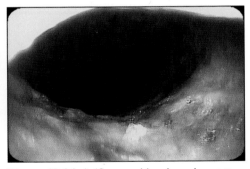

Figure 13.24 A 63-year-old male underwent emergent reintubation post cardiac surgery, then tracheotomy, with posterior glottic stenosis and tracheomalacia. View of trachea from end of tracheotomy tube during inspiration.

TREATMENT

For anterior glottic stenosis, lysis of the web and prevention of recurrence with medication, microflaps, or a stent improves the voice, although it will rarely be perfectly normal (Figures 13.3 through 13.8).

Posterior glottic stenosis may be more difficult to treat. Milder cases (type 1, synechia between the vocal processes) are treated with lysis of the scar tissue, which usually restores normal vocal fold motion and a normal airway. More severe cases (types 2–4) are often treated in a similar manner to bilateral vocal fold paralysis with excision of vocal fold tissue or the arytenoid cartilage to improve the airway, but at a cost to the voice (Figures 13.10 and 13.11) (see also "Vocal Fold Paralysis" section in Chapter 12). Tracheotomy is often necessary, permanently or temporarily, while other surgeries are done to improve the airway. Augmentation of the posterior glottis with a rib cartilage graft is sometimes necessary and usually successful.

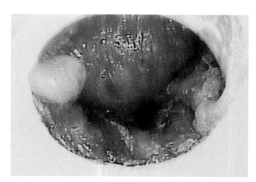

Figure 13.25 Complete collapse of trachea with cough, as seen from tracheotomy tube. Also, significant drying and crusting of mucosa.

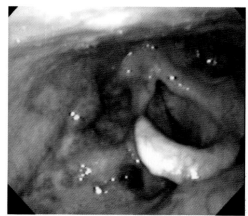

Figure 13.27 A portion of a hemangioma or vascular malformation in the hypopharynx, part of a much larger lesion throughout the neck, the lower portion causing airway obstruction.

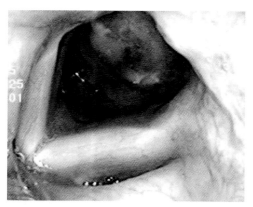

Figure 13.26 A 54-year-old woman with low-grade chondrosarcoma of posterior cricoid cartilage, obstructing airway. Tumor is submucosal.

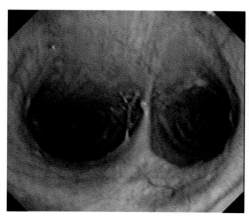

Figure 13.28 Carina in a 41-year-old woman with chronic cough.

Treatment of supraglottic stenosis may involve tracheotomy, excision and/or incision of scars, dilation, placement of stents, and various local flaps.

Most cases of subglottic stenosis respond to incision of the scar tissue and dilation with balloons and application of mitomycin (Figures 13.17 through 13.21). For the traumatic cases, one surgery may be enough. The idiopathic cases, however, tend to recur at an unpredictable rate. More severe or recurrent cases of subglottic stenosis may require a more aggressive, open surgery,

either an anterior or posterior cricoid augmentation with rib cartilage grafts, or a cricotracheal resection. For the idiopathic subglottic stenosis, resection has been more successful in the long term than augmentation. Cricotracheal resection carries with it the risk of injury to one or both recurrent laryngeal nerves.

For tracheal stenosis: if the outer contour of the trachea is normal and there is

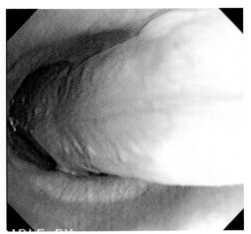

Figure 13.29 Bronchomalacia with complete collapse of right mainstem bronchus with cough in the same patient.

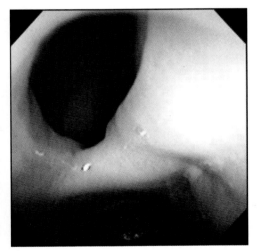

Figure 13.30 Tracheo-esophageal fistula at the site in the posterior tracheal wall where the tracheotomy tube tip had been. Patient had had tracheotomy tube in place for 2 months. View is through the stoma with the tube out.

scarring within the lumen, the problem may be remedied with incisions and dilation. If the outer walls of the trachea are collapsed, then the endoscopic incisions

are unlikely to work and violation of the tracheal wall may occur, leading to tracheomalacia, bleeding, pneumomediastinum, or pneumothorax. Some patients can be managed with placement of a tracheal stent for several months, while others will require resection of the stenosed segment with primary reanastamosis (Figures 13.22 and 13.23). As with cricotracheal resection, there is risk of injury to the recurrent laryngeal nerves.

Keep in mind that tracheotomy can achieve an adequate and safe airway in almost all these situations and should always be considered as a possible permanent solution. Patients with scar above the tracheotomy tube may require a tracheal T-tube to maintain a laryngeal voice.

Sarcoidosis

DEFINITION
Sarcoidosis is a poorly understood disease in which noncaseating granulomas form in various tissues.

CLINICAL FEATURES
The lungs are most commonly involved by sarcoidosis. The region of the larynx most commonly affected by sarcoidosis is the supraglottis. The epiglottis thickens and seems to curl onto itself, eventually taking on a turban shape. The supraglottic airway becomes narrow, causing inspiratory stridor and dyspnea (Figure 13.31). The glottis can also be involved by sarcoidosis. The tissue has an irregular, but not quite ulcerated appearance (Figures 13.32 through 13.36). In the head and neck, sarcoidosis may cause dryness and crusting in the nasal cavity and masses in the skin, lymph nodes, and salivary glands.

DIFFERENTIAL DIAGNOSIS
Cancer and other autoimmune and inflammatory conditions must be ruled out.

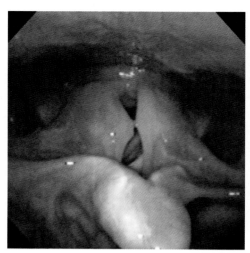

Figure 13.31 Classic turban shaped epiglottis in a 59-year-old woman with sarcoidosis. Note floppy aryepiglottic folds, which cause intermittent inspiratory stridor. Glottis is normal.

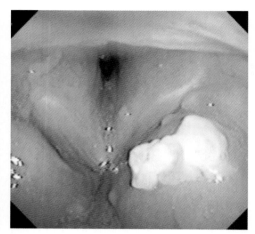

Figure 13.33 Disease progression requiring tracheotomy.

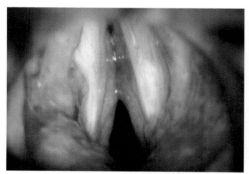

Figure 13.34 Intraoperative photo of same patient with sarcoidosis affecting the glottis prior to steroid injections, after tracheotomy.

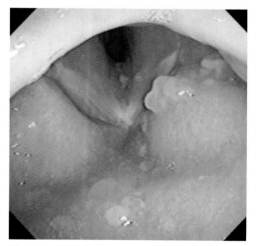

Figure 13.32 A 41-year-old woman with sarcoidosis affecting the glottis and supraglottis. She has dyspnea and dysphonia.

WORKUP

Biopsy reveals noncaseating granulomas. Angiotensin-converting enzyme levels are often high. The lungs must be imaged looking for hilar adenopathy and pulmonary lesions. The workup is often carried out by pulmonologists.

TREATMENT

Supraglottic involvement sometimes requires excision of a portion of the epiglottis or aryepiglottic folds. The mainstay of treatment, however, is systemic medical therapy.

Involved tissues can also be injected with steroids, which may result in a fairly long improvement (Figures 13.34 through 13.36).

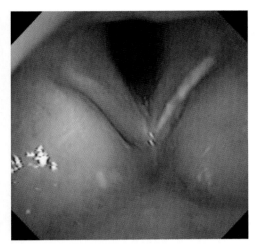

Figure 13.35 Laryngeal examination 9 days after steroid injections.

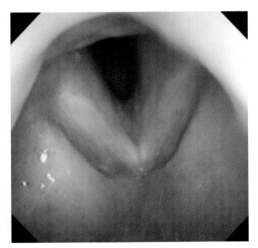

Figure 13.36 Airway 10 months post injection.

Cicatricial pemphigoid

DEFINITION

This is a rare chronic autoimmune blistering disease that can affect any mucous membrane in the head and neck, including the conjunctiva, mouth, nasal cavity, and the supraglottis.

CLINICAL FEATURES

Blisters develop in the aforementioned locations, which lead to scarring. The supraglottis may scar and cause airway obstruction with inspiratory stridor and dyspnea (Figures 13.37 through 13.39).

DIFFERENTIAL DIAGNOSIS

Other autoimmune and inflammatory causes of stenosis should be ruled out.

WORKUP

Biopsy of the affected tissue may yield a diagnosis, but is often inconclusive. Autoimmune laboratory workup should be pursued.

TREATMENT

Maintaining the airway often requires tracheotomy. Epiglottectomy and various endoscopic surgeries to enlarge the airway with incisions, mitomycin application, and steroid injections may be necessary (Figure 13.40).

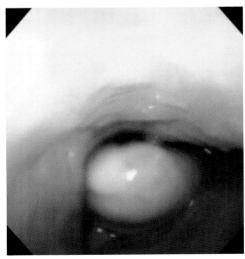

Figure 13.37 A 33-year-old male with cicatricial pemphigoid affecting his nose and larynx. Note the turban-shaped epiglottis.

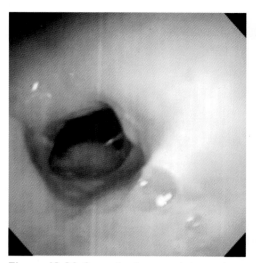

Figure 13.38 Supraglottic stenosis beyond the turban-shaped epiglottis. Bulge in center of view is the right false vocal fold. The true vocal folds are normal, but not seen well in this image.

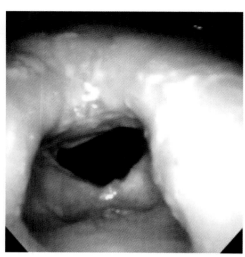

Figure 13.40 Final airway at time of decannulation.

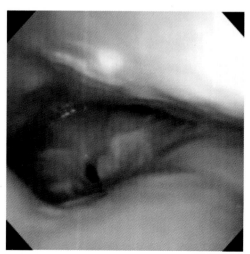

Figure 13.39 Progressive worsening of the airway led to tracheotomy and later epiglottectomy and surgical enlargement of the airway and decannulation.

Other Neuromuscular Causes of Dysphonia and Trauma

Glendon M. Gardner and Michael S. Benninger

- **Muscle tension dysphonia**
- **Vocal fold bowing**
- **Paradoxical vocal fold motion**
- **Laryngeal trauma**
- **Suggested reading**

Muscle tension dysphonia

DEFINITION

Muscle tension dysphonia (MTD) refers to dysphonia due to improper tension in muscles of phonation affecting the vibration of the vocal folds. It is not directly due to an organic lesion, although it may be compensating for one.

CLINICAL FEATURES

Many patients will present with variable dysphonia, the voice often returning to normal, with rapid changes in voice. Some will report inciting events such as changes in temperature (walking into an air-conditioned room), exposure to fumes and scents, or a true case of viral laryngitis. Examination will reveal otherwise normal looking vocal folds, but with phonation, various abnormalities may become evident, all reflecting improper technique. The most common situations include the true vocal folds adducting too forcefully, causing a very tight strained voice, or no voice at all; closure of the supraglottis, resulting in a very rough voice; or lack of closure, with a weak whispery voice (Figures 14.1 through 14.11). The excessive muscle strain will often cause soreness of the muscles in and around the larynx, as well.

DIFFERENTIAL DIAGNOSIS

Adductor spasmodic dysphonia presents with tight voice breaks with the spasm occurring at the level of the glottis. It does not respond to voice therapy. Abductor spasmodic dysphonia has breathy voice breaks with the vocal folds suddenly bursting open during vowels. It also does not respond to voice therapy.

WORKUP

While most cases of MTD are due to incorrect technique in an otherwise normally functioning larynx, sometimes the hyperfunction is compensating for an underlying organic problem, such as

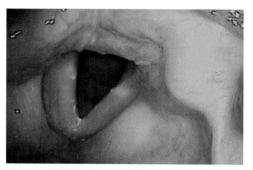

Figure 14.1 A 62-year-old woman with dysphonia for 3 years post hysterectomy.

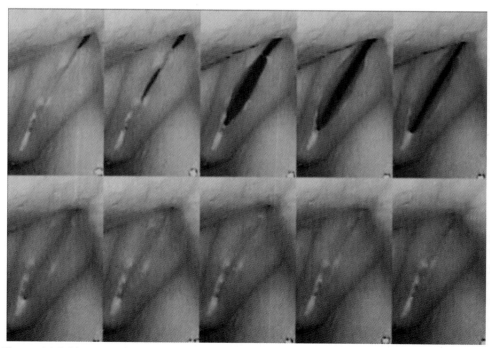

Figure 14.2 Montage of glottic cycle showing prolonged closed phase, suggesting tight closure. Mucosal waves are normal.

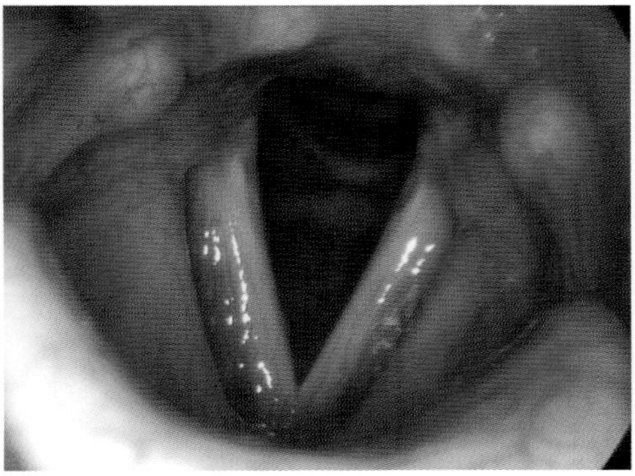

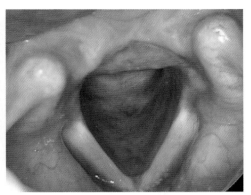

Figure 14.3 A 31-year-old woman with intermittent aphonia or severe whisper dysphonia over 7-year period. Rapid onset with no predisposing factors. Normal vocal fold motion.

Figure 14.5 A 14-year-old girl with loss of voice after bout of laryngitis. Normal motion.

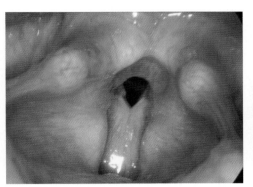

Figure 14.4 Classic whisper posture with arytenoids rotated slightly with posterior glottic gap. Musculomembranous vocal folds adducted tightly and not vibrating. Voice is only a whisper.

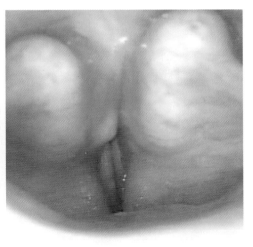

Figure 14.6 Able to achieve complete closure at times.

incomplete glottic closure due to vocal fold bowing, vocal fold paresis, or paralysis. With supraglottic compression, sometimes referred to as dysphonia plica ventricularis, the glottis cannot be seen during phonation and the clinician does not know if the patient is actually able to achieve complete glottic closure (Figures 14.9 and 14.11). Asking the person to phonate while inhaling will cause the supraglottis to relax, providing a clear view of the glottis (Figure 14.12). Also a cough will cause closure and the glottis may still be in view. If the glottis is incompetent, correcting that problem will usually resolve the compensatory MTD. Voice therapy may result in relaxation of the supraglottis providing a view of the glottis during phonation and revealing an underlying glottic abnormality.

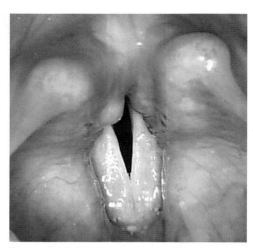

Figure 14.7 Whisper posture while phonating with large posterior glottic gap.

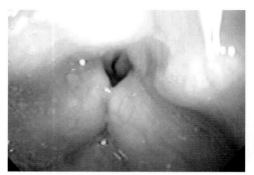

Figure 14.9 Tight closure of false vocal folds with phonation, consistent with "dysphonia plica ventricularis" form of MTD.

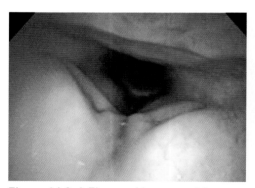

Figure 14.8 A 71-year-old woman with 4-month history of dysphonia following upper respiratory infection with severe cough. Much edema of undersurface of glottis and posterior commissure suggestive of LPR. Also possible bilateral saccular cysts.

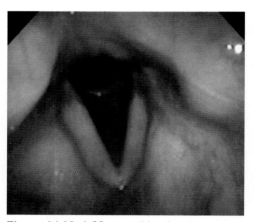

Figure 14.10 A 35-year-old male who experiences severe dysphonia 5 times per year, each episode lasting 2–3 weeks.

voice possible. Those topics are addressed in other sections.

Vocal fold bowing

DEFINITION
Bowed vocal folds are no longer straight and taut and are unable to approximate completely during phonation.

CLINICAL FEATURES
As we age, muscles weaken, ligaments slacken, joints stiffen, and neural conduction slows.

TREATMENT
Voice therapy is the mainstay of treatment for MTD with the vast majority of patients having a normal voice at the conclusion of therapy. If there is an underlying cause of a compensatory MTD, such as vocal fold bowing, paresis, or paralysis, that problem may need to be remedied to achieve the best

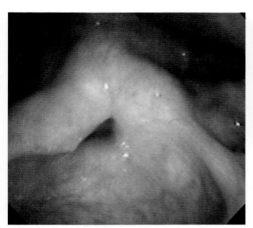

Figure 14.11 Severe closure of supraglottis with phonation.

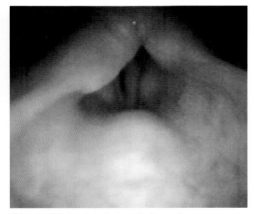

Figure 14.12 Inhalational phonation demonstrates normal vocal motion and ability to achieve closure of glottis.

The voice also normally changes as we age and most listeners can predict the approximate age of a speaker based on the voice without seeing that person. Exceptions exist, of course, and many singers are successful well into their later years.

For some elderly and not-so-elderly people, the vocal folds weaken to the point that they become bowed and unable to

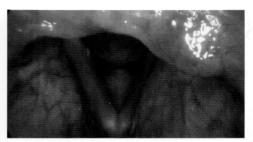

Figure 14.13 A 91-year-old man with several-year history of gradually worsening dysphonia primarily characterized by a weak voice. Subtle vocal fold bowing bilaterally.

approximate adequately (Figures 14.13 through 14.16). Early on the person will note that as the day goes on, and with more use, the voice fatigues and weakens. Later, the voice is persistently softer and lacks volume. In severe cases, especially if the person has Parkinson's disease, they may be almost aphonic.

DIFFERENTIAL DIAGNOSIS
Vocal fold paresis, vocal fold paralysis, sulcus vocalis, Parkinson's disease.

WORKUP
Laryngoscopy is usually adequate to rule out the other causes of an incompetent glottis. If paralysis is suspected, the appropriate workup for that problem must be undertaken as described in another section.

TREATMENT
Initial treatment is voice therapy, which helps many patients. If that is not successful, improving closure by injecting a substance into the vocal folds to increase their volume, or medializing them with implants, will improve the voice (Figures 14.15 through 14.19). Deciding which to pursue depends on the patient's age, overall health and life expectancy, vocal needs, and the surgeon's experience.

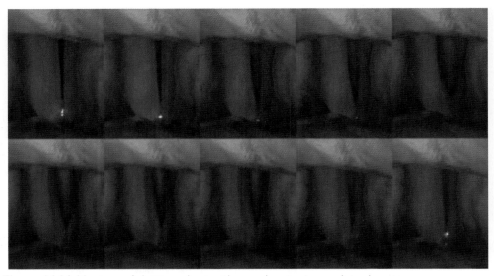

Figure 14.14 Montage of glottic cycle at midrange showing incomplete closure.

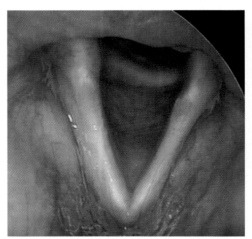

Figure 14.15 An 80-year-old with a 2-year history of dysphonia with bilateral vocal fold bowing.

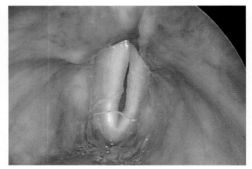

Figure 14.16 Incomplete closure.

The classic description of this condition also includes opening of the vocal folds while attempting phonation causing aphonia, but this latter situation is rarely observed and the voice is usually normal in these patients (Figure 14.22).

Paradoxical vocal fold motion

DEFINITION
Paradoxical vocal fold motion (PVFM) refers to closure of normally mobile vocal folds during inspiration, which causes inspiratory stridor and dyspnea (Figures 14.20 and 14.21).

CLINICAL FEATURES
The typical patient is a teenage girl, although any age or sex may be affected. The episodes are sporadic and may occur during physical exertion; asthma exacerbations; exposure to smoke, fumes, and scents; episodes of LPR;

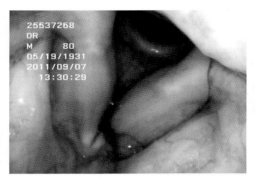

Figure 14.17 Bilateral vocal fold injections performed percutaneously in the office with local anesthesia with Radiesse voice gel causing swelling of both vocal folds as a test to determine if improved closure would improve voice significantly.

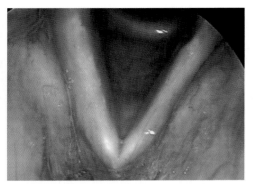

Figure 14.19 Vocal folds straight. Voice remained improved despite temporary nature of injected material and patient had no further intervention.

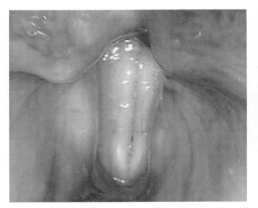

Figure 14.18 Closure and voice improved 1 month post injection.

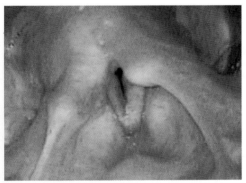

Figure 14.20 Vocal folds adduct during inspiration.

and emotional stress. It may be associated with an anxiety disorder and panic attacks. Because most patients and many clinicians will refer to stridor as "wheezing," many of these patients are treated for asthma when they do not have that disease, similar to patients with bilateral vocal fold paralysis. However, perhaps 50% of patients with PVFM actually have asthma also.

While the presentation of these patients may be very distressing with loud inspiratory stridor and retractions, the O_2 saturation does not drop very much below the patient's baseline, if at all. The patient will not lose consciousness.

DIFFERENTIAL DIAGNOSIS
Bilateral vocal fold paralysis, laryngeal or tracheal stenosis, respiratory dystonia.

WORKUP
Laryngoscopy (best done in these cases with a flexible scope) reveals vocal folds often resting in a paramedian position during "quiet" respiration. With deep inspiration, the vocal folds often come together, either due to the Bernoulli effect or activity of the adductors (Figures 14.20 and 14.21). With a sniff, the

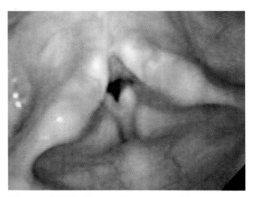

Figure 14.21 Twenty-four-year-old woman. During inspiration, vocal folds adducted, but with patent posterior glottis (whisper posture), causing inspiratory stridor, but allowing adequate air passage.

vocal folds usually abduct, except in the most severe cases. If they do not, asking the patient to cough will cause the folds to open widely either before or after the cough. Sometimes the vocal folds will eventually open normally if watched long enough (Figures 14.23 and 14.24). If the stridor resolves when the vocal folds abduct, the obstruction is at the glottis and is consistent with PVFM. If it persists with an open glottis, the source of the stridor must be in the subglottis or trachea and must be investigated further. If none of the above maneuvers result in an open glottis, the patient may have bilateral vocal fold paralysis, which is much more serious. Various neurologic disorders have also been reported to cause PVFM and should be evaluated if there are other neurologic signs or the condition does not respond to the usual treatment.

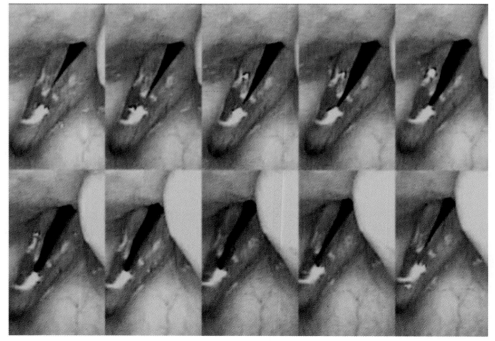

Figure 14.22 Incomplete closure with gap posteriorly during phonation and resultant weak, breathy voice.

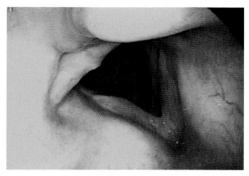

Figure 14.23 Full abduction between coughs demonstrating normal vocal fold motion and normal airway.

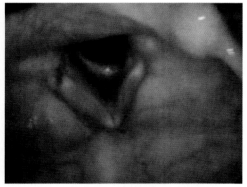

Figure 14.24 Normal abduction seen at times during respiration, showing normal motion and airway.

TREATMENT

Treatment of PVFM is "voice therapy," which is aimed at relaxation techniques to help the patient relax the adductors and allow the vocal folds to open. This is successful the majority of the time. In recalcitrant cases, psychological evaluation should be considered. There are also very rare cases of a respiratory dystonia, which is a focal dystonia causing the same condition described earlier. This may be seen in patients with other dystonias, such as blepharospasm and spasmodic dysphonia. This true dystonia does not respond to voice therapy and may be responsive to botox injections. There are also cases of patients with Munchhausen's syndrome who present with inspiratory stridor and are frequently intubated and sometimes even undergo tracheotomy.

It should be noted that the pulmonary and allergy community refer to PVFM as "vocal cord dysfunction," an unfortunate phrase that is very general and not at all descriptive. The otolaryngology community continues to use the much more accurate term "paradoxical vocal fold motion."

Laryngeal trauma

DEFINITION

Laryngeal trauma may be external (blunt or penetrating) or internal. External is usually the result of accidents (motor vehicle, bicycle, various sports including those with sticks, bats, racquets, and many different sizes of balls) or assaults (guns, knives, fists, feet, pipes, and the same implements used in sports). Internal trauma is often iatrogenic (intubation, poorly performed laryngeal surgery, rigid bronchoscopy, laryngoscopy, or esophagoscopy) or due to inhalation of caustic fumes, fire, or smoke, or ingestion of caustic chemicals.

CLINICAL FEATURES

External trauma can be as mild as a vocal fold hemorrhage after being struck in the larynx with a baseball, with no fractures, or a life-threatening crush injury of the laryngeal cartilages from striking the larynx on the edge of a counter when falling (Figures 14.25 through 14.28). Patients may present with a mildly hoarse voice or may be in severe respiratory distress (Figure 14.29). Many cases of severe laryngeal trauma never make it to a medical facility, dying at the scene of the trauma.

Iatrogenic internal trauma is usually not life threatening, but can still cause significant voice problems. Vocal folds have been

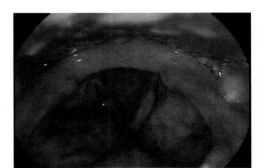

Figure 14.25 Blunt external trauma (struck on neck) 2 weeks prior to presentation in a 22-year-old football player resulting in hemorrhage of the right side of the larynx (false and true vocal folds). Patient experienced pain and hoarseness.

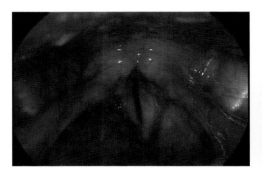

Figure 14.26 No impairment of mucosal wave.

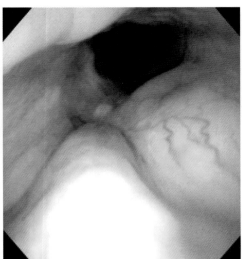

Figure 14.27 A 28-year-old male with self-inflicted laceration of thyroid cartilage and detached anterior commissure, 2 weeks post open reduction with internal fixation.

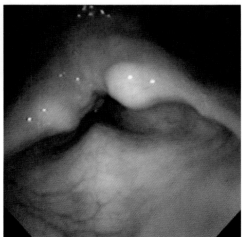

Figure 14.28 Phonation, supraglottic compression, 2 weeks post open reduction with internal fixation.

lacerated and the arytenoid cartilage can be dislocated, although this is a very controversial subject. Patients may have voice complaints immediately after a surgical procedure with endotracheal intubation, or it may develop over the next few weeks.

DIFFERENTIAL DIAGNOSIS

Onset of symptoms immediately at the time of trauma makes the etiology clear. The history may be less clear-cut if the patient is unconscious or if intervention (intubation, exploration of the neck) has occurred between the time of the trauma and the evaluation by the clinician who is assessing the larynx.

WORKUP

If the airway is stable, the patient should be assessed with awake laryngoscopy (Figures 14.25 and 14.26) and, in the case of external trauma, CT scan, to assess the extent of injury

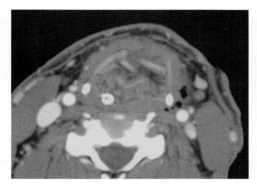

Figure 14.29 Axial CT scan (done after emergent tracheotomy done at outside hospital, prior to repair) demonstrating multiple fragments of thyroid cartilage pushed posteriorly into the laryngeal lumen.

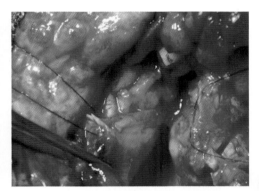

Figure 14.30 Larynx open through laceration. 4-0 prolene sutures through anterior vocal ligaments bilaterally. Sutures later placed through anterior aspects of false vocal folds and petiole.

and plan treatment (Figure 14.29). If the airway is not stable, the patient should undergo an awake tracheotomy and exploration of the larynx without any imaging (Figure 14.33).

TREATMENT

For a mild hemorrhage, simple observation and relative voice rest suffices, while for the more severe injury with impending loss of airway, an awake tracheotomy is recommended. Attempting to intubate the patient with a severe injury can result in complete obstruction. Once the airway is secured, direct

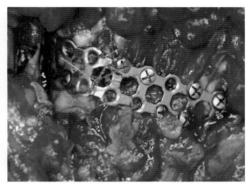

Figure 14.31 After reduction of lacerated thyroid cartilage, sutures from within larynx tied around plate on the outside.

laryngoscopy is performed to assess internal injuries. Definitive treatment is aimed at restoring the larynx to its original configuration by repairing mucosal injuries with absorbable suture and the laryngeal framework with sutures or miniplates. Careful attention should be paid to reestablishing the anterior commissure (Figures 14.30 through 14.35). If there is severe mucosal injury and the framework is unstable, stenting may be necessary for a couple weeks.

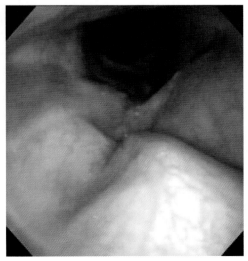

Figure 14.32 Six months post injury with normal airway.

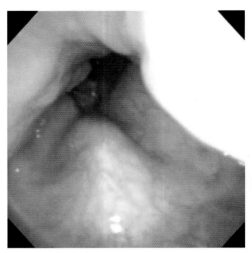

Figure 14.33 Closure not quite complete.

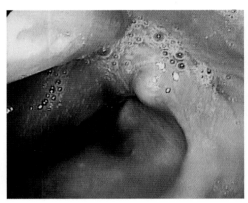

Figure 14.34 Right laryngeal hematoma in a 66-year-old male who fell, striking the larynx against the edge of a counter top, fractured the thyroid cartilage, and presented with worsening airway obstruction due to the hematoma. Underwent awake tracheotomy, open reduction, and fixation of fracture with miniplates and screws. Picture taken 4 days after injury and surgery.

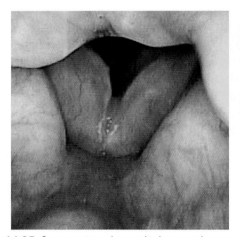

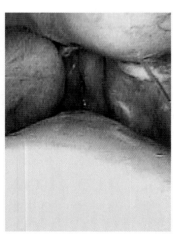

Figure 14.35 Same patient 6 months later with patent airway and good closure.

Conservative care often results in healing of mucosal injuries, but scarring may result, which is very difficult to treat. Caustic ingestion is potentially life threatening, with strong acids and bases causing acute edema and chronic scarring. The esophagus is also at risk.

Suggested reading

Belafsky PC, Postma GN, Koufman JA. 2001. The validity and reliability of the reflux finding score (RFS). *Laryngoscope* 111: 1313–1317.

SECTION 4

OTOLOGY AND NEUROTOLOGY

CHAPTER 15

Normal Ear Examination and External Ear Disorders

Anthony Chin-Quee, Foluwasayo E. Ologe, and Michael D. Seidman

- **Normal ear examination**
- **Normal inner ear**
- **Hearing loss and hearing aid options**
- **Auricular hematoma**
- **Chronic nodularis helicis**
- **Otitis externa**
- **Osteoma**
- **Exostosis**
- **Necrotizing otitis externa (previously known as malignant otitis externa)**

Normal ear examination

The auricle is a cartilaginous framework that serves to collect and direct sound waves to the external auditory canal (EAC) (Figure 15.1).

The middle ear converts sound waves to mechanical energy and amplifies sound before it is transmitted to the inner ear. This takes place by way of the delicate relationships among the tympanic membrane, the ossicles, and the oval window (Figure 15.2).

The tympanic membrane is composed of three layers: the lateral squamous cell epithelial layer; the medial mucosal layer, which faces the middle ear; and the fibrous layer or tunica propria, which lies between the two and is comprised of both circular and radiating fibers. The majority of the tympanic membrane consists of these three layers (pars tensa), with the exception of a

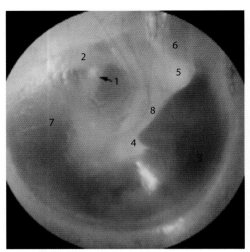

Figure 15.2 Normal right middle ear as seen by otoscopy. 1—posterior crus of stapes, 2—long process of the incus, 3—pars tensa, 4—umbo, 5—lateral process of the malleus, 6—pars flaccida, 7—round window, 8—manubrium of the malleus.

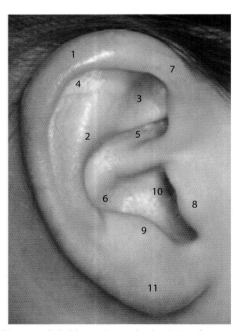

Figure 15.1 Normal auricle. 1—helix, 2—antihelix, 3—triangular fossa, 4—scaphoid fossa, 5—conchal cymba, 6—conchal cavum, 7—helical crus, 8—tragus, 9—antitragus, 10—external auditory meatus, 11—lobule.

small triangular portion of the membrane located superior to the lateral process of the malleus, which is missing the fibrous layer (pars flaccida).

Problems with the external ear and middle ear can often be diagnosed by physical examination. Further evaluation with an audiologic examination is often necessary. This typically includes an audiogram, tympanogram, and acoustic reflexes. Additional workup, such as CT or MRI, can be important in the evaluation.

Normal inner ear

The inner ear is housed within the petrous temporal bone. It is composed of a continuous bony labyrinth, within which there is a membranous labyrinth. The structures within this labyrinth include the cochlea; the superior, posterior, and lateral semicircular canals; the endolymphatic sac and duct; and the vestibule (including the utricle and saccule). The cochlea is the organ of hearing, while the remainder of the inner ear structures functions to maintain balance and equilibrium. The inner ear organs receive innervation from the nerves that travel through the internal auditory canal. These nerves include the superior and inferior vestibular nerves, and the cochlear nerve, all of which are derived from cranial nerve 8. The facial nerve also courses through the internal auditory canal, however it does not directly innervate any of the aforementioned structures (Figure 15.3).

Disorders of the inner ear can often cause hearing loss and/or vertigo. The term "dizziness" is often used by patients to describe a sensation of "room spinning," lightheadedness, unsteadiness, wooziness, confusion, giddiness, a sensation of being pulled, a sensation of walking on a waterbed, a floating sensation, a feeling of being on a boat or just getting off a roller coaster, etc. Typically, describing the sensation that they are experiencing is very difficult for most people with balance problems. Vertigo is a term that describes an abnormal sense of motion, and can be quite difficult for patients to describe. True vertigo is often distinguished on history as a sense of the "room spinning" before a patient's eyes. A generalized sense of imbalance, or lightheadedness, is not often due to inner ear pathology. Because the sense of *balance* is maintained by complex interactions between the inner ear, the somatosensory proprioception system, and the visual system, it is essential that the physician determine the source of the balance abnormality with a thorough history and physical exam. Associated ear symptoms such as hearing loss or fluctuation, tinnitus, ear fullness, or pressure should raise suspicion for an otologic cause. A history of recent infection, trauma, ototoxic medications, or polypharmacy is also vital to obtain. Prior to evaluation by an otolaryngologist, an extensive workup on nonotologic causes of vertigo should be performed by a primary care physician.

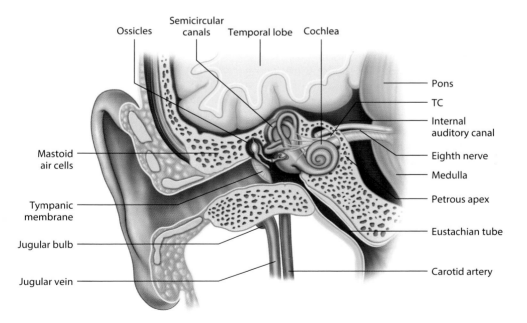

Figure 15.3 Coronal cut of the temporal bone, with normal external, middle, and inner ear structures.

Evaluation by the otolaryngologist will include a complete otolaryngologic head and neck examination and a directed neurotologic exam that will include tests of the cranial nerves, eye movements, and balance testing. Other objective tests that may be done are a comprehensive audiologic examination, auditory brainstem response, ENG, rotational chair testing, platform posturography, and electrocochleography. If after completing the extensive evaluation the source of the balance abnormality remains unclear, imaging by way of CT or MRI may be obtained.

Hearing loss and hearing aid options

For patients who suffer from chronic hearing loss, there are several options for amplification devices. The process by which patients can obtain hearing aids typically consists of a hearing test demonstrating hearing loss (typically valid for obtaining hearing aids within a 6-month window), medical clearance from a physician, followed by a hearing aid selection appointment with an audiologist who will review the myriad in-ear hearing aid options. In addition to the traditional hearing aid options, there is also the option of the SoundBite hearing aid. This aid is designed for patients with unilateral hearing loss. It works by transmitting sound from a microphone in the ear to a dental appliance, which amplifies the sound through vibration.

There are several surgically implantable hearing aids available as well. For unilateral hearing loss, the bone-anchored hearing aid (BAHA) may prove a suitable option. Sometimes patients do not like the idea of the requisite metal abutment sticking out of the skin, in which case the BAHA Attract, or Sophono hearing aids, may be considered—these use magnets to connect the processor instead of the abutment. There is also a fully implantable surgical option,

the Envoy Esteem, which entails implantation of a *driver* in between the ossicles and provides amplification using the eardrum as a natural microphone.

Patients who suffer from severe to profound hearing loss in both ears, and receive little to no benefit from hearing aid use, may be candidates for cochlear implantation. Criteria for implantation include age of at least 12 months, either pre- or postlingual onset deafness in adults or children, bilateral moderate to profound hearing loss (if older than 2 years old), and bilateral profound hearing loss (younger than 2 years old). Audiologic exam must show a three-frequency pure tone loss of an average of 70 dB or worse in the better hearing ear, a speech discrimination score of less than 50% in the ear to be implanted (typically the better hearing ear), and a speech discrimination score of less than 60% when aided with hearing aids. Prior to the operation, high-resolution scan of the temporal bones is obtained to assess for complete cochlear agenesis and abnormalities of the cochlear nerve. Additionally, due to the increased risk of postoperative meningitis in cochlear implant patients, vaccination against *Streptococcus pneumoniae* is generally required prior to surgery. Other risks of the surgery include surgical site infection, facial paralysis, and CSF leak (Figures 15.4 and 15.5).

Auricular hematoma

DEFINITION AND CLINICAL FEATURES
An auricular hematoma is a collection of blood between the auricular cartilage and its associated perichondrium. This is typically secondary to blunt trauma to the external ear and is often seen in athletes who wear poor-fitting protective headgear or no headgear at all. The hematoma forms when tangential force is applied to the auricle. The outer surface of the auricle lacks layers of subcutaneous tissue; thus, when tangential force is applied to the auricle, it is directly

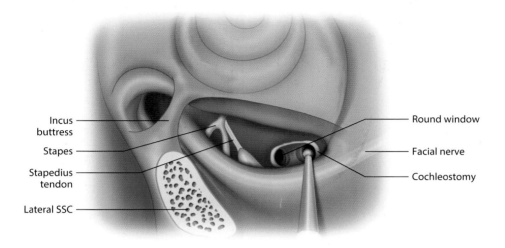

Figure 15.4 Facial recess approach for implantation of cochlear implant.

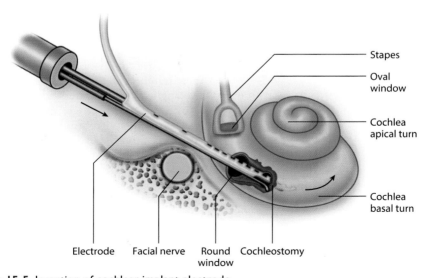

Figure 15.5 Insertion of cochlear implant electrode.

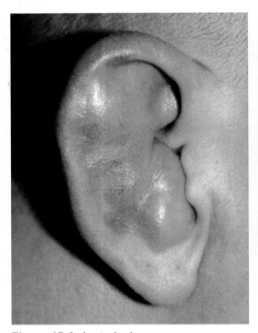

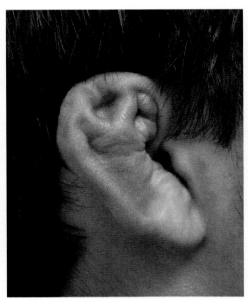

Figure 15.7 Cauliflower ear.

Figure 15.6 Auricular hematoma.

transmitted to the perichondrium and the underlying cartilage. Small blood vessels of the perichondrium are ruptured, leading to leakage of blood and subsequent elevation of the perichondrium off the cartilage.

The patient typically presents with a soft, warm, fluctuant painful mass on the outer surface of the auricle with a recent history of trauma (Figure 15.6).

DIFFERENTIAL DIAGNOSIS
Subperichondrial abscess, perichondritis, cauliflower ear.

WORKUP
No diagnostic testing is currently recommended in the workup of auricular hematoma.

TREATMENT
Treatment of auricular hematoma includes evacuation of the hematoma and prevention of reaccumulation. Although needle aspiration is widely practiced, it is not the recommended mode of evacuation due to a high risk of reaccumulation and infection. Incision and drainage is most commonly performed following local injection of lidocaine with a small retroauricular skin incision. This incision should be carried down through the perichondrium to the level of the cartilage, with complete evacuation of blood. Reaccumulation can be prevented in a number of ways including noninvasive application of plaster molds or silicone splints, bolster dressings, drain placement, and through-and-through suturing. Oral antibiotic prophylaxis is commonly administered for several days following the procedure. The patient should be reevaluated in at least 3 days' time to examine for reaccumulation, and perichondritis. The long-term complications of auricular hematoma include formation of neocartilage (cauliflower ear), cartilage necrosis, chondritis, erythema, hearing loss, and increased risk of otitis externa (Figure 15.7).

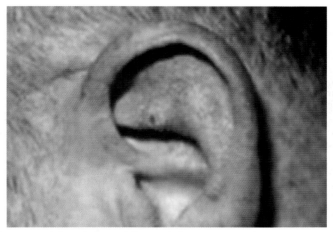

Figure 15.8 Chronic nodularis helicis of the antihelix.

Chronic nodularis helicis

DEFINITION AND CLINICAL FEATURES
Chronic nodularis helicis is a chronic, benign disorder of the helix or antihelix of the external ear. It typically presents as a painful nodule that enlarges rapidly to a maximum size and then remains stable. The onset is precipitated by exposure of the most prominent projection of the ear to pressure, trauma, or cold. Lesions are typically unilateral, and the patient often admits to sleeping on the affected side. Nodules are firm, tender, and round with a raised edge and a central ulcer.

DIFFERENTIAL DIAGNOSIS
Actinic keratosis, atypical fibroxanthoma, basal cell carcinoma, squamous cell carcinoma, Merkel cell carcinoma, cystic chondromalacia, elastotic nodule, keratoacanthoma, perforating dermatoses, pseudocyst of the auricle.

WORKUP
A biopsy is typically performed to establish diagnosis.

TREATMENT
Medical treatment of chronic nodularis helicis centers on symptom relief. Topical antibiotics, topical or intralesional steroids, collagen injections, and cryotherapy have been used to relieve pain and discomfort. Additionally, custom pillows and pressure-relieving prosthesis are available to relieve symptoms. If symptoms cannot be relieved conservatively, surgical treatment is necessary. Wedge excision, curettage, electrocauterization, CO_2 laser ablation, and excision of affected skin and cartilage have all been used in the treatment of these nodules. The recurrence rate is high unless all damaged cartilages are removed and pressure is relieved (Figure 15.8).

Otitis externa

DEFINITION AND CLINICAL FEATURES
Otitis externa is an inflammatory, and oftentimes infectious, disorder of the EAC. The inciting event is disruption of the EAC epithelium, which allows for bacterial infection leading to progressive erythema and edema of the epithelial and subcutaneous layers. Fungal infection is also occasionally seen as

an opportunistic infection following treatment of a preceding bacterial infection. The patient typically presents with symptoms of itching, otalgia, hearing loss, aural fullness, granulation tissue, and otorrhea. On physical exam, typical findings include squamous debris, otorrhea, canal edema, and, in the setting of necrotizing external otitis (in the past known as malignant otitis externa), cranial neuropathies.

DIFFERENTIAL DIAGNOSIS

Necrotizing external otitis, otitis media, cerumen impaction, foreign body, trauma, exostoses.

WORKUP

Generally speaking, cultures are not routinely indicated; however, in the setting of persistent or refractory infection, it is reasonable to consider evaluating for the type of bacteria or fungus present.

TREATMENT

Debridement of the EAC is the initial treatment, as it facilitates clearance of infectious agents, as well as allows for uptake of topical medications. Following debridement, the mainstay of treatment is an antibiotic drop with coverage for *Pseudomonas aeruginosa* (the most common type of bacteria seen). Fungal otitis externa can be treated with debridement and topical antifungals. Complications include cellulitis, perichondritis, medial canal fibrosis, tympanic membrane perforation, and necrotizing otitis externa (in the past, referred to as malignant otitis externa) (Figures 15.9 and 15.10).

Osteoma

DEFINITION AND CLINICAL FEATURES

Osteomas are benign, slow-growing, bony neoplasms that can be found in the EAC. They often arise as single, pedunculated lesions from the tympanomastoid or tympanosquamous suture lines. These masses are

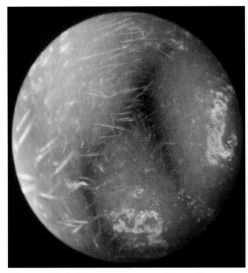

Figure 15.9 Otitis externa with significant EAC edema.

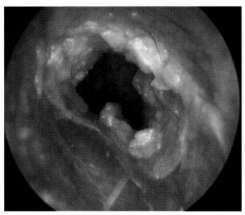

Figure 15.10 Otitis externa demonstrating squamous debris of the EAC.

often found incidentally but can cause symptoms related to the degree of obstruction of the EAC. Patients may complain of hearing loss, or recurrent otitis externa, due to inability of squamous epithelial cells to migrate laterally and subsequent infectious colonization. Exostoses, while histologically the same, are typically multiple unlike osteoma, which is typically a single bony growth.

DIFFERENTIAL DIAGNOSIS
Exostoses, osteosarcoma, Gardner's syndrome.

WORKUP
If hearing loss is suspected, an audiogram should be obtained. A CT scan can be obtained to evaluate the origin and extent of the lesion prior to any consideration for surgical removal (rarely necessary).

TREATMENT
Symptomatic osteomas can be removed surgically, with the surgical approach being determined by the location and extent of the mass. These approaches typically include canaloplasty via transmeatal or retroauricular approach. The approach that the surgeon determines will afford the best exposure of the mass given its size and location in the EAC is chosen. Complications of surgical intervention include recurrent otitis externa, canal stenosis, and damage to surrounding structures (i.e., the temporomandibular joint, facial nerve, tympanic membrane, ossicular chain) (Figures 15.11 and 15.12).

Exostosis

DEFINITION AND CLINICAL FEATURES
Exostoses are the result of hyperplasia of the periosteum and underlying bone of the EAC. These lesions are multiple, smooth, broad-based, and covered in epithelium. These lesions are most often seen in patients who have a history of exposure to cold, wet, and windy conditions, and is commonly known as "surfer's ear." Symptomatic exostoses present similar to osteomas—patients may have hearing loss or pain secondary to recurrent otitis externa.

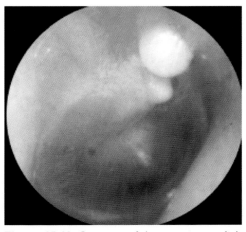

Figure 15.11 Osteoma of the superior medial EAC.

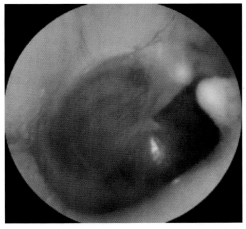

Figure 15.12 Osteoma of the anterior medial EAC.

DIFFERENTIAL DIAGNOSIS
Osteoma, osteosarcoma.

WORKUP
Identical workup to osteoma: If hearing loss is suspected, an audiogram should be obtained. A CT scan can be obtained to evaluate the origin and extent of the lesion prior to surgical removal (Figures 15.13 and 15.14).

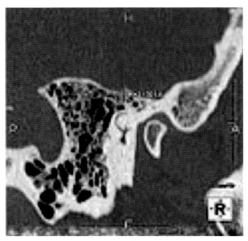

Figure I5.I3 CT temporal bone demonstrating exostoses.

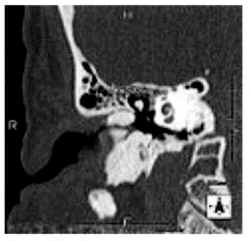

Figure I5.I4 CT temporal bone demonstrating exostoses.

TREATMENT

Surgical removal of exostoses is similar to the removal of osteomas. The surgical approach, either transcanal or postauricular, is determined by the location and extent of the mass. Complications of surgical intervention include recurrent otitis externa, canal stenosis, and damage to surrounding structures (i.e., the

temporomandibular joint, facial nerve, tympanic membrane, ossicular chain). Extreme care is required when drilling the abnormal bone away, so as not to inadvertently contact the ossicular chain. If the ossicular chain is contacted by a high speed drill, the patient may experience sensorineural hearing loss. If the ear is continually exposed to cold, wet conditions, the disorder may recur.

Necrotizing otitis externa (previously known as malignant otitis externa)

DEFINITION AND CLINICAL FEATURES

Necrotizing otitis externa is a very aggressive and potentially fatal infection of the EAC that is most often seen in immunocompromised patients. Patients often present with long-standing otalgia and otorrhea. Classically, there is granulation tissue seen in the floor of the EAC at the bony–cartilaginous junction. The infection progresses from the soft tissues of the ear canal, to the bony structures of the temporal bone, and to the intracranial cavity, or along the skull base to involve the cranial nerves. Intracranial involvement often presents as headache, altered mental status, fever, and nuchal rigidity. The facial nerve is the most commonly involved cranial nerve and presents as unilateral facial paralysis.

DIFFERENTIAL DIAGNOSIS

Otitis externa, temporal bone neoplasm.

WORKUP

Bacterial and fungal cultures of otorrhea should be obtained. CT scans can show evidence of bony erosion, while MRI scans are superior for detecting soft tissue changes and enhancement of the dura, if present. Technetium-99m bone scans detect osteoblastic activity, and are very specific to active infection, should the CT

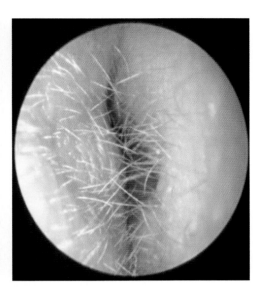

Figure 15.15 Malignant otitis externa with significant EAC edema.

scan be inconclusive. Gallium-67 citrate- and indium-111-labeled leukocyte scans show inflammatory cell activity and have high sensitivity for monitoring resolution of disease.

TREATMENT

Treatment of necrotizing otitis externa is primarily medical. Early infections are often treated with oral antipseudomonal antibiotics (i.e., fluoroquinolones), while more progressive infections are treated initially with IV antibiotics. On occasion, surgical debridement may become necessary, but usually, the surgeon is "chasing" a diffusely spreading disease and surgical intervention may prove futile. Hyperbaric oxygen therapy may be used to facilitate the management of the bone infection (Figure 15.15).

CHAPTER 16

Middle Ear Disorders

Anthony Chin-Quee, Foluwasayo E. Ologe, and Michael D. Seidman

- **Tympanic membrane perforation**
- **Otitis media**
- **Mastoiditis**
- **Paraganglioma**
- **Cholesteatoma**
- **Otosclerosis**
- **Cholesterol granuloma**

Tympanic membrane perforation

DEFINITION AND CLINICAL FEATURES
A tympanic membrane perforation is a hole that develops in the tympanic membrane as a result of chronic infection or trauma. Patients commonly present with otalgia, otorrhea, hearing loss, tinnitus, and a sensation of fullness. Perforations are classified as central (involving the pars tensa, sparing the annulus), marginal (involving the pars tensa and the annulus), and attic (involving the pars flaccida) (Figures 16.1 and 16.2).

DIFFERENTIAL DIAGNOSIS
Retraction pocket, cholesteatoma, tympano-sclerosis, monomeric tympanic membrane.

WORKUP
When evaluating a tympanic membrane perforation, hearing loss and compliance of the middle ear mechanism are quantified by obtaining an audiogram and tympanogram.

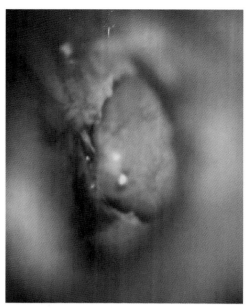

Figure 16.1 Marginal tympanic membrane perforation.

TREATMENT

The majority of traumatic perforations will heal spontaneously over the course of weeks to months. In order to promote healing of perforations associated with chronic otitis media, dry ear precautions and antibiotics are the mainstay of treatment. If the perforation persists, surgical intervention through myringoplasty with autologous cartilage or fat graft for small perforations, and formal tympanoplasty with autologous fascia graft may be required for larger perforations. The approach to the tympanoplasty (transmeatal vs. postauricular, graft underlay vs. lateral graft overlay) is determined by the size and location of the perforation, as well as surgeon preference.

Otitis media

DEFINITION AND CLINICAL FEATURES

Otitis media is defined as an inflammatory condition of the middle ear and mastoid space and is an extremely common disorder of childhood. A middle ear effusion may or may not be present. Inflammation may be acute, subacute, or chronic. Eustachian tube dysfunction is the most important pathological factor. Patients with acute otitis media often present with fever, irritability, otalgia, and hearing loss. In the case of advanced disease, patients may present with tinnitus, vertigo, facial paralysis and

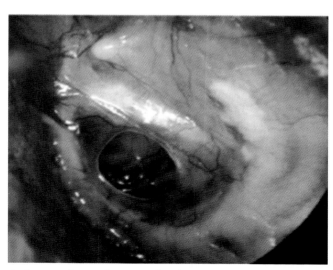

Figure 16.2 Central tympanic membrane perforation.

swelling, and pain behind the ear. In the case of otitis media with effusion, the only presenting symptom may be hearing loss or speech delay. In the case of chronic suppurative otitis media, persistent purulent drainage is observed through a tympanic membrane perforation or tympanostomy tube (Figures 16.3 and 16.4).

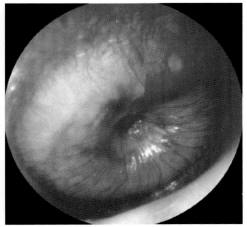

Figure 16.3 Acute otitis media, demonstrating hyperemia and bulging of membrane.

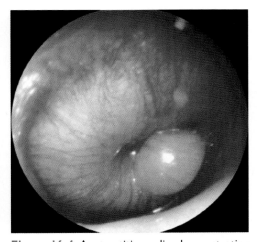

Figure 16.4 Acute otitis media, demonstrating progression of infection, membrane in danger of perforation.

DIFFERENTIAL DIAGNOSIS

Mastoiditis, otitis externa, otosclerosis, cholesteatoma.

WORKUP

A careful examination of the tympanic membrane with pneumatic otoscopy is essential to initial evaluation. An audiogram with tympanometry should be performed for any patient with complaint of hearing loss. If there is suspicion of intracranial complications, a CT scan can be considered.

TREATMENT

Otitis media may be treated with observation, medically with analgesics and antimicrobials agents targeting the most common causative agents of acute otitis media: *Streptococcus pneumoniae, Haemophilus influenzae, Moraxella catarrhalis,* and group A Streptococci. Disease refractory to medical management can be treated with myringotomy with tympanostomy tube placement, as well as adenoidectomy with or without tonsillectomy.

Mastoiditis

DEFINITION AND CLINICAL FEATURES

Mastoiditis can be defined as an inflammatory process of the mastoid air cells. Mastoiditis may be acute, associated with acute otitis media, or chronic, associated with chronic suppurative otitis media. In addition to presenting with symptoms of acute otitis media (fever, hearing loss, otorrhea), pain as well as erythema and swelling in acute mastoiditis may be localized to the postauricular area and is typically worse at night.

DIFFERENTIAL DIAGNOSIS

Deep neck space infection, lymphadenopathy, cellulitis, basilar skull fracture, parotitis, otitis externa, trauma, neoplasm.

WORKUP

Seeing as mastoiditis often arises when there is inefficacy of antimicrobial therapy for acute otitis media; a CBC as well as tympanocentesis/

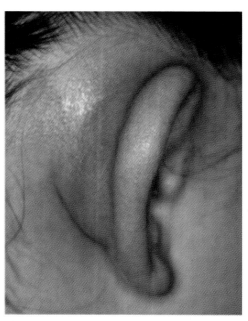

Figure 16.5 Mastoiditis, demonstrating postauricular swelling and erythema.

myringotomy may be performed for both therapeutic pain relief and bacterial cultures. CT scan of the temporal bone is the mainstay of imaging evaluation and can be used to identify signs of need for surgical intervention, including coalescence of air cells, enhancing areas of abscess formation, dehiscence of the tegmen or mastoid cortex, and elevation of the mastoid periosteum (Figures 16.5 and 16.6).

TREATMENT

Acute mastoiditis without evidence of osteitis or periosteitis may be treated medically with antibiotics. If there is evidence of periosteitis, IV antibiotics as well as high-dose steroids (with encapsulated bacteria, steroids may be contraindicated) and tympanostomy tube insertion are recommended. With evidence of osteitis, surgical treatment with mastoidectomy with tympanostomy tube placement is required.

Paraganglioma

DEFINITION AND CLINICAL FEATURES

Paragangliomas are the most common benign tumors of the middle ear. The two most common paragangliomas of the head and neck, glomus tympanicum and glomus jugulare, can be distinguished by their sites of origin. Glomus tympanicum tumors arise from paraganglia on the cochlear promontory in the middle ear, while glomus jugulare tumors arise from the paraganglia of the jugular bulb. Patients often present with hearing loss, pulsatile tinnitus, and aural fullness. Patients may also present with unilateral lower cranial nerve palsies and symptoms of sympathetic system activation (i.e., hypertension, palpitations, diaphoresis, flushing). On physical examination, the common finding is a reddish-blue pulsatile mass in the middle ear space. A bruit may

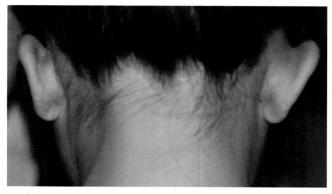

Figure 16.6 Mastoiditis, comparing infection on the right with a normal examination on the left.

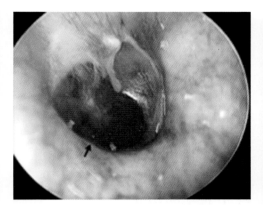

Figure 16.7 Paraganglioma as viewed using microostoscopy.

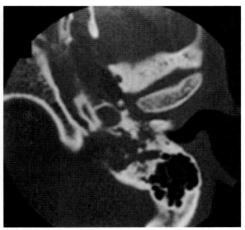

Figure 16.8 CT of right paraganglioma, demonstrating bony erosion of the temporal bone.

be appreciated on auscultation over the mastoid (Figure 16.7).

DIFFERENTIAL DIAGNOSIS

Otitis media, hemotympanum, cholesteatoma, meningioma, neurofibroma, carcinoma, aneurysm.

WORKUP

There is a role for several imaging modalities in the evaluation of the paraganglioma. A CT scan should be obtained to evaluate for patterns of bony erosion and to aid in surgical planning by identifying aberrant anatomy. MRI scan can help delineate tumor from native soft tissues, as well as identify dural involvement in the case of intracranial extension. Angiography is useful to identify vessels for preoperative embolization. Laboratory tests should be performed to assess the secretory status of the tumor, including serum and urine catecholamines, metanephrines, and vanillylmandelic acid. The likelihood of secretion is approximately 3%; however, if this is not known preoperatively, you may experience life-threatening anesthetic complications (Figures 16.8 and 16.9).

TREATMENT

Surgical excision is the definitive treatment in majority of cases. In the event of an incomplete resection or a poor surgical

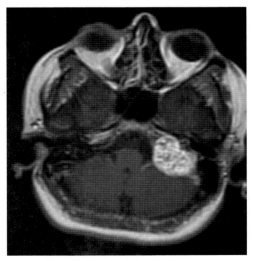

Figure 16.9 MRI of a right-sided paraganglioma.

candidate, angiography with embolization and/or radiotherapy may be used.

Cholesteatoma

DEFINITION AND CLINICAL FEATURES

Cholesteatoma is a benign overgrowth of keratinized squamous epithelium in the

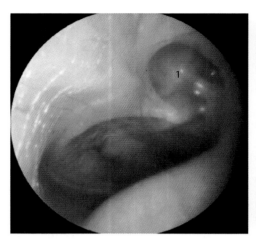

Figure 16.10 Demonstration of a superior retraction pocket, the depths of which can still be appreciated. 1—retraction of the tympanic membrane onto the long process of the incus.

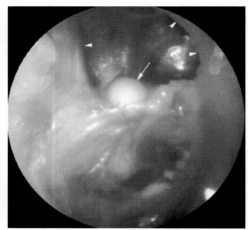

Figure 16.11 Demonstration of a superior retraction pocket, the depths of which can no longer be appreciated (short arrows), with development of cholesteatoma pearl (long arrow).

middle ear, leading to the replacement of middle ear mucosa and resorption of underlying bone. Cholesteatoma can be congenital or acquired in nature. Patients often present with persistent foul smelling otorrhea and hearing loss. Physical examination will often reveal granulation tissue in the external auditory canal, as well as an attic retraction pocket of the tympanic membrane. A white-yellow mass may be seen in the middle ear space (Figures 16.10 and 16.11).

DIFFERENTIAL DIAGNOSIS
Otitis media, otitis externa, tympanic membrane perforation, malignant neoplasm.

WORKUP
Initial workup of cholesteatoma includes physical examination, audiogram, and CT scan of the temporal bone. The senior author (MDS) rarely obtains CT scans for chronic ear issues, reserving the use for some revision procedures, or if the patient

has symptoms suggestive of inner ear or facial nerve involvement (i.e., lateral canal fistula, dizziness, or facial paresis). Typical imaging findings include blunting of the scutum, bony erosion of the lateral attic wall, superior external auditory canal, and ossicles. In the case of advanced cholesteatoma, nonenhancing mass with smooth borders can be appreciated eroding surrounding bone.

TREATMENT
Surgical management of cholesteatoma with mastoidectomy is the mainstay of treatment. In the event that a canal wall up mastoidectomy is performed, a "second-look procedure" may be performed in 9–12 months to evaluate for recurrence of the disease. Generally speaking, the past teaching is that cholesteatoma recurs in approximately 40% of patients; however, in the senior author's experience (MDS), it is approximately 5%. If there is recurrent disease, the canal wall

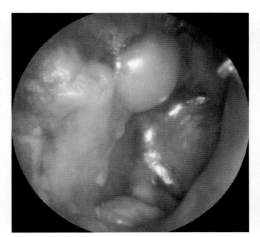

Figure 16.12 Cholesteatoma pearl.

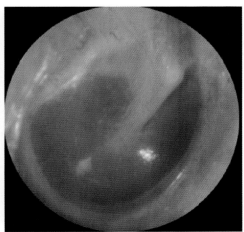

Figure 16.13 Schwartze's sign in a patient with otosclerosis.

may need to be taken down, and the patient is then managed with outpatient mastoid debridement and aural toilet (Figure 16.12).

Otosclerosis

DEFINITION AND CLINICAL FEATURES

Otosclerosis is an autosomal-dominant disorder with variable penetrance. It is characterized by abnormal alternating phases of bone resorption and formation in the bony otic capsule. This will most commonly result in fixation of the stapes footplate and conductive hearing loss. Rarely, otosclerosis can affect other areas of the otic capsule, resulting in sensorineural hearing loss. The most common presenting symptom is a conductive hearing loss. On physical examination, otoscopy can demonstrate a focus of reddish-blue discoloration on the cochlear promontory (Schwartze's sign) (Figure 16.13).

DIFFERENTIAL DIAGNOSIS

Fibro-osseous footplate fixation, congenital footplate fixation, ossicular discontinuity, fixed malleus–incus syndrome, crural atrophy, congenital cholesteatoma, Paget's disease, osteogenesis imperfecta.

WORKUP

Initial workup includes otologic exam including micropneumotoscopy to assess for malleus mobility, tuning fork testing, and audiogram, which will typically show a fictitious conductive loss at 2000 Hz (Carhart's notch). Stapes reflex testing is also appropriate. A high-resolution CT scan of the temporal bone is rarely helpful or necessary (Figures 16.14 through 16.16).

TREATMENT

Medical treatment includes daily doses of sodium fluoride, though it is rarely used; bisphophanates have been tried with limited success. Due to typically good speech discrimination, these patients may be suitable hearing aid candidates. Surgical intervention is the preferred treatment and consists of stapedectomy or stapedotomy using KTP laser, with replacement of the ossicle with a prosthesis.

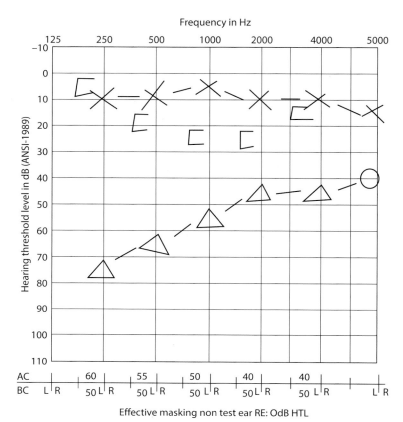

Figure 16.14 Carhart notch in a patient with otosclerosis.

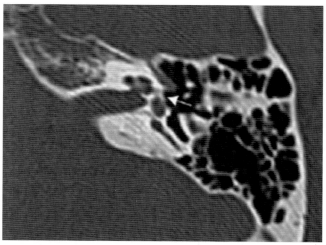

Figure 16.15 CT of otosclerosis demonstrating thickening of the fissula ante fenestram, right ear.

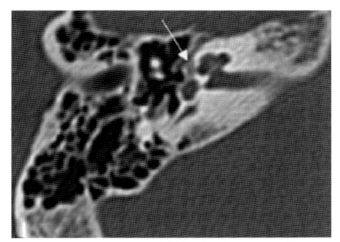

Figure 16.16 CT of otosclerosis demonstrating thickening of the fissula ante fenestram, left ear.

Cholesterol granuloma

DEFINITION AND CLINICAL FEATURES

Cholesterol granuloma of the temporal bone is an expansile lesion incited by an inflammatory response with subsequent hemorrhage in an area of impaired aeration. This results in formation of cholesterol crystals (as the heme resorbs), which in turn stimulate an inflammatory response. Within the temporal bone, cholesterol granuloma may arise from the tympano-mastoid compartment, or the petrous apex. The former is often found in patients with chronic otitis media and is rarely symptomatic. Cholesterol granulomas of the petrous apex can present with chronic deep ear pain, or retro-orbital pain. Patients may also present with hearing loss, dizziness and neuropathies of the trigeminal, abducens, and facial nerves.

DIFFERENTIAL DIAGNOSIS

Cholesteatoma, epidermoid cyst, encephalocele, mucocele, petrous apicitis, meningioma, schwannoma, chondrosarcoma, chordoma, plasmacytoma, metastatic disease, internal carotid artery aneurysm, Langerhans cell histiocytosis, asymmetric fat in the petrous apex.

WORKUP

Diagnosis relies primarily on imaging. A CT with fine cuts of the temporal bone characteristically shows a lesion with smooth borders, little if any rim enhancement, and bony changes secondary to lesion expansion. Relationships between the lesion and surrounding structures can be appreciated on CT images in preparation for surgical treatment. On MRI, the lesion is hyperintense on both T1- and T2-weighted images and does not display enhancement with the addition of contrast. Diffusion-weighted imaging may also offer assistance in the preoperative diagnosis. Prior to treatment, an audiogram should be obtained as well (Figures 16.17 and 16.18).

TREATMENT

Asymptomatic lesions can be managed expectantly with serial MRI examinations. For symptomatic lesions, surgical drainage is the primary treatment modality.

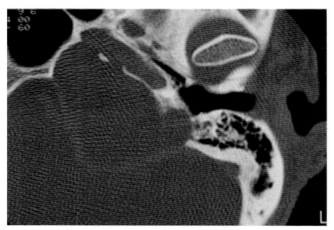

Figure 16.17 Preoperative CT temporal bone of a cholesterol granuloma.

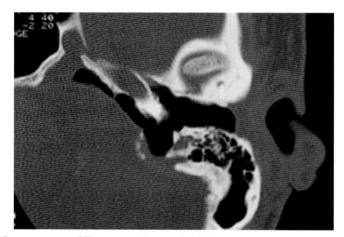

Figure 16.18 Postoperative CT temporal bone of a cholesterol granuloma.

The approach to the lesion is determined by the patient's degree of hearing loss in the affected ear, as well as the complexity of the anatomical relationships between the lesions and other temporal bone structures. In the author's experience, the petrous apex can most often be exposed by using either a retrocochlear or retrofacial approach with the aid of neuronavigation (Figures 16.19).

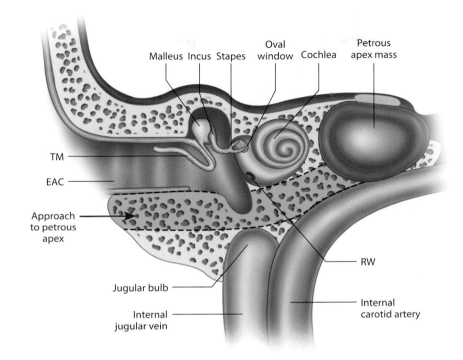

Figure 16.19 Anatomy of the retrocochlear approach to the petrous apex.

Inner Ear Disorders

Anthony Chin-Quee, Foluwasayo E. Ologe, and Michael D. Seidman

- **Schwannoma**
- **Meningioma**
- **Benign paroxysmal positional vertigo**
- **Meniere's disease**
- **Bell's palsy**
- **Ramsay Hunt syndrome**
- **Temporal bone fractures**
- **Superior semicircular canal dehiscence**

Schwannoma

DEFINITION AND CLINICAL FEATURES

A schwannoma is a benign proliferation of Schwann cells within the nerve sheath of a peripheral nerve. In the head and neck, these occur most frequently in the cerebellopontine angle (CPA) and may involve the vestibulocochlear, facial, and trigeminal nerves. Patients often present with unilateral hearing loss, tinnitus, vertigo, disequilibrium, facial numbness, and facial weakness. Less commonly, patients may present with decreased visual acuity, dysphagia, hoarseness, and headache.

DIFFERENTIAL DIAGNOSIS

Meningioma, epidermoid cyst, arachnoid cyst, glioma, hemangioblastoma, papilloma, glomus tumor, primary bone tumor, metastatic lesion.

WORKUP

Workup should begin with an audiogram, which may demonstrate sloping high-frequency hearing loss and "rollover"—decreased speech discrimination as speech decibel level increases. Auditory brainstem reflex (ABR) testing should be performed and will often show a decreased, or absent, response. High-resolution CT scan of the

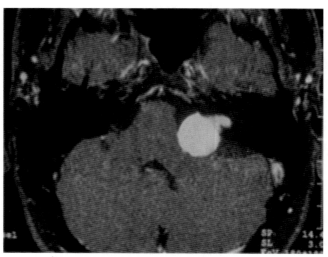

Figure 17.1 MRI of a left vestibular schwannoma, T2-weighted image, demonstrating progression of the lesion, with surrounding edema of the brain parenchyma.

temporal bone may be obtained for evaluation of bony erosion and surgical planning; however, the gold standard for diagnosis of schwannoma is MRI with contrast. The schwannoma characteristically appears iso-/hypointense on T1-weighted images and heterogeneously hyperintense on T2-weighted images. The lesion enhances with contrast (Figures 17.1 through 17.3).

TREATMENT

Schwannomas of the CPA can be treated with surgery, radiation, or observation. Lesions are often observed when very small in size and in elderly patients and followed with yearly MRI scans. If the patient is deemed a poor surgical candidate, treatment with stereotactic radiation therapy (i.e., Gamma Knife, Cyber Knife) is an option. There are three main surgical approaches considered when evaluating a vestibular schwannoma for removal. The *translabyrinthine* approach is typically the first considered. Although it poses the least theoretical risk to the facial nerve, the main downside is that hearing will be obliterated with this approach. The *retrolabyrinthine* (or *suboccipital*) approach

is typically used for tumors that are closer to the brainstem, with the bulk of the tumor in the cerebellopontine angle (as opposed to within the internal auditor canal). Hearing can be saved in this approach, depending on the size of the mass. The *middle cranial fossa* approach is typically used for tumors of the IAC that are less than 10–14 mm in size. Again, hearing can be saved in this approach; however, there is a higher incidence of meningitis, encephalopathy, and seizures given the degree of exposure and retraction on the brain required. Postoperative function of the facial nerve ranges from 50% to 90% depending on the size of the tumor (Figures 17.4 and 17.5).

Meningioma

DEFINITION AND CLINICAL FEATURES

Meningioma is a neoplasm arising from the endothelial cells of the arachnoid villi. Patients with meningioma of the cerebellopontine angle present in a similar manner to those with schwannoma—unilateral hearing loss, tinnitus, vertigo, disequilibrium, facial numbness, and facial weakness.

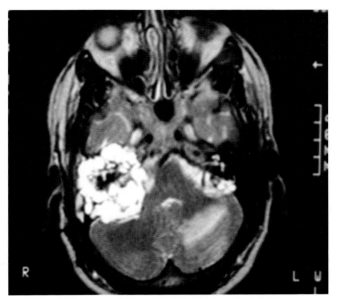

Figure 17.2 MRI of an advanced right vestibular schwannoma, T2-weighted image, demonstrating heterogeneity.

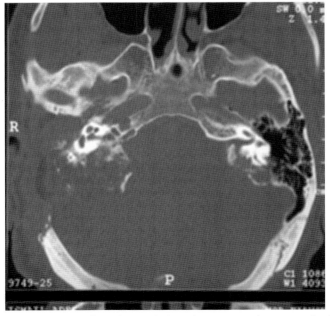

Figure 17.3 CT temporal bone of a right vestibular schwannoma, demonstrating bony erosion.

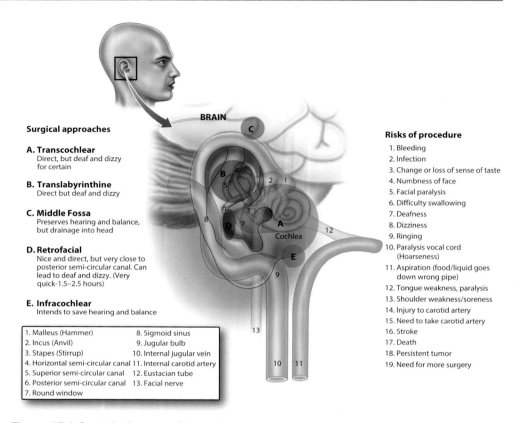

Surgical approaches

A. Transcochlear
Direct, but deaf and dizzy
for certain

B. Translabyrinthine
Direct but deaf and dizzy

C. Middle Fossa
Preserves hearing and balance,
but drainage into head

D. Retrofacial
Nice and direct, but very close to
posterior semi-circular canal. Can
lead to deaf and dizzy. (Very
quick-1.5–2.5 hours)

E. Infracochlear
Intends to save hearing and balance

1. Malleus (Hammer)	8. Sigmoid sinus
2. Incus (Anvil)	9. Jugular bulb
3. Stapes (Stirrup)	10. Internal jugular vein
4. Horizontal semi-circular canal	11. Internal carotid artery
5. Superior semi-circular canal	12. Eustacian tube
6. Posterior semi-circular canal	13. Facial nerve
7. Round window	

Risks of procedure

1. Bleeding
2. Infection
3. Change or loss of sense of taste
4. Numbness of face
5. Facial paralysis
6. Difficulty swallowing
7. Deafness
8. Dizziness
9. Ringing
10. Paralysis vocal cord
    (Hoarseness)
11. Aspiration (food/liquid goes
    down wrong pipe)
12. Tongue weakness, paralysis
13. Shoulder weakness/soreness
14. Injury to carotid artery
15. Need to take carotid artery
16. Stroke
17. Death
18. Persistent tumor
19. Need for more surgery

Figure 17.4 Sagittal schematic of the right temporal bone, outlining multiple approaches to the CPA, and associated risks.

DIFFERENTIAL DIAGNOSIS

Schwannoma, pituitary macroadenoma, craniopharyngioma, hemangiopericytoma, sarcoidosis, tuberculosis, idiopathic hypertrophic pachymeningitis, Paget's disease, fibrous dysplasia.

WORKUP

Workup should begin with an audiogram, which may demonstrate sloping high-frequency hearing loss and "rollover." A decreased, or absent, response on ABR testing is common. High-resolution scan of the temporal bone will typically show a homogenous, contrast-enhancing mass

with a well-defined border and associated edema. The meningioma typically appears isointense on T1-weighted images, hyperintense on T2-weighted images, and enhances brightly with gadolinium. A "dural tail" is typical (Figures 17.6 and 17.7).

TREATMENT

Definitive treatment of meningiomas includes surgical resection of the tumor, dural attachment, and involved bone. Though meningiomas can be variable in their locations, the otolaryngologist will often be consulted prior to the removal of tumors of the petro-clival region. These tumors can

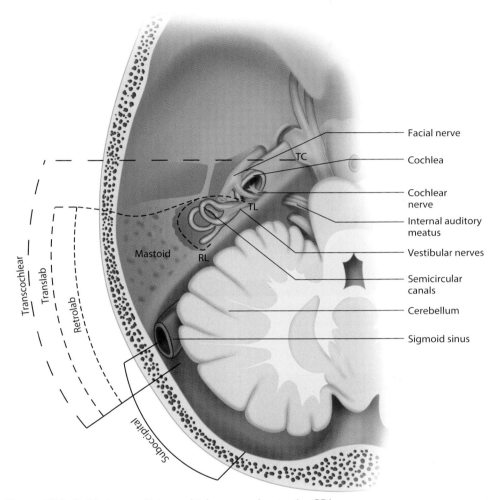

Figure 17.5 Axial view, outlining multiple approaches to the CPA.

typically be removed using a combination of presigmoid and postsigmoid transtemporal and transpetrosal approaches to the skull base. These approaches require craniotomies, complete mastoidectomy, and middle cranial fossa approach. In the case of inoperable tumors, incomplete resection or malignant meningioma radiation therapy is indicated. Regular follow-up with MRI is indicated, as meningiomas have a high recurrence rate (Figures 17.8 and 17.9).

Benign paroxysmal positional vertigo

DEFINITION AND CLINICAL FEATURES

Benign paroxysmal positional vertigo (BPPV) is a very common balance disorder, which is characterized by short-lived spells of vertigo lasting 15–60 seconds provoked by rapid changes in head positioning. Although there may be a history of head trauma or recent infection, the cause is usually unknown.

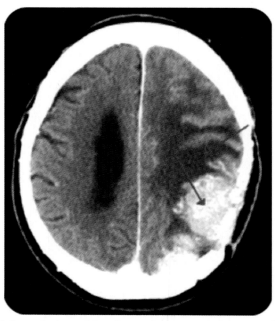

Figure 17.6 CT of a left meningioma (closed arrow), demonstrating mass effect, and surrounding edema of the brain parenchyma (open arrow).

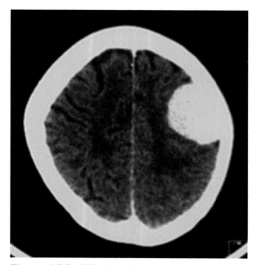

Figure 17.7 CT of a left meningioma.

DIFFERENTIAL DIAGNOSIS

Meniere's disease, vestibular neuronitis, labyrinthitis, superior semicircular canal dehiscence.

WORKUP

The Dix–Hallpike maneuver is pathognomonic for this condition. A positive test will reveal a delayed and then fatigable rotatory, and geotropic nystagmus when the head is turned to the affected side.

TREATMENT

The mainstay of treatment for BPPV is the particle repositioning (Epley) maneuver. Following this maneuver, patients are encouraged to sleep upright for 48 hours and avoid positions that evoke dizzy spells. For persistent symptoms, Cawthorne exercises

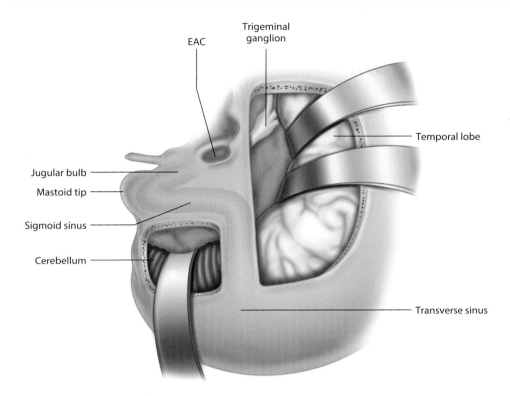

Figure 17.8 Demonstration of the combination approach to a petroclival mass.

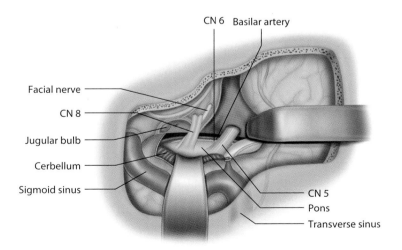

Figure 17.9 Anatomy of the petroclival approach.

(designed to stress the balance system by evoking dizziness) may be performed by the patient at home. If conservative treatments fail, surgical options include singular neurectomy and semicircular canal occlusion.

Meniere's disease

DEFINITION AND CLINICAL FEATURES

Meniere's disease, also known as endolymphatic hydrops, is thought to arise secondary to expansion of the endolymphatic compartment due to increased pressure. There appears to be a strong association with allergic disorders. Patients present with the constellation of episodic vertigo lasting up to several hours, fluctuating hearing loss, sensation of fullness in the affected ear, and tinnitus.

DIFFERENTIAL DIAGNOSIS

BPPV, perilymphatic fistula, vertebral/basilar artery insufficiency, migraine, vestibulopathy, vestibular neuronitis, labyrinthitis, vestibular schwannoma, central nervous system lesion.

WORKUP

During a Meniere's attack, audiogram can typically show a low-frequency hearing loss. This loss can change on subsequent testing when the disease is not active. Electrocochleography during an attack can show a summating potential of greater than 50%, which is indicative of increased inner ear pressure; some suggest anything greater than 40% is significant. Vestibular testing, including electronystagmography, and VEMP testing play a role in ruling out other causes of vertigo. CT and MRI scan can be used to rule out other causes of symptoms, should clinical suspicion for a lesion be high (Figures 17.10 and 17.11).

TREATMENT

Treatment is primarily medical, with use of diuretics and dietary modification, which

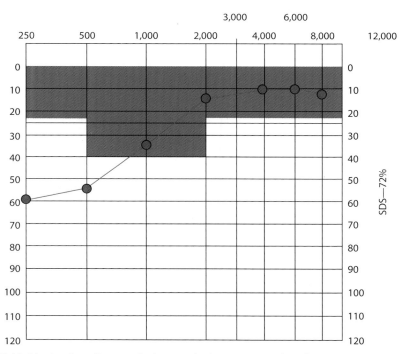

Figure 17.10 Meniere's audiogram during attack, demonstrating low-frequency sensorineural hearing loss.

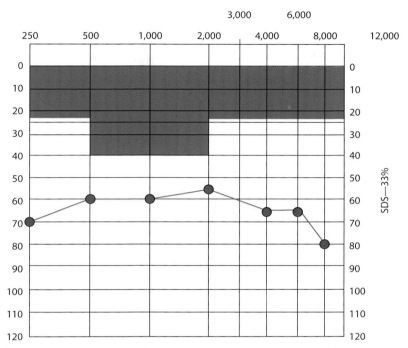

Figure 17.11 Meniere's late stage audiogram, demonstrating sensorineural hearing loss across several frequencies.

includes low sodium diet, caffeine, alcohol, and tobacco avoidance. Some patients are sensitive to dietary modification, and some have no such relationship. Management of allergies, seen in up to 50% of patients with Meniere's disease, may be very helpful. In the event of failure of medical management (oral steroids for 1–2 weeks, transtympanic gentamicin, beta-histidine [not approved by the U.S. FDA; frequently used in Canada and the United Kingdom with 80%–85% improvement]), surgical options include endolymphatic sac decompression, vestibular nerve section, and labyrinthectomy (Figure 17.12).

Bell's palsy

DEFINITION AND CLINICAL FEATURES
Bell's palsy is defined as an acute-onset idiopathic facial nerve weakness/paralysis. It is a diagnosis of exclusion after other potential causes of facial nerve damage have been ruled out. Aside from the characteristic acute onset (24–48 hours) of unilateral upper and lower facial weakness, patients may also present with blurred vision secondary to decreased tearing and eyelid closure, ear pain, hyperacusis, taste disturbance, and dry mouth.

DIFFERENTIAL DIAGNOSIS
The differential diagnosis of facial paralysis is extensive, and includes infection—otitis externa/media, mastoiditis, Ramsey Hunt syndrome, Lyme disease; neoplasm of temporal bone or cerebellopontine angle, diabetes mellitus, hyperthyroidism, trauma, congenital birth defect, intoxication, and vascular malformation.

WORKUP
Workup is limited but could include lab work (rarely needed), imaging (MRI indicated if

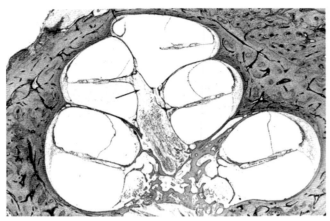

Figure 17.12 Human temporal bone section, endolymphatic hydrops, and organ of Corti (arrow).

no recovery in 3 months, but is often done earlier to reassure both the patient and the physician), and audiologic testing to aid in ruling out all other causes of facial paralysis. In the case of complete paralysis, ENoG testing may be done within the first 14–21 days of paralysis onset to assess the degree of neural degeneration.

TREATMENT
Medical treatment is the first line, consisting of systemic corticosteroids and possibly antivirals, as there is much evidence supporting the idea that herpes simplex virus type 1 is a causative agent in Bell's palsy. Protective eye care should also be instituted. In the case of complete paralysis and evidence of 90% nerve degeneration or greater on ENoG testing, surgical decompression of the nerve may be considered (Figures 17.13 and 17.14).

Ramsay Hunt syndrome

DEFINITION AND CLINICAL FEATURES
Ramsay Hunt syndrome, or herpes zoster oticus, is caused by a reactivation of latent varicella zoster infection, and is defined as a herpetic vesicular rash of the concha, external auditory canal, or pinna with an

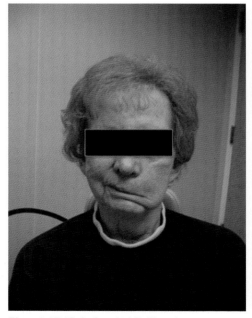

Figure 17.13 Left-sided Bell's palsy, at rest.

ipsilateral facial nerve palsy. Patients typically present with severe, paroxysmal deep ear pain, and herpetic lesions of the ear and mouth. Vertigo, tinnitus, hearing loss, fever, headache, and cervical adenopathy may also be present.

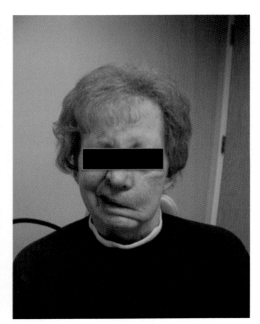

Figure 17.14 Left-sided Bell's palsy, during attempted smile.

DIFFERENTIAL DIAGNOSIS
Bell's palsy, trigeminal neuralgia, postherpetic neuralgia, temporomandibular joint disorder.

WORKUP
In addition to the pathognomonic physical examination findings, an infectious laboratory workup could be performed, including CBC, ESR, electrolytes, and viral studies. An audiogram should be obtained if there is any complaint of hearing loss. Imaging is usually not necessary to make the diagnosis; however, an MRI with contrast can help to evaluate inflammation of the facial nerve.

TREATMENT
Treatment of Ramsay Hunt syndrome is typically medically and includes systemic steroids, antivirals, vestibular suppressants, and pain control. Surgery has no role in management (Figures 17.15 and 17.16).

Temporal bone fractures

DEFINITION AND CLINICAL FEATURES
Temporal bone fracture is defined as the clinical condition in which there is a complete or incomplete break in the temporal bone, induced by impact with a blunt surface, penetrating missiles, or sharp objects. These patients may present with hearing loss, vertigo, otorrhagia, and CSF leak. Physical examination may reveal lacerations of the EAC, Battle's sign, Raccoon sign, hemotympanum, tympanic membrane perforation, and otorrhea on otoscopic exam.

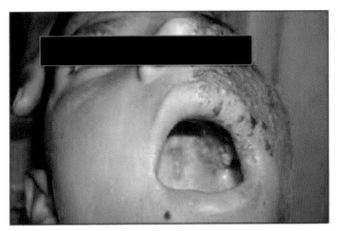

Figure 17.15 Ramsay Hunt, demonstrating vesicles of the face and oral cavity.

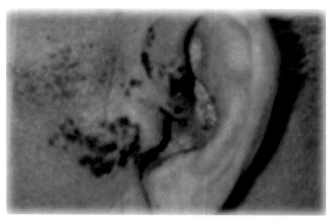

Figure 17.16 Ramsay Hunt, demonstrating vesicles of the external ear and preauricular skin.

DIFFERENTIAL DIAGNOSIS

The differential diagnosis of temporal bone trauma includes ossicular chain discontinuity, tympanic membrane perforation, cerebrospinal fluid leak, perilymphatic fistula, and vascular injury/anomaly.

WORKUP

In addition to the physical examination, the primary imaging modality is high-resolution CT scan with thin cuts through the temporal bone. Fractures are classified as longitudinal, transverse, or oblique. Longitudinal fractures are far more common; however, transverse fractures are more likely to violate the otic capsule.

TREATMENT

The majority of temporal bone fractures are observed. Surgical intervention is indicated in the setting of immediate onset facial nerve injury. Oftentimes, given the severity of the trauma, this may not be initially assessable. Surgery may also be appropriate for conductive hearing loss secondary to ossicular chain dislocation or tympanic membrane perforation, and persistent CSF leak (Figures 17.17 through 17.19).

Superior semicircular canal dehiscence

DEFINITION AND CLINICAL FEATURES

Superior semicircular canal dehiscence is defined as a thinning and dehiscence of the bony superior aspect of the superior canal. Patients typically complain of vertigo brought on by loud sounds (Tullio's phenomenon) or aural pressure (Hennebert's sign). Pneumatic otoscopy may also reveal nystagmus in the plane of the superior semicircular canal.

DIFFERENTIAL DIAGNOSIS

BPPV, labyrinthitis, Meniere's disease, ototoxicity, perilymphatic fistula, otosclerosis, migraine.

WORKUP

A thin-cut CT of the temporal bone is one of the first steps in confirming a diagnosis. Additionally, audiogram and vestibular-evoked myogenic potentials may be used to confirm the diagnosis (Figures 17.20 through 17.22).

TREATMENT

SSCD can be treated conservatively with observation and avoidance of stimuli. Surgical interventions include placement of myringotomy tubes, canal resurfacing, and canal occlusion.

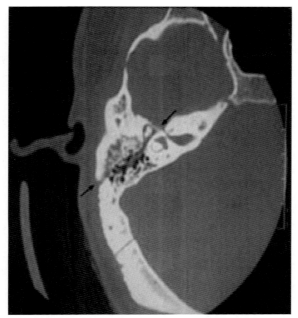

Figure 17.17 Longitudinal temporal bone fracture (arrows).

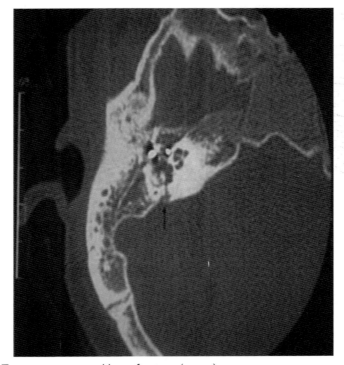

Figure 17.18 Transverse temporal bone fracture (arrow).

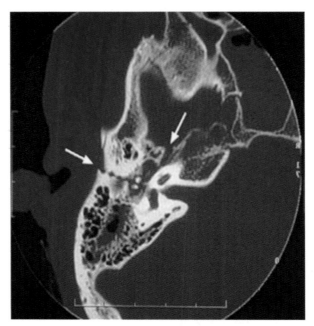

Figure 17.19 Complex temporal bone fracture with an oblique component (left arrow), and a longitudinal component (right arrow).

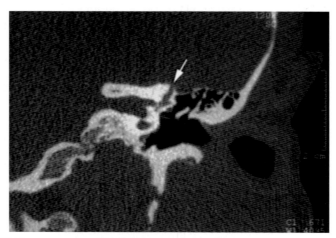

Figure 17.20 CT demonstrating SCC dehiscence, coronal view.

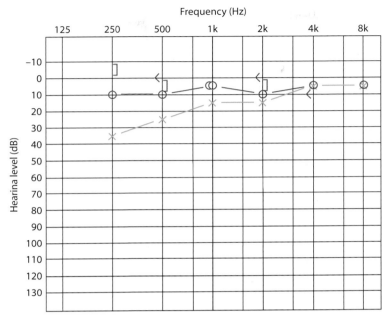

Figure 17.21 Audiogram with low-frequency conductive hearing loss typical of SCC dehiscence.

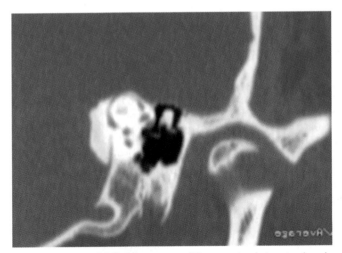

Figure 17.22 CT demonstrating SCC dehiscence, oblique sagittal view in the plane of the superior canal.

SECTION 5

FACIAL PLASTICS

CHAPTER 18

Normal Facial Analysis

Celeste Gary and Laura T. Hetzler

- **Photographs**
- **Facial aesthetic units**
- **Forehead and brow**
- **Periorbital region**
- **Perioral region and chin**
- **Suggested reading**

Assessment of the face for facial plastic surgery requires an understanding of the aesthetic ideal in relation to age, sex, body type, and cultural and contemporary trends. Once one understands what makes a face attractive, then an analysis can be performed to determine the problem areas and determine the priorities of surgery. Key concepts include balance, proportion, symmetry, and harmony.

Photographs

Photographs should be obtained prior to facial aesthetic surgery. Photos should be taken with the patient in the Frankfort horizontal position, and the supratragic notch should be on a level with the infraorbital rim. At a minimum, a frontal view, left and right lateral views, and left and right oblique views should be obtained. Other additional views include lateral with smile, frontal with smile, basal, and close-ups of planned operative sites.

FACIAL ANATOMIC LANDMARKS

Trichion: Midline at hairline

Glabella: Prominence in midsaggital plane, superior to the root of the nose

Nasion: Nasofrontal suture

Sellion: Deepest soft tissue point within the nasofrontal angle

Radix: Root of the nose, which contains the sellion and nasion

Rhinion: Cartilaginous–bony junction

Supratip break: Just cephalic to the tip-defining point

Tip-defining point: Two points representing the highest point on the crural arch

Infratip lobule: Portion of the lobule inferior to the tip-defining point, superior to the nostril

Infratip break: Junction of the columella and the lobule

Alar crease: Most posterior portion of the nose

Stomion: Embouchure of the lips

Pogonion: Anterior most border of the chin

Menton: Inferior most portion of the chin

Cervical point: Menton and neck intersection

Tragion: Supratragic notch of the ear

SKIN

The skin has a key role in facial appearance. The texture, thickness, elasticity, and degree of sun damage should be assessed by inspection and palpation. Skin lesions, scars, rhytids, and pigmentation should also be noted.

Pigmentation is assessed with the Fitzpatrick's sun-reactive skin types:

Skin type	Skin color	Tanning response
I	White	Always burns, never tans
II	White	Usually burns, tans with difficulty
III	White	Sometimes mild burn, tan average
IV	Brown	Rarely burns, tans with ease
V	Dark Brown	Very rarely burns, tans very easily
VI	Black	Never burns, tans very easily

Aging skin results in a thinned epidermis, decreased subcutaneous fat, loss of dermis elasticity, decreased melanocytes, decreased mounts of type I collagen, and reduced vascular supply.

HAIR

The position of the hairline, temporal recession, and density of hair follicles should be taken into account when considering surgical incisions.

Facial aesthetic units

FACIAL THIRDS

Facial height is divided into three equally spaced segments, demarcated by the trichion, glabella, subnasale, and menton (Figure 18.1).

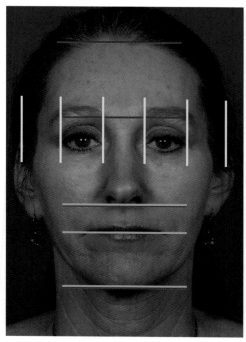

Figure 18.1 Facial height divided into thirds (red), lower face further subdivided into thirds (blue), and vertical face divided into fifths (yellow).

LOWER FACIAL THIRDS

Lower third is further divided into 1/3, subnasale to stomion, and 2/3, stomion to menton (Figure 18.1).

VERTICAL FIFTHS

Facial width is divided into five equally spaced segments demarcated by the lateral auricle, lateral canthus, medial canthus, medial canthus, lateral canthus, and lateral auricle (Figure 18.1).

Forehead and brow

Considered the upper third of the face.
   Classically described brow position in the female

1. Brow begins medially at a vertical line drawn perpendicular through the alar base.
2. Brow terminates laterally at an oblique line drawn through the lateral canthus of the eye and the alar base.
3. The medial and lateral ends of the eyebrow lie at approximately the same horizontal level.
4. The medial end of the eyebrow is club shaped and this gradually tapers down laterally.
5. The apex of the brow lies on a vertical line drawn directly through the lateral limbus of the eye.

MALE BROW

1. The apex of the brow lies on a vertical line through the lateral limbus of the eye.
2. The entire complex is minimally arching.
3. The brow is positioned at or just above the supraorbital rim.

Two main age-related changes to the upper third of the face are brow ptosis and hyperdynamic facial lines.

1. Brow ptosis can cause lateral hooding over the upper eyelids, which is a problem of the upper third of the face and not an eyelid issue. Assess whether the patient has limited superiolateral visual fields as this is a functional indication for surgical intervention of the upper third of the face.
2. Hyperdynamic facial lines are caused by repeated pull on the skin by the underlying facial muscles.

Periorbital region

This includes the upper and lower eyelids, the medial and lateral canthal regions, and the globe.
   Intercanthal distance should be approximately equal to the width of one eye. In Caucasian patients, the intercanthal distance should be equal to the interalar width of the nasal base.
   The snap test assesses lower lid laxity. The lower lid is grasped between the thumb and forefinger and pulled away from the globe. An abnormal result is delayed return to the globe surface or return only after blinking. Scleral show should be addressed.
   The eyelids often show the earliest signs of aging. Problems include skin laxity, pseudoherniation of the orbital fat through the septum, prominent fat pads, and orbicularis muscle hypertrophy. Other periorbital problems such as lid ptosis, enophthalmos, proptosis, exophthalmos, lower lid laxity or malposition, and lateral hooding should be assessed.
   Hyperdynamic lines in this region are known as "crow's feet."

CHEEK

The aesthetic unit that extends from the preauricular crease laterally, to the nasolabial fold medially, from the zygomatic arch and inferior orbital rim superiorly, to the inferior border of the mandible. The most noticeable landmark is the malar eminence, which consists of the zygomatic arch and the maxillary bones. A prominent malar eminence is considered both youthful and beautiful.

The buccal fat pad should be assessed. Aging in his area causes a weakening in the supportive matrix between the SMAS (superficial muscular aponeurotic layer) and the underlying buccal fat pad. This results in deepened nasolabial creases and jowling. Hollow cheeks can occur with lack of buccal fat bulk.

Hypertonic facial muscles can result in festooning and facial rhytids.

NOSE

This is considered the most noticeable of the facial aesthetic units. It is typically described in terms of its length, width, projection, and rotation.

Aesthetic subunits of the nose, nine total (Figures 18.2 and 18.3)

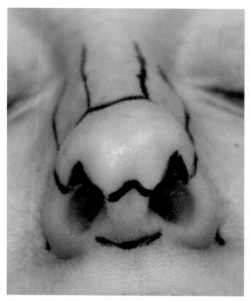

Figure 18.3 Nasal aesthetic subunits, base view: columella, paired soft tissue triangles.

1. Paired/bilateral subunits include alar, soft tissue triangle, and nasal sidewall.
2. Central subunits include nasal dorsum, nasal tip, and columella.

Nasal thirds

1. Upper third: nasal bones and skin
2. Middle third: upper lateral cartilages, septum, and skin
3. Lower third: lower lateral cartilages and septum

General aesthetics

1. Dorsum follows a smooth curve downward from the medial aspect of the brows to the supratip region.
2. The tip should show a double break and supratip break, which separates the dorsum from the

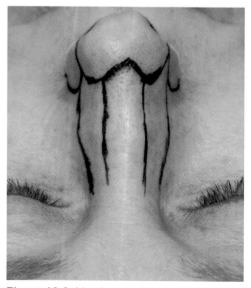

Figure 18.2 Nasal aesthetic subunits: dorsum, tip, bilateral sidewall, and bilateral alar subunits.

lobule and is located 1–3 mm above the tip-defining point and an infratip break between the infratip lobule and columella.

3. Columellar show of 2–4 mm is ideal.
4. Frontonasoorbital line should be smooth from the eyebrows along the lateral edge of the nasal dorsum and then slightly diverge at the tip.
5. Nasofrontal angle (Figure 18.4):
   a. Angle between the external nose and forehead
   b. Approximately 120°
6. Nasolabial angle (Figure 18.4):
   a. Determines tip rotation
   b. Male: 90°–105°
   c. Female: 95°–110°

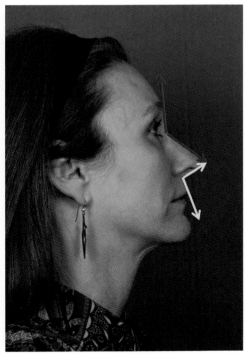

Figure 18.4 Nasofrontal angle (red) and nasolabial angle (yellow).

7. Tip projection:
   a. Distance between the facial plane and the tip of the nose
8. Lobular height:
   a. Should be 1/3 of the total height on the basal view

Perioral region and chin

This includes the region from the subnasal and nasolabial folds to the menton. The contour of the chin is determined by the shape and position of the mandible as well as the soft tissue overlying it. The chin should align with a vertical line from the vermillion border of the lower lip to the chin. If the line is anterior to the pogonion, then the patient is microgenic or possibly micrognathic.

Full lips are favored. The upper lip should be fuller and project slightly anterior to the lower lip in profile.

With aging, there is lengthening of the upper lip, thinning of the red lip portions, and midface retrusion.

Perioral rhytids should be assessed. Marionette lines can appear.

NECK

Addressing cervicomental definition is an important part of facial aesthetics. A youthful neck has a well-defined mandibular line that casts a submandibular shadow. A cervicomental angle of 90° or less is considered youthful. The location of the hyoid bone should be noted. If it is at the level of the fourth cervical vertebra, it is considered ideal. If it is lower, an obtuse angle results.

Cervical fat volume and redundancy of neck skin should be noted as well.

Aging results in jowling, chin ptosis, ptotic submandibular glands, and platysmal banding.

EARS

The top of the auricular helix should be at the level of the lateral eyebrow. The inferior attachment of the earlobe should be at the level of the alar-facial junction. The width to length ratio of the ear is about 0.6:1. The ear should protrude from the posterior scalp <30° and mid-ear should be no more than 2 cm from the head.

Suggested reading

Bailey BJ, Johnson JT, Newlands SD. 2006. *Head and Neck Surgery-Otolaryngology*, 4th ed. Philadelphia, PA: Lippincott Williams & Wilkins, pp. 2481–2498.

Papel I. 2009. *Facial Plastic and Reconstructive Surgery*, 3rd ed. New York: Thieme Medical Publishers, Inc., pp. 177–186, 477–486.

Nose

Krishna Patel and Laura T. Hetzler

- ## Rhinoplasty: Nasal bone deformity/nasal tip deformity
- ## Postrhinoplasty complications: Inverted-V deformity, pollybeak
- ## Nasal valve collapse
- ## Rhinophyma
- ## Nasal Mohs defects and reconstruction
- ## Suggested reading

Rhinoplasty: Nasal bone deformity/nasal tip deformity

Krishna Patel

NASAL BONE DEFORMITY
Definitions and clinical features
While planning rhinoplasty procedures, critical pre-assessment of the nasal dimensions in all standardized views is critical. By profile, the ideal nasal projection can be defined by a ratio measuring the height of the nasal tip to the length of the nasal dorsum, which should equal 0.67. Additionally, on the lateral view or profile, the nasal dorsum should lie along or slightly lower than a line drawn from the nasion to the nasal tip. If nasal bones protrude significantly over this line, there exists nasal bone deformity in the form of a dorsal hump (Figure 19.1).

On frontal view, the nasal dorsum should be straight with the width of the bony sidewall base equaling 75% of the width of the alar base. If the nasal dorsum is not straight, there exists a nasal bone deformity in the form of a *crooked nose* (Figure 19.2).

Both dorsal humps and crooked noses may involve distortion of the nasal bones, upper lateral cartilages, and septum. Determining the underlying cause is imperative for surgical correction.

Differential diagnosis
Etiology of nasal bone deformities may be genetically predisposed or induced by trauma or surgery. If congenital, often the

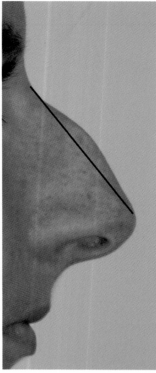

Figure 19.1 Lateral view of a dorsal hump nasal bone deformity. Nasal shape should ideally follow a straight plane from the nasion to the nasal tip depicted by the black line.

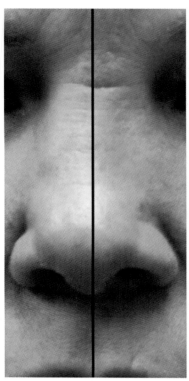

Figure 19.2 Frontal view of a crooked nose nasal bone deformity induced by trauma. The nasal bones are severely deflected to the right of midline, which is depicted by the black line.

deformity becomes more pronounced during puberty when the nasal bones are growing and achieving mature form.

The splaying of the nasal bone or midline creasing may be a sign of larger craniofacial anomalies such as frontonasal dysplasia, midline clefting, or the mass effect of a dermoid or nasal/septal mass.

Workup

Physical examination with thorough inspection, palpation, and anterior rhinoscopy is sufficient. Nasal endoscopy may aid in diagnosing if septal deviations are contributing to the nasal bone deformity. In the setting of trauma, computed tomography (CT) scans may be helpful, although not indicated for isolated nasal bone deformities. Photography of frontal, oblique, lateral, and base views enables objective measurements of the nasal dimensions.

If a more unusual nasal bone shape is present, CT scans aid in detecting larger craniofacial anomalies such as frontonasal dysplasia, midline clefting, or the mass effect of a dermoid or nasal/septal mass.

Treatment

Surgical correction of the nasal dorsal hump often requires rasping the nasal bony dorsum and performing medial and lateral osteotomies. The crooked nasal bone deformity also involves osteotomies but should be tailored to address the asymmetry with any combination of medial, lateral, and/or intermediate osteotomies.

NASAL TIP DEFORMITY
Definitions and clinical features
Like nasal bone deformities, critical analysis of the nasal tip dimensions is necessary. 50%–60% of the nasal tip should lie above a horizontal line drawn from the upper lip. As stated previously, the nasal height/length ratio should equal 0.67. The tip should appear symmetric with two light-reflecting points at the domes. On lateral view, the columella should have 2–4 mm of show, and ideally, the contour reveals an infratip and supratip break. The nasolabial angle ranges from 90° to 115°, with preferentially higher angles for females. Disruption of these dimensions may manifest as a nasal tip deformity.

When asymmetry exists at the tip, this most often generates a nasal tip deformity. The asymmetry may be genetically predisposed or may be caused by trauma or previous nasal surgery. Regardless, the most common underlying etiology is due to the irregular shape and contour of the lower lateral cartilages.

If the nasal skin is very taut and thin revealing the lower lateral cartilages as knoblike, this is defined as *bossae* (Figure 19.3). Bossae are typically a sequela of previous rhinoplasty, where the lower lateral cartilages become weakened from resection and buckle unpredictably.

Differential diagnosis
The most common underlying etiology of nasal tip deformities is due to irregularly shaped lower lateral cartilages. However, skin diseases that manifest with growth protuberances may also present as asymmetrical tip deformities.

Workup
Physical examination with thorough inspection, palpation, and anterior rhinoscopy is sufficient. Photography of frontal, oblique,

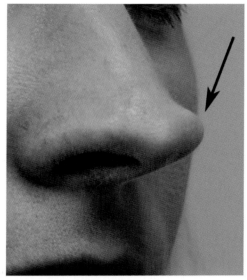

Figure 19.3 Oblique view of bossae nasal tip deformity. Tip appearance is knoblike and overprojected.

lateral, and base views enables objective measurements of the nasal dimensions.

Treatment
Correction can be achieved by surgically exposing the lower lateral cartilages and correcting the source of the deformity. If the deformity is due to asymmetry, then goals should be directed toward achieving symmetrically shaped cartilages, which may be performed through suture and camouflage grafting techniques. If the deformity is due to weakened or buckling cartilages (Figure 19.4), then structural grafting is necessary.

Postrhinoplasty complications: Inverted-V deformity, pollybeak

Krishna Patel

DEFINITIONS AND CLINICAL FEATURES
A risk of rhinoplasty is an undesirable result that causes physical and/or functional compromise. Two classic complications of

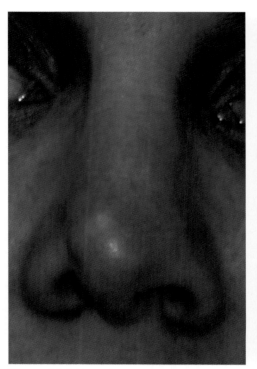

Figure 19.4 Frontal view of a nasal tip deformity that is pinched and asymmetric.

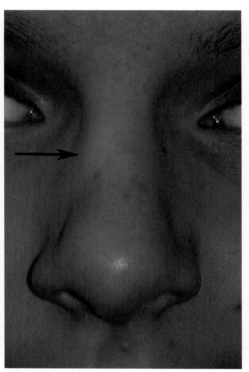

Figure 19.5 Frontal view of a subtle inverted-V deformity caused by a dorsal hump reduction. The arrow denotes the bony-cartilaginous junction revealing an inverted-V shadowing and a disruption to the brow-tip aesthetic line.

rhinoplasty surgery are the inverted-V and pollybeak deformities.

The inverted-V deformity is identified on frontal view as visibility of the caudal edges of the nasal bones, with disruption of the brow-tip aesthetic line. Classically, the inverted V occurs at the bony-cartilaginous junction where the upper lateral cartilages collapse underneath the nasal bones (Figures 19.5 through 19.7). This may happen after any surgical technique that disrupts the bony-cartilaginous junction, such as a dorsal hump reduction or aggressive septal resection resulting in loss of structural support to the upper lateral cartilages.

The pollybeak deformity (Figure 19.8) is seen as fullness in the supratip region, best seen on lateral view. Etiology of the pollybeak deformity can be multifactorial. Causes include poor tip support causing loss

of tip projection, inadequate cartilaginous dorsal hump reduction, overresection of the bony dorsal hump, excess dead space, and scar formation at the supratip region.

DIFFERENTIAL DIAGNOSIS

Congenital nasal deformities may share similar appearances as postrhinoplasty deformities. Trauma and oncologic radiation treatments may also induce similar deformities as those caused by surgical rhinoplasty.

WORKUP

A positive history of previous nasal surgery and physical examination with thorough inspection, palpation, and anterior rhinoscopy are

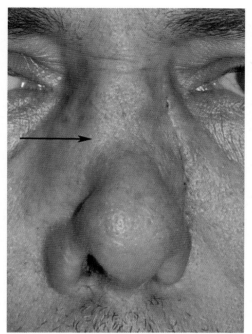

Figure 19.6 Frontal view of a severe inverted-V deformity caused by surgical loss of septal support and radiation effects. The arrow denotes the bony-cartilaginous junction revealing an obvious inverted-V deformity.

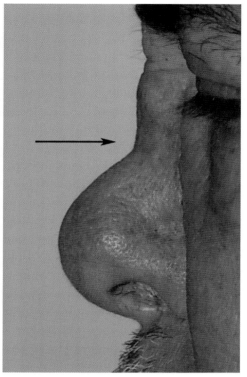

Figure 19.7 Lateral view of a severe inverted-V deformity caused by surgical loss of septal support and radiation effects. The arrow denotes the bony-cartilaginous junction.

sufficient. Photography of frontal, oblique, lateral, and base views enables objective measurements of the nasal dimensions.

TREATMENT
Secondary revision rhinoplasty is necessary to correct the deformity.

To correct the inverted-V deformity, reestablishing support to the bony-cartilaginous junction is commonly performed through placement of spreader grafts.

Surgical correction of the pollybeak deformity relies on properly identifying the etiologic cause. Techniques should be tailored to address the underlying cause of the deformity. For loss of tip support, a columellar strut graft or caudal septal extension graft can recreate proper support and projection of the nasal tip. If there was

inadequate cartilaginous hump reduction, then further cartilage resection is required. If overresection of the bony dorsal hump occurred, grafting of the bony dorsum may be necessary. If scar is causing the supratip deformity, then conservative steroid injection with Kenalog or taping may improve healing and reduce fullness.

Nasal valve collapse

Krishna Patel

DEFINITIONS AND CLINICAL FEATURES
The internal and external nasal valves represent the cross-sectional area of the nasal cavity with the greatest resistance to airflow.

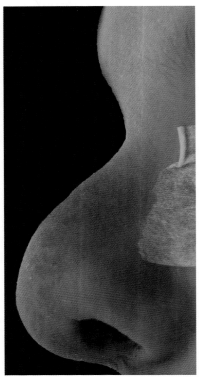

Figure 19.8 Lateral view of a pollybeak deformity caused by inadequate cartilaginous dorsal hump reduction.

Narrowing of these areas can cause nasal airway obstruction during respiration. The internal valve boundaries are the caudal margin of the upper lateral cartilage, the septum, the anterior head of the inferior turbinate, and the nasal floor. The internal valve angle measured at the junction of the septum and the upper lateral cartilage normally is 10°–15°. The external valve is defined as the nasal vestibule. The borders include the area under the ala, the caudal septum, the medial crura of the lower lateral cartilage, the nasal sill, and the nasal rim.

The terminology of nasal valve "collapse" typically implies that the narrowing is caused by the dynamic process of soft tissue collapsing under the negative pressure generated by airflow during inspiration. The dynamic collapse of the valves commonly is due to an inherent weakness within the cartilage structure of the upper lateral cartilages (for the internal valve) or lower lateral cartilages (for the external valve). Additionally, if the lateral crus of the lower lateral cartilage is cephalically malpositioned, the nasal sidewalls are weaker, which exacerbates external valve collapse. Aggressive resection of the lower or upper lateral cartilages during cosmetic rhinoplasty may cause compromised structural support and postoperative nasal valve collapse.

DIFFERENTIAL DIAGNOSIS

An inflammatory process such as allergic rhinitis can generate a dynamic narrowing of the nasal valves through fluctuating mucosal edema. Anatomic obstructions, such as septal deviation, can statically narrow the nasal valves and generate similar nasal obstructive symptoms.

WORKUP

Perform anterior rhinoscopy to inspect the shape and strength of the lower/upper lateral cartilages. During normal respiration, observe for visible collapse of the valves on anterior rhinoscopy exam or collapse of the supra-alar creases on external nasal inspection. Improvement of nasal obstructive symptoms with valve stabilizing maneuvers (Cottle, modified Cottle) can confirm existence of collapse.

Physical findings suggestive of valve compromise include deepened supra-alar grooves, pinched nasal tip, narrowed middle nasal third, or "parentheses" deformity caused by a cephalically malpositioned lateral crus of the lower lateral cartilage (Figures 19.9 through 19.11).

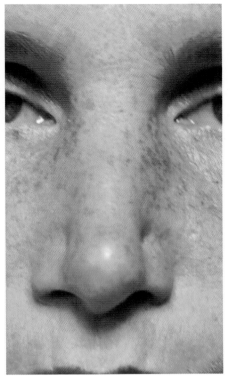

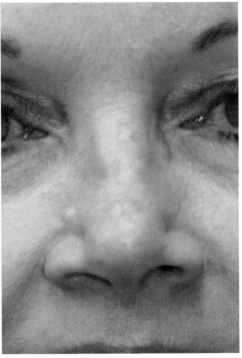

Figure 19.10 Frontal view of external valve collapse translating on external exam as deepened supra-alar grooves.

Figure 19.9 Internal valve collapse translating on external exam as a narrowed middle nasal third caused by aggressive cartilage resection during a rhinoplasty.

TREATMENT

Nonsurgical intervention includes use of nasal cones or Breathe Right® strips, which support the weakened cartilages and open the nasal valves.

Surgical correction for internal valve collapse includes spreader grafts, butterfly grafts, and flare sutures. Surgical correction for external valve collapse includes batten grafts, strut grafts under the lateral crus of the lower lateral cartilage, or caudal repositioning of the lateral crus of the lower lateral cartilage. Placement of synthetic implants has been described to strengthen the valves.

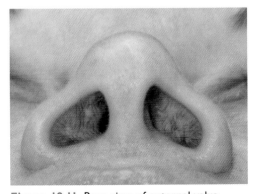

Figure 19.11 Base view of external valve collapse revealing narrowing of the nasal passageway from recurvature and collapse of the lower lateral cartilages.

Rhinophyma

Krishna Patel

DEFINITIONS AND CLINICAL FEATURES

Rhinophyma is a chronic progressive skin disease caused by overgrowth of sebaceous glands. Nasal skin is porous, oily, and thickened, with a ruddy-reddish discoloration. In milder forms, the nose appears bulbous; however, in severe forms, the nose may be completely distorted with tumorlike irregularities that obstruct the nasal vestibule (Figures 19.12 through 19.14). This presents typically over 40 years of age. It affects men more than women, and it may represent a severe progression of long-standing rosacea.

Postulated infectious pathogenesis suggests that the mite species, *Demodex folliculorum*, incites an abnormal hyperplasia of the sebaceous glands. Historically, excess

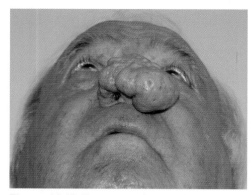

Figure 19.13 Base view of severe form of rhinophyma, causing nasal obstruction.

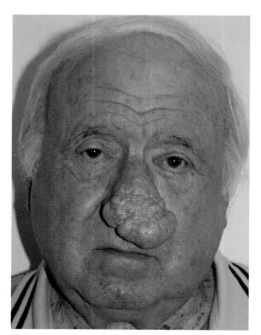

Figure 19.12 Frontal view of severe form of rhinophyma.

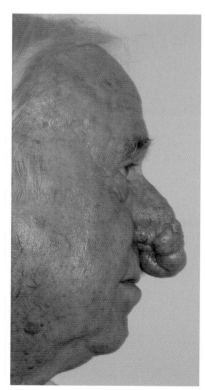

Figure 19.14 Lateral view of severe form of rhinophyma.

alcohol was speculated to cause the disorder; however, this has been disproven.

DIFFERENTIAL DIAGNOSIS
Rosacea, lymphoma, or other lymphoproliferative diseases.

WORKUP
This is often diagnosed by clinical evaluation alone. Skin biopsy may confirm diagnosis.

Patient often has previous medical history of rosacea.

If not classical in appearance, biopsies should be performed because more serious diseases may mask as rhinophyma, such as lymphoma, other lymphoproliferative diseases, or angiosarcoma.

TREATMENT
Surgical intervention for physically distorted noses involves debulking the excess tissue with a scalpel, electrocautery, or laser (CO_2 or erbium/YAG). Dermabrasion and skin grafting are less frequently employed as well. Care must be taken to remove only the dermal tissue plane, so that the open wound will reepithelialize without causing scarring of the deeper subcutaneous layer or cartilaginous structures.

Medical maintenance to prevent progression is similar to that for rosacea. The medical treatment is used for mild forms of rhinophyma or for postsurgical prevention in severe forms. Daily low-dose tetracycline is commonly used. Alternative oral antibiotics used include erythromycin or minocycline. Topical agents used include metronidazole gel, 15% azelaic acid, benzoyl peroxide, and tretinoin.

Nasal Mohs defects and reconstruction

Laura T. Hetzler

CLINICAL FEATURES AND DEFINITIONS
Nasal reconstruction requires careful preoperative analysis to define the explicit elements of nasal architecture affected. Nasal mucosal lining, structural support such as cartilage and bone, and external nasal skin must be reconstructed individually. Equal importance must be granted to function as well as aesthetic outcome. The transition of contours, color, and texture in the nasal form makes a precise reconstruction extremely difficult.

DIFFERENTIAL DIAGNOSIS
Nasal defects may be the result of traumatic injury or neoplasm, both benign and malignant. Certain nasal deformities can be the result of systemic diseases such as connective tissue disorders, autoimmune and rheumatologic disorders, as well as lymphoma. Diseases such as Wegener's granulomatosis, sarcoidosis, lupus, and others can lead to deformities that may be difficult or imprudent to attempt correction in the presence of active disease.

WORKUP
Considerations must be given to the disease course and need for further treatment such as chemotherapy or radiation therapy before embarking on a longer staged reconstructive course. Contraindications to nasal reconstruction include poor overall health status and inability to safely tolerate a procedure. Positive margins or uncertain margins may indicate observation prior to reconstruction. Patients with diabetes mellitus, poor nutritional status, and history of active tobacco use are at an increased risk of poor wound healing.

Patient expectations must be managed prior to nasal reconstruction. Addressing risks for asymmetry, skin mismatch, a prolonged healing period, scars, poor function, graft or flap failure, donor site morbidity, and multiple surgical stages must be openly discussed.

The first step in formulating a reconstructive plan includes the analysis of the defect size, depth, and composition. The condition of the surrounding skin, the local vascular supply, and history of surgery or radiation therapy need to be considered. Adjacent skin with similar texture, color, and thickness should ideally be utilized for superior outcomes. Strict attention should be given to functional insufficiencies and should be addressed prior to formal reconstruction.

PERTINENT ANATOMY

All nasal reconstructions must separately address the three layers of the nose: skin, framework of cartilage and bone, and mucosal lining. The nose is visually perceived as having natural concave and convex surfaces that become apparent as lighted ridges and shadowed valleys, which are the basis of nasal subunits. Five of the nasal subunits are considered convex: the tip, the nasal dorsum, the columella, and the bilateral alar subunits (see Figures 18.2 and 18.3). Four nasal subunits are referred to as concave: the paired soft tissue triangles and nasal sidewalls. If more than 50% of a subunit is involved, it is recommended that the remaining subunit should be resected at the time of reconstruction for an improved aesthetic result. A thorough understanding of these subunits combined with the anticipated healing qualities of certain graft and flaps is fundamental to creating a suitable reconstructive plan of the nasal form.

The upper and middle thirds of the nose are shaped by the nasal bones and by the dorsal septum and upper lateral cartilages, respectively. The overlying skin in this area is thin and mobile. The lower third nasal shape is maintained by the lower lateral cartilages and fibrofatty tissue supporting a more thick sebaceous skin that is fixed to the underlying framework. Precise attention to the 3D structure of the lower third of the nose and strict adherence to the subunits in this area are critical in maintaining the natural shape of the nasal tip.

TREATMENT

Reconstructive decisions are guided by location and size of defect in conjunction with thickness or components to be reconstructed. Reconstruction may vary from simple grafting to extensive multistage approaches. Flaps and grafts that cross subunit lines, particularly the alar crease, may require later revisions to refine aesthetic results.

Nonsurgical therapy for patients intolerant of surgical intervention includes prosthetic application with either bone implant settings or simple adhesive. Healing by secondary intention may be acceptable for small subcentimeter defects and particularly for concave subunits such as the nasal sidewalls, medial canthal portions of nasal root, and alar creases. The defect in these cases must be at least 6 mm from the alar margin to avoid distortion.

External nasal skin reconstruction
Primary closure
Vertical closure of dorsal subunit defects may be performed in smaller defects of 1 cm or less. Wide full thickness undermining may be necessary to achieve tensionless closure.

Grafting
Skin grafts are generally full thickness when used in superficial nasal reconstruction. Donor site is selected based on recipient location. The thin skin of the nasal dorsum and sidewall is best reconstructed with thin postauricular skin. Preauricular donor skin is best for nasal tip or alar grafting due to similar thickness and sebaceous quality. Supraclavicular donor sites are medium thickness with less sebaceous quality than the preauricular site but are a good source for larger skin-only defects. The columellar subunit may be reconstructed with a skin graft if the underlying medial crural support is still intact. The principle of delayed grafting may be employed for

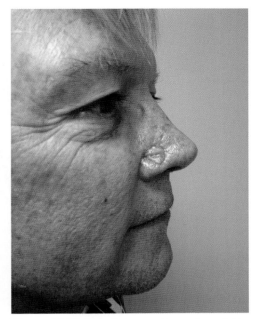

Figure 19.15 Full-thickness skin graft to right nasal sidewall and alar defect, 1 month post procedure.

deeper defects that need to granulate prior to grafting (Figure 19.15).

Composite grafts composed of auricular skin and cartilage may be used in alar rim full-thickness defects that are 1 cm or less. The helical root is the most common site of harvest for composite grafts.

Local flaps

Local flaps may be used for soft tissue coverage and are used throughout all subunits of the nose. These may be used in conjunction with structural or lining flaps in composite reconstructions. Glabellar flaps are employed in upper nasal third reconstruction. Simple nasofacial flaps can be used for sidewall or alar subunits. Larger sidewall unit defects are amenable to larger superior- or inferior-based meilolabial flaps. All of these transposition flaps may require a second procedure for standing cone deformities at the base of the flap or to refine the alar crease should the subunit line be crossed.

Bilobed flaps as described by Zitelli and Esser may be used in the dorsal, the sidewall, and especially the nasal tip subunit in skin-only defects of 1.5 cm or less. Again full-thickness elevation of the nasal skin will be necessary to close without standing cone deformity.

Pedicle flaps

Larger defects of the nose greater than 1.5 cm are often reconstructed with pedicled flaps that have a named arterial and venous blood supply. The most commonly utilized pedicled flap in nasal reconstruction is the paramedian forehead flap based on the supratrochlear artery and vein (Figure 19.16).

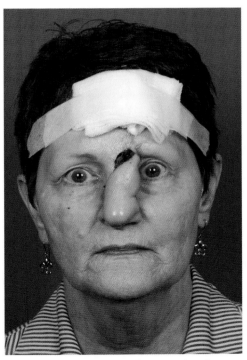

Figure 19.16 Interpolated paramedian forehead flap 3 weeks post-op from first stage.

The supratrochlear neurovascular bundle lies approximately 1.7–2.2 cm from the midline glabella at the level of the medial brow. The meilolabial flap based on the angular artery is also used for alar or columellar subunit reconstruction. Pedicle flaps are routinely a two-staged procedure that requires a division and inset of the flap secondarily. Adjunctive procedures to refine or thin the flap may be necessary to improve upon an initial result.

Structural nasal reconstruction

Cartilage and bone may be harvested from various sites for support in nasal reconstruction. Nasal septal cartilage may be harvested and is ideal for nasal sidewall and columellar support. Auricular cartilage may be harvested from either conchal bowl; however, if alar contour is needed, the contralateral conchal bowl is used (Figure 19.17). Costal cartilage may be used when large stocks of autologous cartilage are needed for robust support or septal and auricular cartilage is not available (Figures 19.18 and 19.19). Irradiated cadaveric costal cartilage is available as an allograft. Calvarial bone for dorsal support may be used as well.

Nasal lining reconstruction

Inadequate nasal lining reconstruction can compromise even the best structural and external nasal restoration. Bipedicle

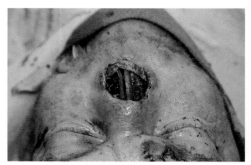

Figure 19.18 Autologous costal cartilage grafts used for total nasal support after rhinectomy.

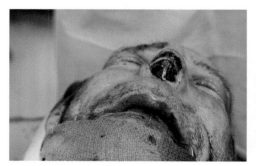

Figure 19.19 Autologous costal cartilage grafts used for total nasal support after rhinectomy.

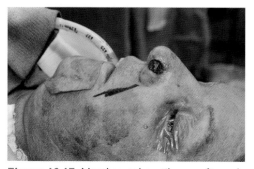

Figure 19.17 Nasal septal cartilage graft used as alar support prior to transposition flap closure.

vestibular skin or mucosal flap can be used with skin grafts filling the donor site if necessary. Septal mucoperichondrial flaps may be based off of the caudal septum ipsilaterally or the contralateral dorsal septum to serve as nasal sidewall or vestibular lining. Inferior turbinate flaps may be used as well and are based off of the anterior turbinate. The same local or pedicle flaps that are used in external nasal reconstruction may be used with the skin facing inward to serve as nasal lining (Figures 19.20 through 19.22). Free tissue transfer with a three paddle radial forearm free flap has been described as well for intranasal lining for total nasal reconstruction.

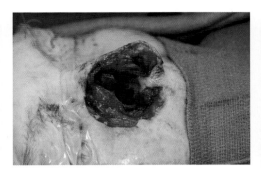

Figure 19.20 Large heminasal defect.

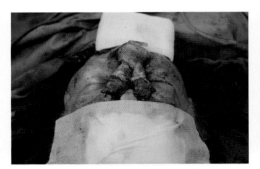

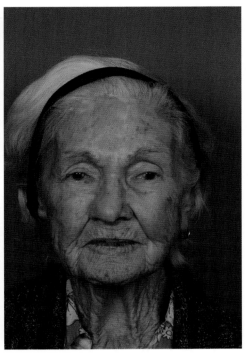

Figure 19.21 Left and right paramedian forehead flaps used as nasal lining and external skin coverage, respectively, for large heminasal defect.

Figure 19.22 Eleven-month postoperative photo of bilateral paramedian forehead flap for full-thickness nasal reconstruction.

Suggested reading

1. Bailey BJ, Johnson JT, Newlands SD. 2006. *Head and Neck Surgery-Otolaryngology*, 4th ed. Philadelphia, PA: Lippincott Williams & Wilkins, pp. 2393–2410, 2421–2452.

2. Baker S. 2007. *Local Flaps in Facial Reconstruction*, 3rd ed. Philadelphia, PA: Elsevier Inc.

CHAPTER 20

Ear

Laura T. Hetzler, Allison M. Holzapfel, and Celeste Gary

- Otoplasty
- Mohs defects and reconstruction of the auricle
- Ear trauma and repair
- References
- Suggested reading

Otoplasty

Laura T. Hetzler

INTRODUCTION

Congenital prominence or malformation of the external ear is one of the more common reasons that the pediatric population undergoes cosmetic surgery. Otoplasty is a surgical procedure designed to give the auricle a more natural anatomic appearance.

ANATOMY

The external ear is a cartilaginous structure with exception of the lobule. The cartilaginous plate of the auricle is covered by tightly adherent skin anteriorly and more mobile skin posteriorly. The morphology of the ear is characterized by smooth undulations and furrows (Figure 20.1). The normal auricle has an angle with the scalp of approximately 20°–30°. When measured from the mastoid skin, the helical edge is ideally 1.5–2.0 cm

lateral to the skull. The average height and width of the auricle are 63.5 and 35.5 cm in a male and 59.0 and 32.5 cm in a female, respectively. The auricle is 85% of adult size by the age of 3% or 4% and 95% of adult size by age 5 or 6. Though younger cartilage is more pliable and otoplasty is most commonly performed on children between 4 and 14 years old, similar corrections can be achieved on patients of all ages.

PREOPERATIVE EVALUATION

The age of 4–6 years old is ideal in that the auricular size is near the adult dimensions as well as an improved ability to tolerate dressing changes and bandaging. This is also the age at which other children will begin teasing each other for perceived differences.

Precise preoperative evaluation by the surgeon requires careful analysis. The ears must first be evaluated separately. Multiple locations of abnormalities can contribute to the deformity and must be corrected

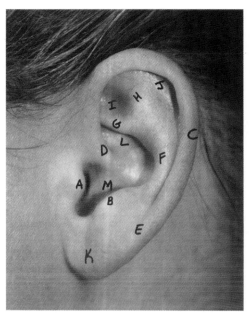

Figure 20.1 Key. A, Tragus; B, Antitragus; C, Helix; D, Helical crus; E, Cauda helicis; F, Common crus of the antihelix; G, Inferior crus of the antihelix; H, Superior crus of the antihelix; I, Triangular fossa; J, Scaphoid fossa; K, Lobule; L, Conchal cymba; M, Conchal cavum.

Objective measures are helpful as well. The helical–mastoid distance should be measured at superior, mid-, and inferior helix or lobule and should be less than 2 cm (Figure 20.4). Preoperative photographs should be taken to include anterior and posterior full face views as well as close-up lateral and oblique views to depict architecture and absent landmarks.

NONSURGICAL MANAGEMENT

The simplest method of nonmedical treatment of auricular deformities is limited to adaptations of hairstyles to cover or camouflage the external ear. If the deformity is noted in the neonatal period shortly following birth, "molding" with ointment-impregnated cotton balls or gauze to recreate the standard folds and furrows of the normal ear is possible. Simple banding or taping may be used to reposition a significant lop or overfolded auricle as well as intrauterine positional deformities. The effects of maternal progesterone for the first 6 weeks of life allow the auricular cartilage to maintain a certain amount of malleability for reshaping.

independently. The most common anatomic abnormality observed in prominent ears has to do with the overgrowth of the conchal cartilage (Figure 20.2). The more frequently talked about deformity has to do with underdevelopment of the antihelix (Figure 20.2). Perceived lobule prominence can also occur secondary to soft tissue excess or helical crus length. These two causes are corrected in different manners as a result of adequate physical exam. Other auricular malformations are described that include lop ear (Figure 20.3) or overfolding of the superior helix; Stahl's ear deformity, which has flattening of the superior helical rim, and antihelical and scaphoid fossa deformities; constricted ear (Figure 20.3); cryptotia; and simply intrauterine positioning deformities.

SURGICAL MANAGEMENT

There are two main techniques employed in otoplasty, cartilage splitting and cartilage sparing. Cartilage-splitting technique involves resection of full-thickness regions of cartilage and subsequent repositioning of the remaining framework to the desired position. This technique can result in disruption of the smooth contours of the auricle or give rise to unfortunate rippling in the auricular skin. This technique is sometimes necessary to reduce a significantly overprojected conchal bowl.

Cartilage-sparing techniques use sutures and/or partial-thickness weakening of the cartilage for reshaping the existing framework to a more ideal conformation maintaining smoother contours and a more natural appearance. A postauricular

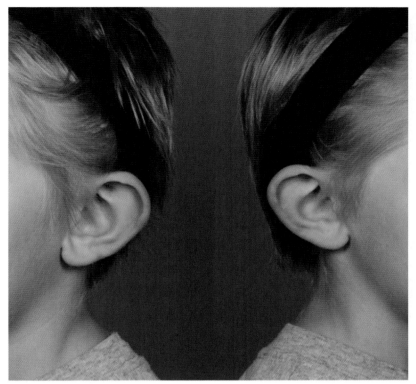

Figure 20.2 A 4-year-old male with overgrowth of conchal bowl and ill-defined antihelical fold.

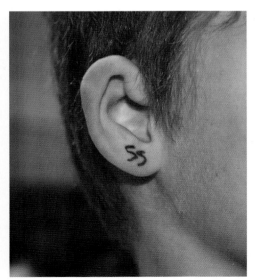

Figure 20.3 Congenital constricted ear with lop deformity.

skin incision is created in an elliptical or hourglass fashion just lateral to the post-auricular crease. Dissection is performed laterally toward the helical edge if antihelical refinement is to occur or if a lop deformity needs to be corrected. A conchal setback and reduction requires resection of the soft tissue from the postauricular crease to include the posterior auricular muscle and allow little interface between your conchal bowl and the mastoid.

CONCHAL PROTUBERANCE CORRECTION

The conchal bowl can be anatomically enlarged or only relatively prominent if it rests at an increased angle from the mastoid skin. The standard technique to improve the conchomastoid position is a conchal setback or Furnas-type suture. Cartilage-modifying

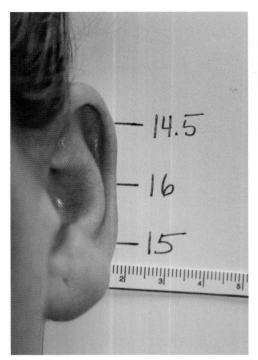

Figure 20.4 Helical rim to mastoid distance should be less than 2 cm.

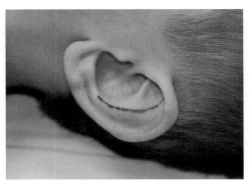

Figure 20.5 Preoperative marking of proposed antihelical fold of left ear.

methods utilized include both cartilage cutting and sparing techniques. A full-thickness strip of the concha cavum can be excised to reduce the size of the cartilaginous bowl or the posterior surface of the conchal bowl can be shaved in a partial-thickness fashion to allow scarring and contraction of the conchal bowl in the direction of the mastoid. Conchomastoid sutures can then be placed to allow repositioning of the conchal bowl closer to the skull. Care must be taken not to place the mastoid stitch too anteriorly or the external auditory canal could be compromised. The author prefers 4-0 mersilene for this maneuver and has little trouble with suture complications in this region.

ANTIHELIX CORRECTION

The anticipated contour of the antihelix is often identifiable in preoperative analysis.

The antihelical common crus and superior crus are marked in the preoperative area or prior to injection in the operating room (Figure 20.5). The neoantihelix is then marked by passing a 25 gauge needle through the cartilage anterior to posterior with methylene blue. The Mustarde suture technique of antihelix formation utilizes between three and four horizontal mattress sutures to create the proposed shape. Suture placement is paramount to create a smooth contour. The suture is placed through the posterior surface of the auricle extending through the anterior perichondrium exiting posteriorly resulting in an approximately 10 mm bite. The author prefers 4-0 nylon though mersilene has also been described. Placement of the medial and lateral limbs of each horizontal mattress stitch must be far enough apart, roughly 15 mm, so that pinching does not occur. The individual mattress stitches need to be no more than 1–2 mm apart to avoid buckling (Figure 20.6). Overcorrection is recommended as the suture will often relax with time to allow the helical rim to be visible lateral to the antihelix.

LOBULE IRREGULARITIES

Lobule prominence can be a soft tissue or cauda helicis phenomenon. Correction is performed by soft tissue reduction or trimming of excess cartilage, respectively.

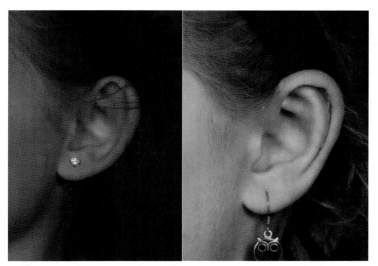

Figure 20.6 Pre-op and 1-year post-op photo demonstrating improved contour of antihelical fold left ear.

CONTRAINDICATIONS

Contraindications would include any patient with unrealistic expectations. A thorough discussion of preexisting asymmetries and limitations of surgery are imperative. History of bleeding disorders should be noted as postsurgical hematomas can be catastrophic to the healing process and can cause significant deformity. Patients with a history of keloids or hypertrophic should be advised that these may occur following otoplasty.

COMPLICATIONS

Complications can be divided into early and late complications. Hematoma and infection are typically heralded by atypical amounts of pain. Asymmetry or incomplete correction is the most common complaint. Management of expectations during preoperative discussions allows the surgeon to point out preexisting asymmetries that will be difficult to correct for. Overcorrection resulting in telephone ear or reverse telephone ear deformity may occur. Suture webbing or bridging as well as delayed suture complications can be an issue as well.

Mohs defects and reconstruction of the auricle

Allison M. Holzapfel

INTRODUCTION

The projection of the auricle and, therefore, its significant exposure to the sun make the auricle a common site for the development of skin malignancies. Nonmelanoma skin cancer of the auricle represents 6%–10% of all cutaneous neoplasms. The relative frequency of squamous cell carcinoma, basal cell carcinoma, and melanoma of the auricle has been reported with variation but ranges from 35% to 60% for squamous cell carcinoma, 30% to 60% for basal cell carcinoma, and 2% to 6% for malignant melanoma.[1–5] The helix, antihelix, and posterior surfaces of the auricle are the most common locations for cutaneous malignancies.[6] Mohs micrographic surgery aims to evaluate 100% of the margins of the specimen to reduce the risk of recurrence. The tissue-sparing nature of Mohs surgery is of great advantage on the ear due to its limited amount of tissue available for reconstruction. A smaller defect allows easier reconstruction and a better cosmetic outcome.[3]

The goal of reconstruction of defects of the auricle is to retain the approximate size, shape, and projection of the ear. As both ears are not readily visible at the same time, some small differences in size and shape are quite acceptable. When planning reconstruction, the defect size and location and the availability and condition of the adjacent skin, as well as the health and aesthetic desires of the patient, are all taken into consideration. Reconstructive options include healing by secondary intention, primary linear closure, skin grafting, chondrocutaneous advancement flaps, cartilage grafting, and local transposition flaps. Proper planning is essential to create an acceptable ear with minimal scarring and a minimal number of procedures.

DEFECTS OF THE LATERAL SURFACE OF THE AURICLE

Defects within the lateral surface of the auricle itself are readily repaired with secondary intention healing or full- or split-thickness skin grafts. Concave surfaces of the ear, including the concha, cymba, and triangular fossa, are ideal candidates for healing by secondary intention (Figure 20.7). The scar contraction forces help fill in the defect and decrease the size of the final scar. Any exposed cartilage may be excised to allow granulation tissue from the opposite side to speed healing.[7] If a well-vascularized tissue bed, such as perichondrium or subcutaneous tissue, is present within the

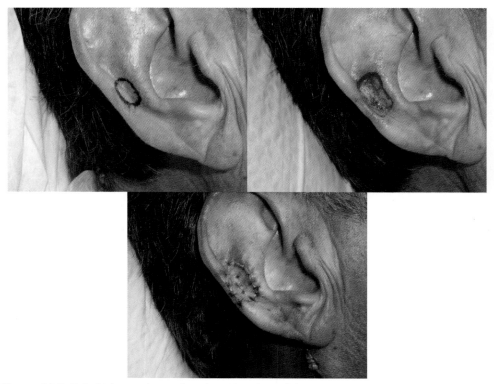

Figure 20.7 Full-thickness skin graft to lateral surface of the ear.

defect, a full- or split-thickness skin graft may be the most advantageous reconstructive option. The contralateral postauricular skin is an excellent full-thickness skin graft source. Immobilizing the graft with a bolster-type dressing decreases the buildup of serosanguinous fluid beneath the graft and improves the chances of graft survival.

DEFECTS OF THE HELIX AND HELICAL RIM

Defects of the helical rim can involve skin only or skin and cartilage. Treatment of defects with intact cartilage can be treated by simple linear closure (Figure 20.8). This can create a depression or flattening of the helical rim that can be camouflaged by extending the linear closure or significant undermining of the skin on the medial side

of the ear. This closure usually works best with smaller defects. For larger defects in a patient in which complicated repair is not warranted, cartilage can be trimmed and the anterior and posterior wound edges sewn together or oversewn.

Helical rim defects that do not extend deeply into the antihelix can be repaired with a sliding chondrocutaneous advancement flap (Figure 20.9). In this flap, the skin along the helical rim is undermined both superiorly and inferiorly. The flap has two possibilities. In the first, the flap is detached both anteriorly and posteriorly. The flap is relatively narrow in this version, which can limit its available length. In the second, the posterior skin is left intact and advanced with a much broader flap base. The skin is advanced and repaired to reconstruct

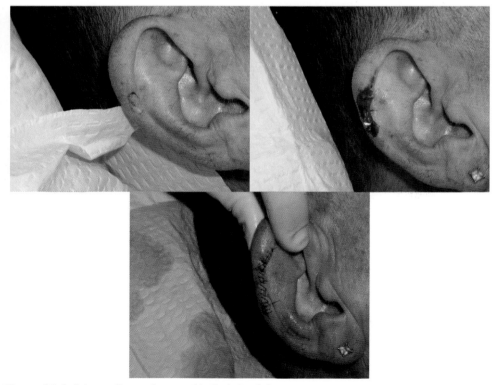

Figure 20.8 Primary linear closure of helical rim defect.

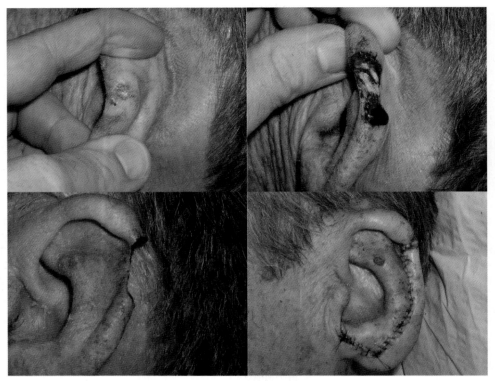

Figure 20.9 Chondrocutaneous helical rim advancement flap.

the natural contour of the helix. Mattress sutures are mandatory to prevent helical notching. Burrows triangles are removed on the posterior surface of the ear. This flap is usually limited to defects 2.5 cm or less.[8]

The banner transposition flap based on either the pre- or postauricular skin is an excellent tool for reconstruction of anterior superior helical rim defects.[9] Figure 20.10 demonstrates a posteriorly based flap. As these transposition flaps carry their own blood supply, they can also be used to cover autogenous cartilage grafts placed for structural support.

Defects that involve the cartilage of the helical rim and extend into the scaphoid fossa can be repaired with a full-thickness wedge excision. This excision allows the ear to maintain its overall shape and alignment but decreases the ear's overall size. Care must be taken in defects greater than one-fifth of the helix, as closure can place undue tension on the ear and cause cupping of the residual cartilage. Larger defects of the skin and cartilage may require large Burrow's triangles in a star-shaped pattern to repair the defect without distorting the relative shape of the ear but do cause a significant decrease in the size of the ear.[10]

A staged postauricular advancement flap can also be used in lateral helical rim and scaphoid fossa defects to maintain the overall size of the ear. Autogenous cartilage grafting may be included to maintain the contour of the auricle. In this flap, the mastoid skin is undermined toward the scalp and a pedicle is maintained while advancing the edges to the lateral side of the defect. The pedicle is divided 2–4 weeks later with flap trimming and possible reconstruction

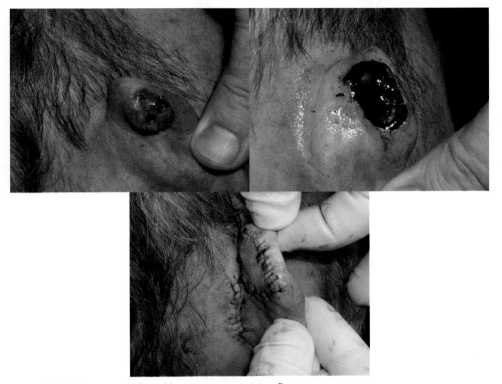

Figure 20.10 Posteriorly based banner transposition flap.

of the donor defect or healing by secondary intention (Figures 20.11 and 20.12).

Larger defects measuring over one-third of the auricle require the use of cartilage, a temporoparietal fascia flap (TPFF), and a skin graft for reconstruction. The TPFF is based on the posterior branch of the superficial temporal artery. The TPFF is a thin and mobile flap that provides a robust blood supply to the underlying cartilage graft and nourishes the overlying skin graft. Structural cartilage grafts can be harvested from the ipsilateral or contralateral conchal bowl, the nasal septum, or the rib cartilage. These grafts are secured to the existing cartilage for structural support. Awareness of the anatomical location of the temporal branch of the facial nerve immediately deep to the temporoparietal fascia is very important.

Dissection anteriorly and inferiorly at the level of the zygomatic arch should be limited to avoid damage. The TPFF is draped over the cartilage and sutured in place. A full-thickness skin graft is placed over the flap. The donor skin graft is typically harvested from the contralateral postauricular skin.[10–14]

DEFECTS OF THE LOBULE

Lobular defects can usually be closed with a full-thickness wedge excision and simple closure. This will decrease the size of the ear but maintain the overall shape. Defects involving the entire lobule can be reconstructed with staged local flaps from the postauricular skin, including a tubed single-pedicle flap or a posterior–inferior-based chondrocutaneous flap.[15,16]

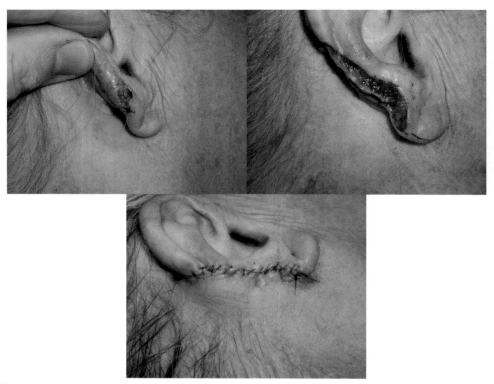

Figure 20.11 Pedicled flap development and inset.

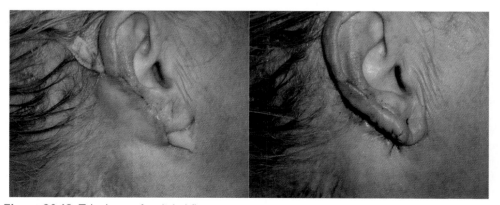

Figure 20.12 Takedown of pedicled flap.

DEFECTS OF THE POSTAURICULAR AREA

Due to the mobility and relative excess of skin in the postauricular area, rotational and transpositional flaps are easily executed for repair (Figure 20.13). Full-thickness skin grafts are also a viable option in defects with nutritious wound beds. Defects that lie in the postauricular sulcus can easily be allowed to heal by secondary intention without the distortion of the auricle.

DEFECTS OF THE PREAURICULAR SULCUS

Due to the laxity of the cheek skin, defects in the preauricular sulcus can usually be repaired with simple cheek advancement flaps. The flaps can extend all the way to the helical root and across the tragus. This scar can rarely be seen from a frontal view and hides well within the traditional facelift scar.

CONCLUSIONS

The surgeon's approach to auricular reconstruction must focus on maintaining the size and shape of the auricle so that it appears similar to the contralateral ear. The reconstruction should be performed with similar tissues providing support and maintaining function while providing the best possible aesthetic outcome.

Ear trauma and repair

Celeste Gary and Laura T. Hetzler

DEFINITIONS AND CLINICAL FEATURES

The ear has unique anatomy that centers around a cartilaginous framework with a

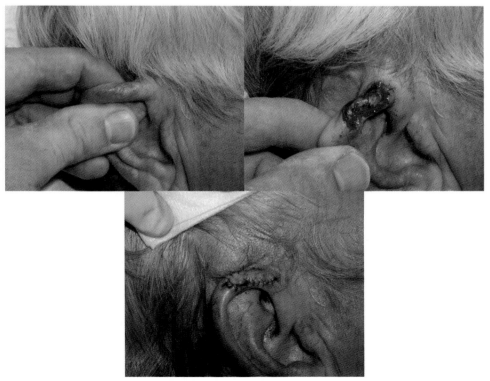

Figure 20.13 Postauricular transposition flap. (Photo by Scott Nelton, Crestview Hill, KY.)

tightly adherent skin envelope anteriorly with more loosely adherent skin posteriorly.

Ear lacerations should be divided into two categories:

1. Defects of cutaneous coverage
   a. With intact cartilage
   b. With disrupted cartilage
2. Full-thickness defects

Auricular hematomas can occur with contact sports, especially wrestling. Shearing forces disrupt the connections between the cartilage, perichondrium, and skin and cause microvascular disruption. Blood accumulates in the space between the perichondrium and the cartilage.

DIFFERENTIAL DIAGNOSIS
Auricular skin lesions including skin malignancies can present as nonhealing auricular ulcers and lacerations.

WORKUP
Adequate investigation of the extent of a laceration including the involvement of damage to the perichondrium and cartilage is paramount.

Timing of the injury should be considered. Most lacerations can be repaired primarily but lacerations over 24 hours old and human or dog bites over 5 hours old may need delayed closure after several days of treatment with antibiotics. Though this is good practice, due to the robust auricular blood supply, late closure is often safe.

TREATMENT
When repair of the ear is needed, an ear block is a helpful approach for anesthesia in a patient who is not sedated or under general anesthesia. This technique involves infiltration of the soft tissues surrounding the attachment of the auricle with a local anesthetic, 1% lidocaine or 0.5% bupivacaine. If performed properly, the need for local anesthetic infiltration at the laceration site may be avoided as this can distort the thin and adherent tissues of the auricle.

The ear and surrounding soft tissue should be thoroughly irrigated with saline and should be prepared with an antiseptic solution. A sterile drape should be placed (Figures 20.14 and 20.15).

AURICULAR HEMATOMA MANAGEMENT
Either needle aspiration or incision and drainage can be performed.

After adequate evacuation of the hematoma is performed and irrigation of the wound is completed, a compression dressing or bolster of antibiotic-coated dental rolls, Xeroform gauze, or thermoplastic splinting material should be secured to the hematoma site with a through and through suture (usually a 3-0 nonabsorbable suture) to prevent reaccumulation. This bolster can be removed in 7–10 days.

LACERATION REPAIR
Focus should be on retaining the normal position and contour of the helical rim and conchal bowl.

Defects of cutaneous coverage with intact cartilage can be managed with primary skin repair with a fine suture, commonly a 5-0 or 6-0 absorbable or nonabsorbable suture. If avulsion of the skin alone has occurred, a full-thickness skin graft can be placed over intact perichondrium or the wound can be left to heal by secondary intention.

Defects of cutaneous coverage with disrupted cartilage should be addressed by coverage of the cartilage with vascularized tissue or excision of the denuded cartilage.

Full-thickness defects up to 5 mm can be closed primarily. A three-layer closure is ideal and involves repair of the cartilage with anterior and posterior skin (Figures 20.16 and 20.17).

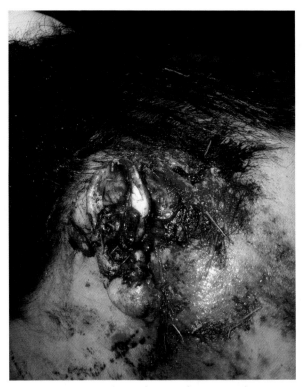

Figure 20.14 Right auricular trauma with significant soft tissue avulsion.

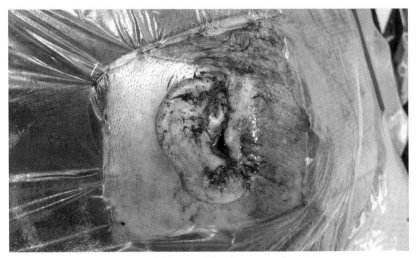

Figure 20.15 Right auricular trauma following debridement and repair.

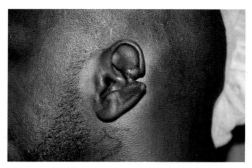

Figure 20.16 Left posttraumatic healing of helical rim laceration.

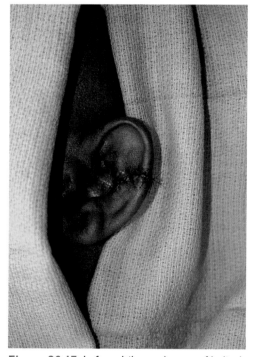

Figure 20.17 Left multilayer closure of helical rim defect.

If the laceration involves the canal, placement of antibiotic-coated gauze or a wick should be considered as a management option.

Ear lacerations can be managed with many types of suture material. A 4-0 or 5-0 absorbable suture should be used to close the cartilage and/or perichondrium. The auricular skin can be closed with a 5-0 or 6-0 absorbable or nonabsorbable suture. To avoid helical notching, the eversion of the skin should be considered a high priority or a Z-plasty.

COMPLICATIONS

Auricular hematoma post laceration repair requires exploration of the wound, hemostatic control, irrigation, and closure. Untreated hematomas can result in cartilage loss secondary to pressure necrosis and subsequent auricular deformity. Infection can occur as well. This should be treated with drainage and antibiotics to cover gram-positive cocci and *Pseudomonas*. The goal is to prevent perichondritis and chondritis that can result in cartilage necrosis or thickening and deformity.

References

1. Arons MS, Savin RD. 1971. Auricular cancer: Some surgical and pathological considerations. *American Journal of Surgery* 112:770–776.
2. Ahmad I, Das Gupta AR. 2001. Epidemiology of basal cell carcinoma and squamous cell carcinoma of the pinna. *Journal of Laryngology and Otology* 115:85–86.
3. Bumsted RM, Ceilley R, Panje W, Crumley R. 1981. Auricular malignant neoplasms: When is chemotherapy (Mohs technique) necessary? *Archives of Otolaryngology* 107:721–724.
4. Duffy KL, McKenna JK, Hadley ML et al. 2009. Nonmelanoma skin cancers of the ear: Correlation between subanatomic location and post-Moh's micrographic surgery defect size. *Dermatologic Surgery* 35:30–33.
5. Gustaityte-Larsen D, Illum P. 2013. Nonmelanoma skin cancer of the auricle is treated according to national guidelines. *Danish Medical Journal* 60(3):A4587.

6. Songcharoen S, Smith RA, Jabaley ME. 1978. Tumors of the external ear and reconstruction of defects. *Clinics in Plastic Surgery* 5:447–457.
7. Vuyk HD, Cook TD. 1997. Auricular reconstruction after Mohs' surgery. A review. *FACE* 5(1):9–21.
8. Antia NH, Buch VI. 1967. Chondrocutaneous advancement flap for the marginal defect of the ear. *Plastic and Reconstructive Surgery* 39(5):472–477.
9. Masson JK, Mendelson BC. 1977. The banner flap. *American Journal of Surgery* 134(3):419–423.
10. Park SS, Hood RJ. 2001. Auricular reconstruction. *Otolaryngology Clinics of North America* 34(4):713–738.
11. Cheney ML, Hadlock TA, Quatela VC. 2007. Reconstruction of the auricle. In: Baker, SR (ed.), *Local Flaps in Facial Reconstruction.* Edinburg, TX: Elsevier Mosby, pp. 581–624.
12. Park C, Chung S. 1998. A single-stage two-flap method for reconstruction of partial auricular defects. *Plastic and Reconstructive Surgery* 102(4):1175–1181.
13. Ruder RO. 1994. Injuries of the pinna. In: Gates, GA (ed.), *Current Therapy in Otolaryngology: Head and Neck Surgery.* Philadelphia, PA: Mosby, pp. 127–131.
14. Armin BB, Ruder RO, Azizadeh B. 2011. Partial auricular reconstruction. *Seminars in Plastic Surgery* 25(4):249–256.
15. Cook TA, Miller PJ. 1995. Auricular reconstruction. *Facial Plastic Surgery* 11(4):319–329.
16. Yotsuyanagi T. 1993. Ear lobe reconstruction using a chondrocutaneous flap. *Plastic and Reconstructive Surgery* 94(7):1073–1078.

Suggested reading

Bailey BJ, Johnson JT, Kohut RI et al. 2006. *Head and Neck Surgery-Otolaryngology*, 4th ed. Philadelphia, PA: Lippincott Williams & Wilkins, pp. 935–948.

Papel I. 2009. *Facial Plastic and Reconstructive Surgery*, 3rd ed. New York: Thieme Medical Publishers, Inc., pp. 421–434.

Papel I. 2009. *Facial Plastic and Reconstructive Surgery*, 3rd ed. New York: Thieme Medical Publishers, Inc., pp. 907–918.

Quatela V, Cheney M. 1995. Reconstruction of the auricle. In: Baker, SR and Swanson, NA (eds.), *Local Flaps in Facial Reconstruction.* St. Louis, MO: Mosby-Year Book, pp. 443–479.

Aging Face

Bradford Terry, Laura T. Hetzler, Blake Raggio, Aditi Bhuskute, Lane D. Squires, and Jonathan Sykes

Neuromodulators

Bradford Terry and Laura T. Hetzler

INTRODUCTION

Injection of botulinum toxin has become the most frequent aesthetic procedure performed in the United States. It is versatile and outstandingly safe when used properly by experienced practitioners. Botulinum toxin products are derived from two serotypes of neurotoxins produced by *Clostridium botulinum*. Botulinum toxin temporarily improves dynamic rhytids caused by muscle contraction.

MECHANISM OF ACTION

Botulinum toxin works at the neuromuscular junction to prevent muscular contraction by inhibiting the release of acetylcholine. Presynaptic neurons harbor vesicles with the acetylcholine neurotransmitter inside, which are ready to release when signaling occurs. The toxin enters the terminal end of the presynaptic neuron and inhibits acetylcholine release.

FORMULATIONS AND EFFICACY

There are several approved formulations of botulinum toxin that are derived from two serotypes: type A and type B. Type A derivatives are more prevalent and have various brand options. OnabotulinumtoxinA is the most common and most studied brand of type A. Newer type A formulations include abobotulinumtoxinA and incobotulinumtoxinA. At this time, rimabotulinumtoxinB is the only type B agent that is FDA approved. It is a primary agent for cervical dystonia and has also been studied to a lesser degree for cosmetic use.

The generally accepted clinical effectiveness of onabotulinumtoxinA begins to appear in 1–3 days, peaks in 1–4 weeks, and gradually declines after 3 months. Some patients may have longer response, especially if they have received multiple treatments to the same area. Rare occurrences of antibody formation arise, which causes decreased efficacy of treatments.

CONTRAINDICATIONS

Absolute contraindications to usage are known hypersensitivity to any component of the product and allergy to cow's milk protein should not be given abobotulinumtoxinA. Injections should not be administered to patients with current infections at site of injection. Relative contraindications are neuromuscular disorders including myasthenia gravis, Eaton–Lambert syndrome, myopathies, and amyotrophic lateral sclerosis. Caution should be used for patients taking drugs that can interfere with neuromuscular transmission such as aminoglycosides, cholinesterase inhibitors, quinidine, magnesium sulfate, succinylcholine, and curare-type nondepolarizing blockers. Most botulinum toxins are pregnancy class C agents; thus, injection is avoided in pregnant women.

PREPARATION

As with most cosmetic procedures, photo documentation before and after treatment is useful for assessing individual patient improvement. Potential adverse effects, benefits, anticipated duration of treatment, and need for retreatment should be addressed and discussed with the patient. Realistic expectations and psychosocial factors should be evaluated.

Type A botulinum toxins must be reconstituted in saline prior to use. Recommendations for dilution vary by formulation and between practitioners from 1cc to 4cc's of nonpreserved saline. The reconstituted solution must be refrigerated if not used immediately and has a limited shelf life of 4–24 hours according to package inserts, but many clinicians keep solution for longer periods. Anesthesia of treatment areas is often performed by holding an ice pack to anticipated areas and applying topical anesthetics.

TREATMENT TIPS

Small-volume syringes and a fine needle such as 30 gauge are used for injection. Men typically have more musculature in their face and require more per injection site than women. The dosage for each location is dependent on the number of injection sites per muscle, size of muscle, and desired outcome for paralysis or milder weakening of the muscle. Patients may be instructed to sit upright for 2–4 hours after injection and to not rub the areas for 24 hours. Schedule a follow-up appointment for 2–3 weeks to perform touch-up injections for unsatisfactory areas.

SIDE EFFECTS

Cosmetic application of botulinum toxin is relatively safe when appropriately dosed and administered by properly trained personnel. The most common side effects are bruising and swelling. Patients can describe mild and transient effects of headache or flulike symptoms. Complications of treatment to the upper face include brow ptosis due to weakness of frontalis muscle, eyelid ptosis due to weakening of the levator palpebrae superioris muscle, and assymetric brow arching. In addition, orbital and periorbital effects include diplopia, ectropion, lower eyelid droop, epiphora, decreased strength of eye closure, and dry eye. In the lower face, complications include asymmetrical smile, flaccid cheek, incompetent mouth, and inability to whistle. The rare but required black-box side warnings include aspiration, dysphagia, pneumonia, anaphylaxis, and death.

RHYTIDS AND TECHNIQUES
Glabellar rhytids
This is the most commonly treated area of dynamic rhytids. The glabellar complex consists of the corrugator supercilii, procerus, depressor supercilii, and orbicularis oculi muscles, all of which function as brow depressors. Glabellar rytids are vertical lines primarily caused by contraction of the corrugator supercilii and horizontal lines caused by the procerus muscle. Five to six sites are commonly targeted that should fall above the supraorbital rim by approximately 1 cm (Figure 21.1, black).

Transverse forehead rhytids
Forehead rhytids are caused by contraction of the frontalis muscle. Treatment of the frontalis should only weaken the muscle in order to preserve some facial animation and avoid brow ptosis. Typically, about 6 sites are injected in a straight or slight "v" pattern (Figure 21.1, white).

Lateral canthal rhytids
Lateral canthal rhytids, or crow's feet, are radial oriented lines formed by contraction of the lateral fibers of orbicularis oculi muscle. The radial contraction of the muscle appearance is exacerbated by smiling. Hyperactive areas are noted when the patient squints and can be targeted as injection sites. Typically, around 3–5 sites are injected at least 1 cm lateral to the orbital rim just beneath the skin. Locations are planned in a radial fashion from canthus and inferior to the eyebrow (Figure 21.1, red).

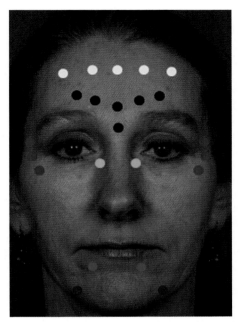

Figure 21.1 Sites of injection for botulinum toxin improvement of kinetic rhytids (black, glabellar rhytids; white, forehead rhytids; red, crow's feet; green, bunny lines; blue, perioral rhytids; purple, frown lines).

Nasal "bunny lines"
Bunny lines are rhytids that originate on the nasal dorsum and radiate laterally toward the nasofacial groove. The treatment of a single injection in bilateral nasofacial groove at least 1 cm inferior to the medial canthus is sufficient for these rhytids (Figure 21.1, green).

Perioral lip rhytids
Also known as smoker's lines or lipstick lines, perioral lip rhytids radiate outward from the lips and are accentuated with puckering the lips. Perioral rhytids are formed by skin pleating from repetitive contraction of the orbicularis oris, photodamage, loss of volume, and pursing of lips. These are difficult to treat with toxin injection alone and often require additional fillers. Target sites are typically one to two locations on each

quadrant of the lips (Figure 21.1, blue). Overweakening of the orbicularis oculi can cause altered lip proprioception, dysarthria, dysphagia, and drooling.

MOUTH FROWN

The rhytids at corner of the mouth traveling inferiorly give the appearance of a frown at rest. The depressor anguli oris pulls the oral commissure inferiorly while opposed by the zygomaticus muscle complex. Target injections to the depressor anguli oris muscle are just anterior to the masseter muscle, essentially at the inferior extent of the marionette lines (Figure 21.1, purple). This can improve the downward position of the commissure at rest as well as improve developing rhytids.

Fillers

Bradford Terry, Laura T. Hetzler, and Blake Raggio

INTRODUCTION

Injectable fillers play an important role in nonoperative cosmetic enhancement. They are utilized to improve many issues from fine rhytids to broad-based volume deficits. The ideal filler has not been discovered yet. It would be biocompatible, noninflammatory, affordable, and durable and not migrate. There are many compositions that last many months, such as hyaluronic acid or collagen fillers to semipermanent fillers like poly-L-lactic acid (Table 21.1).

TYPES OF FILLERS
Hyaluronic acid

Hyaluronic acid (HA) is the most widely utilized filler. HA stabilizes intercellular structures by forming a viscoelastic framework. It avidly attracts water molecules causing volume expansion and hydration of the skin. Some patients remark that periods of dehydration versus adequate hydration make a difference in their result.

Cross-linking was developed to prevent degradation and promote longevity. Larger molecules of HA filler have been designed for a more robust result with deeper injections in areas of greater volume deficits. Benefits of HA include absence of skin test, biodegradability, longevity, easy storage at room temperature, and reversibility if necessary. Placement of HA into the subcutis or deep dermis is recommended but may vary by defect and location. HA is FDA approved for severe facial rhytids and folds such as nasolabial but also used in lip augmentation, brow elevation, tear trough, and chin, cheek, and jowl augmentation. HA is generally well tolerated with normal minor common side effects and rare delayed hypersensitivity and granulomatous reactions.

Collagen

There are three types of collagen available: bovine, human, and porcine. Bovine collagen is made of calf skin composed of mostly type I collagen fibers. Patients must undergo skin testing prior to use. Collagen fillers have the shortest duration of action that may be beneficial for filler trials or other applications. Common side effects include immediate mild bruising, edema, and erythema. Hypersensitivity reactions to bovine collagen are present in about three percent of patients. Rarely local tissue necrosis, abscess formation, and recurrence of herpetic eruptions occur.

Autologous fat

Fat is harvested from other areas and is transplanted to the face. The main advantage is there is no risk for hypersensitivity or foreign body reactions. Fat is partially reabsorbed by the body and reportedly 20%–80% of the injected material is retained. Unpredictable reabsorption can lead to contour irregularities. Complications include donor site morbidity, necrosis, and calcification of the injected fat and rarely fat emboli.

Table 21.1 Semipermanent fillers

Filler	Material/properties	Duration	MOA	Uses	Adverse effects
Collagen	Bovine collagen Human collagen	3–6 months 3–4 months	Space-filling effect	Superficial and deep rhytids	Common—mild bruising, edema, and erythema; hypersensitivity reactions to bovine collagen Rare—localized tissue necrosis and abscess formation
	Autologous collagen	4–6 months			
Hyaluronic acid (HA)	Non–animal HA; cross-linked with butanediol diglycidyl ether (BDDE)	3–6 months	Space-filling effect of HA with water binding to HA molecules	Correction of moderate to severe rhytids and folds	Common—bruising, discomfort, edema, and erythema
	Non–animal HA, cross-linked HA; some contains lidocaine, cross-linked with BDDE	6–12 months	Stimulation of collagen synthesis may contribute	Few forms of HA for lip enhancement, deeper rhytids, and facial sculpting	Infrequent—hypersensitivity reactions, granulomatous reactions, infections, or complications of vascular occlusion
Calcium hydroxylapatite microspheres (CaHA)	Synthetic, uniform, and smooth CaHA microspheres suspended in an aqueous carboxymethylcellulose gel carrier	12 months	Stimulate the local production of endogenous collagen	Correction of moderate to severe facial rhytids and folds	Common—transient erythema, edema, ecchymosis, pain on injection, and pruritus Less common—noninflammatory lip nodules
Poly-L-lactic acid (PLLA)	Microparticles of biocompatible and biodegradable synthetic polymer	12–24 months	Stimulates fibroblast proliferation and collagen formation, leading to a progressive increase in volume of the dermis	Correction of facial lipoatrophy For correction of shallow to deep nasolabial fold contour deficiencies and other rhytids	Common—hematoma, bruising, edema, discomfort, inflammation, and erythema; asymptomatic subcutaneous papules Less common—granulomatous reactions
Autologous fat	Harvesting and reinjection of fat	Months to years (variable)	Space-filling effect	Dermal/lip augmentation	Morbidity in the donor site, prolonged edema, infections, contour irregularities, and necrosis or calcification

Calcium hydroxyapatite

Calcium hydroxyapatite (CaHA) is a longer-acting semipermanent filler. The CaHA formed into microspheres and suspended in a gel carrier. It causes a mechanical filling effect and endogenous production of collagen around the microspheres. CaHA is viscous and therefore injected deeper into the dermal–subcutaneous border. The longevity depends on location but typically at least 12 months and up to 2 years. It is generally well tolerated with rare hypersensitivity reactions. Caution should be used with injection into dynamic areas of the lips.

Poly-L-lactic acid

Poly-L-lactic acid (PLLA) is a semipermanent filler with duration of 9–24 months. PLLA is a synthetic polymer that stimulates an inflammatory response as the product is degraded. In the first couple of weeks, there are a decrease in volume and then gradual increase as the fibrous reaction causes collagen deposition. Full effects may take several months as the filler continues to work. PLLA is utilized for volume filling for broad areas of thinning or depression especially in HIV patients with lipoatrophy.

APPLICATION SITES
Upper face

Superficial application for horizontal forehead rhytids and glabellar rhytids is often combined with botulinum toxin injection. Glabellar rhytids can be injected with filler with either linear threading or serial puncture technique directly beneath the rhytid (Figure 21.2). The temporal fossa can be augmented with deeper filler injections for patients with temporal wasting. Lateral browlift can be accomplished by injecting into the subdermal space at the lateral brow cilia.

Midface

Fillers can be applied for tear trough depression and projection of the malar region that may be difficult to correct with surgery.

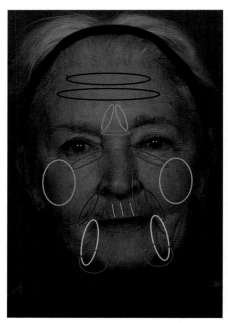

Figure 21.2 Areas amenable to filling: forehead rhytids (black), vertical glabellar rhytids (green), horizontal glabellar rhytids (gray), tear trough (red), malar eminence (orange), nasolabial creases (purple), marionette lines (pink), prejowl sulcus (blue), smokers lines (yellow).

Malar eminence projection needs higher volumes of filler, 1–2 mL, applied with a fanning or cross-hatching method (Figure 21.2). Larger-molecule HA fillers or semipermanent fillers may be used in this region. Fillers may also be used to make minor nose improvements such as tip definition or minor revisions of rhinoplasty; however, these techniques may be too sophisticated for the novis injector.

Lower face

The most common application site is the lower face. Nasolabial folds are augmented with single or multiple layers using either linear threading or serial puncture techniques. Application of filler medial to and under the fold directly can be performed at

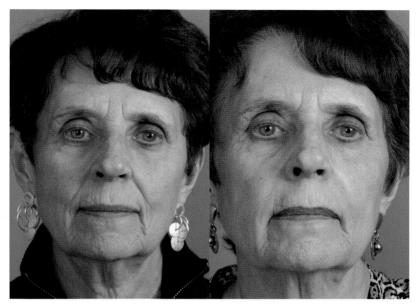

Figure 21.3 Radiesse filler into bilateral nasolabial creases. (Image courtesy of Benjamin Marcus.)

the discretion of the practitioner or may be serially injected in separate settings to avoid overfilling (Figure 21.3). The oral and perioral areas are frequent treatment locations. Lips are augmented with varying amounts depending on patient desire. Filler is placed in the dermal layer. Additional placement in vermillion border or philtrum may also improve results. Perioral rhytids such as marionette lines and prejowl sulcus can be improved with fillers. The prejowl sulcus is an area where deeper, larger molecule depot injections may be beneficial (Figure 21.2). Finally, mental augmentation and mandible projection can be amplified using fillers.

TREATMENT
Preparation
Photo documentation is important before and after each patient. Remove all makeup and clean sites with alcohol. Topical anesthetic or nerve blocks may be performed for added patient comfort. Discuss with patient the risks, benefits, and anticipated duration of action.

Depth of injection
The depth of injection depends on the type of filler, the defect location, or the depth of rhytid. For superficial rhytids, thinner fillers should be used and injected at level of superficial dermis. Filler placed into the mid to deep dermis is appropriate for moderate-depth defects with thicker products in the HA group. For deeper defects, the filler can be placed into the dermal–subcutaneous junction or even supraperiosteal. The deeper the penetration, the less visible a given amount will be.

Injection techniques
Fillers can be applied by several different methods to augment specific target areas. The four common techniques include serial puncture, threading, fanning and cross-hatching. In the serial puncture method, the needle is inserted and small bead of product is delivered and then repeated multiple times along the length of the rhytid. Care must be taken to place the beads of filler close enough to ensure a smooth contour of correction.

To thread filler, the needle is tunneled at the appropriate depth along the length of the needle, and as the needle is withdrawn, the product is applied in a steady stream. Threading is often used for lip augmentation and nasolabial folds. Fanning uses the same technique as threading and is repeated in a radial pattern. Finally, crosshatching uses the fanning technique in two locations that creates threads that are perpendicular to each other. Crosshatching is useful for large and broad-based areas of volume deficit.

Facial rejuvenation and rhytidectomy

Aditi Bhuskute, Lane D. Squires, and Jonathan Sykes

DEFINITIONS AND CLINICAL FEATURES
The face is the central organ of emotion and identity. Defining an individual's unique appearance universally includes a discussion of their facial features. Medical and surgical techniques to rejuvenate facial appearance in patients with facial again can improve self-confidence by bestowing a more youthful appearance. Often patients will seek to change their appearance because of perceived flaws, which can be normal signs of aging including forehead or glabellar creases, ptosis of lateral eyebrow, redundant eyelid tissue, generalized skin laxity, ptosis of malar tissue, perioral wrinkling, deepening of the labiomental creases, jowling, and an excessive submental fat pad.[1]

While facelifting procedures address ptosis and atrophy of facial tissues, they have no predictable effect on the patient's actual skin quality. Skin affected by sun damage, excessive creasing, or irregular pigmentation is best treated via medical therapies or skin resurfacing. Each of these therapies will be addressed separately as outlined in the succeeding text.

PERTINENT ANATOMY
The rhytidectomy procedure involves making a periauricular incision with elevation and tightening of the supportive soft tissues. The type of rhytidectomy procedure is often defined by the plane of dissection used as related to the superficial musculoaponeurotic system (SMAS) (Figure 21.4). The SMAS is a continuous musculofascial sheath housing the anterior midfacial mimetic muscles, arising from the zygomatic arch, extending inferiorly to be continuous with the platysma muscle. Posteriorly, the SMAS forms a separate layer superficial to the parotid/parotidomasseteric fascia. Superficial to the SMAS are skin and subcutaneous fat. Deep to the SMAS, there is a layer of areolar tissue that can inform the surgeon as to the location of the facial nerve branches. Although the facial nerve branches travel deep to the SMAS layer and generally underlie this areolar tissue, more medially, the branches of the facial nerve are located superficially and innervate the overlying muscles and are in danger of direction or traction injury.[2] Another potential danger zone for injury occurs near the zygomatic arch as the soft tissue anatomy is generally tightly compressed in this area (Figure 21.5). Dissection in this region can be performed either superficial to the nerve branches in the subcutaneous plane or deep to the branches on the surface of the deep temporalis muscle fascia.

WORKUP
The management of a facelift patient involves many stages of care before the day of the actual procedure.[3] Even before the initial consultation, each interaction with the physician and office staff is critically measured by the patient to formulate their level of comfort and trust. The initial consultation allows the surgeon and patient to explore a working relationship in which trust is built and true motivations and expectations are explored. While it is important that a cosmetic surgeon learn which patients are good potential candidates, it is equally crucial that each clinician be able to distinguish which patients are poor candidates and are to be avoided. After counseling

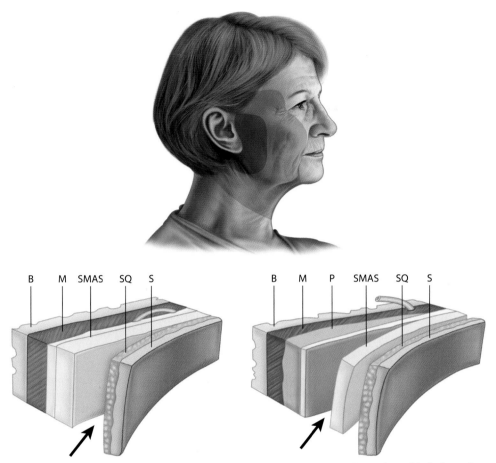

Figure 21.4 The layers of the face. The soft tissue layers of the face are shown here. Underlying the skin and subcutaneous tissue is the superficial musculoaponeurotic system (SMAS). Note that the SMAS lies in a separate layer superficial to the parotidomasseteric fascia, and underlying this fascial layer is the parotid tissue posteriorly and a layer of loose areolar tissue anteriorly. The facial nerve branches travel within this layer. Great care should be taken as the dissection is carried medially as the branches can lie more superficially within this plane. (Adapted from author's personal images/files.)

together, the clinician should decide on the most appropriate surgical therapies to offer. Specific questions evaluating the patient's medications, allergies, medical comorbidities, prior surgeries, and smoking habits must also be explored in the initial consultation. As this surgery is always elective, all attempts should be made to minimize complications by optimizing the patient's medical status prior to the operation.

A preoperative visit should also be offered to allow time to reconnect, ensure appropriate expectations are set, and to answer any and all remaining questions. At this appointment, each surgeon should be forthright with potential complications and direct and honest about the recovery process. A well-informed patient can lead to decreased pre- and postsurgical anxiety and alleviate unreasonable fears. Preoperative photographs should

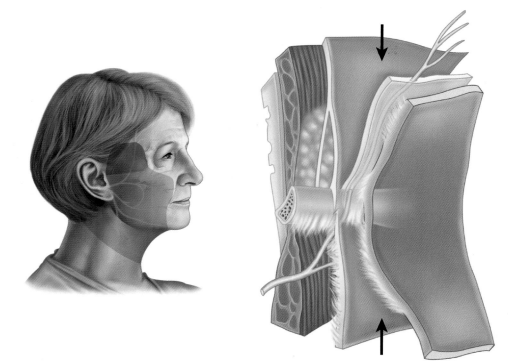

Figure 21.5 Relationship of zygoma with the facial nerve. The relationship of the temporal branch of the facial nerve and the zygoma is shown here. Note that inferior to the zygomatic arch, the temporal branch lies just deep to the superficial musculoaponeurotic system (SMAS) layer, while above the zygomatic arch, this branch is contiguous layer of the SMAS or the temporoparietal fascia. (Adapted from author's personal images/files.)

be taken, as they are essential for preoperative and postoperative patient counseling, intraoperative decision making, and chart documentation.

MEDICAL TREATMENT

The use of these medical techniques as adjunctive therapies to surgical rhytidectomy has been proven to be beneficial in improvement of the aging face. Numerous noninvasive treatment options exist but can be simplified into three technologies: laser ablative therapy, chemical peels, and radiofrequency techniques.

Laser treatment has taken an increasing role in the reduction of facial rhytids through dermal remodeling and the mainstay of laser therapy is the unfractionated CO_2 ablative laser. The use of a laser for resurfacing relies on the properties of the laser to target discrete chromophores in the dermis or the dermal–epidermal junction. Lasers that penetrate deeper into the dermis are more effective at treating rhytids, while more superficial lasers target scars, vascular lesions, and actinic keratoses. Superficial rhytids can be nearly eliminated and dynamic rhytids can be significantly effaced. Lasers are advantageous as they can deliver a precise treatment to a specified area, but the ablative nature of this device can lead to increased risk of scarring, hypopigmentation, and extending postoperative healing and downtime.[4]

Chemical peels have been a mainstay of facial rejuvenation for many years. Unlike laser ablation, chemical peels induce caustic liquefaction of the exposed tissue. In general, chemical peels compare favorably to laser resurfacing. Superficial-depth peels target the epidermis with occasional involvement of the papillary dermis. Medium-depth peels target the papillary and upper reticular dermis. Deep chemical peels penetrate to the mid reticular dermis. Peels cause epidermolysis, protein precipitation, and denaturation of the native tissue. The deeper the peel, the more likely the photodamaged skin can be removed and neocollagenesis begins, although superficial-depth peels are especially effective for solar lentigines and melasma. Solutions for peels include Jessner's trichloroacetic acid peel and Baker–Gordon phenol peels. Disadvantages of chemical peels include lack of laser-like precision to a targeted area, need for neutralization of peel solution, scarring, and infection. However, the healing time after chemical peels is predictable, especially with superficial-depth peels.[5]

Recently, the development of skin resurfacing technologies has emerged that induce dermal injury while maintaining epidermal integrity. Radiofrequency technology applies energy to the skin with concomitant cryogen cooling of the epidermis, which in result causes controlled dermal injury. This injury causes collagen remodeling, shown in clinical and ultrastructure analysis. Early studies have shown that with multiple radiofrequency treatments, an improvement in skin laxity can result.[5]

SURGICAL TREATMENT

Facelift surgery has changed significantly since Lexer described the first subcutaneous rhytidectomy in the early twentieth century. Early facelift surgery involved subcutaneous dissection and redraping of skin with removal of excess skin after redraping. As with the use of any tissue expanders, the skin stretches and becomes lax with time. For this reason, subcutaneous rhytidectomy has not been shown to have longevity. This technique has largely been replaced with SMAS and sub-SMAS techniques. Most facelift surgeries begin with dissection above the platysma muscle and submental lipectomy to improve the contours of the jawline and submental fat pad. The platysma muscle is then included in all suspensions to tighten the aforementioned areas.

The SMAS flap is the mainstay of facelift surgery today. As described in the succeeding text, the SMAS is a layer that is in close proximity to the facial nerve and its branches. Inferior to the zygomatic arch, the facial nerve branches lie just deep to the SMAS layer, while above the zygomatic arch, the temporal branch of the facial nerve lies within the contiguous layer of the SMAS or the temporoparietal fascia (Figure 21.5).

There have been several basic techniques described to address the ptotic SMAS and fat layers. The first is the SMAS plication technique. The safest of the three techniques, the surgeon carries the dissection along the SMAS and subcutaneous tissue. This tissue is then grasped and a nonabsorbable suture is placed to pull the tissue up in a cosmetically pleasing vector. This technique does not violate the SMAS and keeps the facial nerve branches safe. Careful consideration should be made to keep the sutures from penetrating too deeply in order to avoid the nerve injury. Another SMAS technique is called SMAS imbrication. In this technique, a horizontal incision is made in the SMAS inferior to the zygomatic arch and anterior to the skin incision site. The flap is then undermined; a cutback is made in the 90° angle. The SMAS is then pulled and sutured into place. The SMASectomy technique involves excision of a small rectangle in a vector parallel to the nasolabial fold. This allows the pull of the SMAS to be perpendicular to the nasolabial fold to improve and efface the fold. The SMAS rectangle is excised and the proximal and distal borders are sutured, inducing a vector to pull the ptotic SMAS, subcutaneous tissue, and skin vertically upward.

Excellent cosmetic results have been made with a variety of SMAS suspension techniques. However, facial plastic surgeons continually face difficulties adequately addressing the nasolabial fold and promote longevity of the suspension techniques. The deep plane technique involves a composite flap with the skin and SMAS layer being elevated in a single layer before fixation sutures are used to lift the flap superiorly (Figure 21.6). Dissection is taken in a subcutaneous plane initially for 2–3 cm anterior to the tragus. The sub-SMAS plane is then entered immediately superficial to the orbicularis and zygomaticus muscles. Superiorly, the dissection is performed below the facial

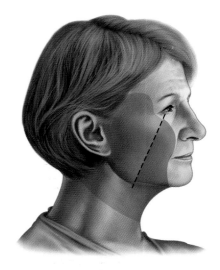

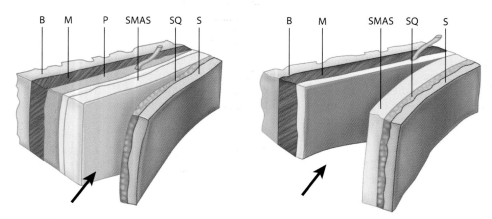

Figure 21.6 The deep plane technique. The relationship of the skin layers in the deep plane rhytidectomy dissection is shown here. The subcutaneous plane is raised initially prior to entering the sub–superficial musculoaponeurotic system plane as noted by the dotted line above. Please note the proximity of the facial nerve during the deep plane dissection. (Adapted from author's personal images/files.)

nerve at the level of the deep temporalis fascia. This creates a large, thick flap, which is then resuspended under tension.

COMPLICATIONS

The face is visible and exposed daily. Therefore, it is essential to prevent complications from facelift surgery as these can have a significant negative impact on the patient's overall satisfaction and outcome of the surgery. Surgical complications can be divided into preoperative, perioperative and postoperative complications. Preoperative complications most often occur due to patient factors, including their medications, smoking status, hypercoagulable state, age, and medical comorbidities (diabetes, emphysema, hypertension). Adequate preoperative evaluation for surgical candidacy is essential in prevention of surgical complications. Perioperative complications are most often associated with general anesthesia and surgical technique. Improper placement of surgical incisions can lead to poor scars and malposition of the hairline. Poor placement of temporal and post auricular incisions can lead to raising of the hairline in an abnormal fashion. Increased wound tension can result in postoperative alopecia. Inappropriate pull of the skin flap can create a vector that creates a "windswept" look. Also, if careful attention is not taken around the tragus and lobule, abnormal ear deformities and a pixie ear deformity can also occur.[6]

Postoperative complications are often multifactorial in nature, but identification and management of these complications in a timely manner are essential for good outcomes in facelift surgery. The most common and potentially serious postoperative complication of facelift surgery is hematoma. This can occur in up to 15% of facelift patients. Meticulous hemostasis during surgery is of the utmost importance. An expanding hematoma can put the facelift flap under pressure and compromise the vascular flow to the flap itself. Most postoperative hematomas are identified at the immediate end of the operation while bandaging or washing the patient's hair. These can be quickly evacuated with pressure or by placing a suction catheter under the skin flap. Immediate placement of a pressure dressing is imperative to prevent accumulation of blood. Minor hematomas are often reabsorbed or can be evacuated in office. Major expanding hematomas often require emergent treatment with removal of the sutures and exploration for bleeding points.

Facial nerve injury can be the most devastating postoperative complication in facelift surgery and can occur in 2%–3% of facelift patients. Common causes of facial nerve injury include direct injury with surgical instruments, neuropraxia by stretching, thermal injury from cautery, and compression injury from suture, edema, or hematoma. The most common site of motor facial nerve injury occurs at the marginal mandibular branch, with the second most common being the temporal branch as it passes just over the zygomatic arch. If facial nerve injury is detected at the time of surgery, immediate repair can be performed. Facial nerve weakness has been shown to regain some function if complete transection has not occurred.

Other potential complications of facelift surgery include seromas and sialoceles, infection, flap necrosis, and hypertrophic scarring. With the recent advent of SMAS and sub-SMAS facelift techniques, postoperative seroma and sialocele can occur. Minor seromas and sialoceles respond very well to aspiration and pressure dressing application. Infection is a rare complication that must be recognized early and treated appropriately with antibiotic therapy. If the skin wound is under tension, flap necrosis and hypertrophic scarring can occur. Flap necrosis most often occurs due to increased pressure or tension on the flap. This most often occurs in the postauricular portion of the facelift flap as the flap is longest and under the most tension in this area. The most important factor to prevent flap necrosis is prevention of perioperative smoking. Stretching or widening of the facelift scar can occur if the flap is placed under tension, in addition to hypertrophy of the scar itself. Intralesional steroids can be used to reduce a poor cosmetic result from hypertrophic scarring.[6]

SUMMARY

In summary, facial rejuvenation procedures range from rhytidectomy to various skin resurfacing techniques as mentioned earlier. The SMAS is an important anatomic landmark for the critical structures of facelift anatomy. Recent advances in medical therapies, including chemical peels, laser resurfacing, and radiofrequency therapy, can be effectively utilized independently or in conjunction with surgical therapy. Each procedure is not without complication, but these can be minimized. It is important to counsel patients for realistic expectations of all facial rejuvenation procedures.

Blepharoplasty

Bradford Terry and Laura T. Hetzler

DEFINITIONS AND CLINICAL FEATURES

The eyes and periorbital area play a crucial role in facial expression and aesthetics. Blepharoplasty is understandably one of the most common facial plastic surgeries performed. It can rejuvenate youthfulness to the face or correct functional eyelid problems. The task of the aesthetic surgeon is to strike the balance between excess soft tissue removal and volume depletion. It is important to consider the surrounding structures in the evaluation and enhancement of the eyelids including the eyebrows, forehead, and cheeks.

AGING PROCESS

The aging process of the face affects the periorbital region primarily through laxity of tissues, redistribution of fat, and hypertrophy or weakening of muscles. There are many factors that contribute to the look of aging including effects of gravity, sun exposure, smoking, stress, and many disease processes. Several characteristic signs of aging include rhytids, descent of the eyebrow, malar descent and subsequent lengthening of the lower lid, and decrease in visible size of the palpebral fissure.

PERTINENT ANATOMY

Eyelid skin is the thinnest skin in the body yet has a rich vascular supply. The orbicularis oculi encircles the orbit, functions as a sphincter, and assists as a pump for tears during blinking. The combination of skin and orbicularis oculi defines the anterior lamella. The tarsus and the conjunctiva comprise the posterior lamella. The tarsus is a stiff cartilage like plate that functions as a major support of the upper and lower eyelid. Conjunctiva is the inner surface of eyelid that reflects at the fornix to cover the globe.

Upper lid retraction (opening) is performed mostly by the levator palpebrae superioris with some contribution by Mueller's muscle. Lower lid retractors, the capsulopalpebral fascia, attach to the inferior tarsus and are an expansion of the inferior rectus.

The orbital septum is an extension of periosteum and contains the orbital fat. It fuses with levator aponeurosis and the dermis to form the upper eyelid crease. In the lower lid, the septum fuses with the capsulopalpebral fascia. In the upper lid, the superior fat compartments lie posterior to the septum and anterior to the levator aponeurosis. The upper lid has a medial and central fat compartment with the lacrimal gland occupying the lateral lid. The central compartment fat pad is larger and more yellow than its dense and whiter medial counterpart. The lower lid contains three fat compartments separated by the inferior oblique between the medial and central fat pads, while the arcuate expansion is between the central and lateral fat pads (Figure 21.7).

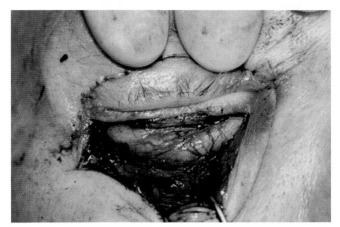

Figure 21.7 Postseptal orbital fat of the lower lid. (Courtesy of Ben Marcus.)

TERMINOLOGY
In order to understand the complexities of preoperative analysis prior to blepharoplasty, a brief review of terminology of facial aging changes with their major causes is in order. Dermatochalasis is often confused with blepharochalasis. Blepharochalasis is an inflammatory condition of the eyelids manifesting as edematous and atrophic eyelid skin that allows for protrusion of fat. It is usually intermittent and recurrent due to histamine response related to increased levels of IgE. Dermatochalasis is the more common "baggy eyes" that occurs with aging due to loss of skin elasticity and apparent excess upper lid skin. Lateral hooding, "droopy eyelids," is caused by dermatochalasis and brow descent or ptosis. Orbital septum weakness allows for steatoblepharon, which is a pseudoherniation of orbital fat. Festoons are redundancies of orbicularis oculi muscle in lower lid and may contain orbital fat protrusion. The tear trough is a crescent-shaped depression between the orbicularis oculi and levator labii superioris medially. Malar bags are skin and fat protruding from the malar prominence.

INDICATIONS
Cosmetic improvement is often the motivation, but there also are some indications for medical conditions. Certain medical indications resulting from eyelid ptosis include impairment of visual fields, eye strain, and impaired reading ability. Lower eyelid blepharoplasty can be combined with tarsal tightening procedures to improve defects causing corneal or conjunctival irritation, for example, entropion, ectropion, epiphora, or corneal exposure. Other medical conditions need to be ruled out for which surgery will not alleviate or could conceivably worsen symptoms including allergic, fluid retention, or metabolic causes. Confounding cosmetic issues need to be screened including lagophthalmos, lower lid laxity, vision loss, dry-eye syndrome, ptosis of lacrimal gland, ptosis of eyebrows, or ptosis of the lid itself.

PREOPERATIVE EVALUATION
Overall: Evaluation of the periorbital region for blepharoplasty should not start with the eyelids. Attention to Fitzpatrick skin type, pigmentation, preexisting scars, and signs of hypertrophic scarring should be noted. Symmetry defines the face and sources of asymmetry should be closely examined and discussed with the patient.

Analysis of the upper face: Includes both the arch and position of the brow. The female brow extends from medially, in a position slightly superior to the orbital rim, to laterally with an arch present at the level of lateral limbus. Males have a flatter arch that is located roughly at the level of the orbital rim.

Analysis of the midface: Includes the volume status, shape, and fold position. The midface should have smooth transitions between the lower lid and cheek.

Direct palpebral analysis: Demonstrates that the lateral canthus rests 2 mm above the medial canthus. The upper eyelid crease should sit 8–10 mm above the lash line. The upper lid should cover 2–3 mm of the superior limbus but not encroach on the pupil. The lower lid should rest on the inferior limbus or 1 mm below. The lower lid should also be examined with eye movement because pseudoherniation becomes more apparent in upward gaze. The snap test for assessing lid tone is performed by pinching, pulling, and releasing the lid that should snap back quickly. The lid distraction test pulls the lower lid inferiorly and should be less than 10 mm.

Ocular testing: Includes visual acuity and visual fields with objective testing. Use the Schirmer test to measure the amount of lacrimation for dry eyes.

UPPER LID BLEPHAROPLASTY

During preoperative evaluation, the patient is marked in the upright position. Mark the supratarsal crease from slightly lateral to medial canthus extending to the lateral canthus and then angled about 30° posterolaterally and superior to the supratarsal crease (Figure 21.8). Pinch the skin with forceps to allow visualization of the predicted result. Local anesthesia is applied, and first, only the skin is incised with a blade. Scissors are then used to remove the skin from underlying muscle. A small amount of orbicularis oculi muscle can be excised to expose the underlying preaponeurotic fat. The eye may be gently pressed to reveal excess fat. The orbital septum may then be incised with judicious removal of excess fat using scissors and cautery. Meticulous hemostasis is achieved to prevent orbital hematoma. Skin closure can be performed with Prolene or fast-absorbing gut suture in a running fashion (Figures 21.9 and 21.10).

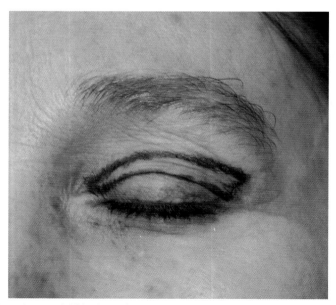

Figure 21.8 Typical upper lid blepharoplasty incision.

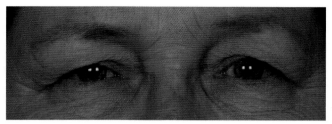

Figure 21.9 Dematochalasis and lateral hooding.

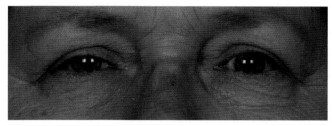

Figure 21.10 Three-month postoperative photo following upper lid blepharoplasty.

LOWER LID BLEPHAROPLASTY

Two common approaches are used for lower lid blepharoplasty. The subciliary approach can be used to treat excess skin, pseudoherniation of fat, and orbicularis oculi hypertrophy. The transconjunctival approach leaves no visible incisions but is primarily to treat pseudoherniation of fat and can be combined with pinch excision of skin for mild amounts of tightening.

SUBCILIARY APPROACH

An incision is created 2 mm inferior to lower lid margin from the punctum medially to roughly 6 mm lateral to the lateral canthus. The skin flap is dissected free of the underlying orbicularis oculi muscle. Dissection through orbicularis is performed in a beveled or stairstep fashion from the skin incision. Small incisions in the orbital septum can be created for each fat compartment. Pressure on the globe reveals excess fat to be removed judiciously with scissors and cautery. Careful skin excision can be judged by having the patient look up and open their mouth if awake.

The incision may be closed with 6-0 absorbable running suture.

TRANSCONJUNCTIVAL APPROACH

Expose the lower lid conjunctiva with a Desmarres retractor. Incise into the conjunctiva inferior to tarsus using monopolar cautery. A submuscular plane can be followed to the orbital rim. Small incisions in orbital septum can be made for each fat compartment with depression of the globe to reveal excess fat. No sutures are needed for closure of the tranconjunctival approach though some surgeons prefer a few fast-absorbing gut simple interrupted sutures.

COMPLICATIONS

The most feared complication of blepharoplasty is retro-orbital hemorrhage with vision loss due to optic nerve compression. Conservative skin resections are made to prevent the major issue of lagophthalmos and lower lid retraction. Other complications include infection, excess skin removal, blepharoptosis due to levator muscle injury, diplopia from superior or inferior oblique muscle damage, ectropion, web formation, and hollowed out appearance.

Brow ptosis and browlift

Laura T. Hetzler

DEFINITIONS AND CLINICAL FEATURES

Brow ptosis is a term used to describe descent of the eyebrow and associated fat pads that occur with aging. Brow ptosis is frequently seen in conjunction with dermatochalasis or age-related eyelid changes, and one cannot accurately improve lid appearance without formally ruling out whether or not brow ptosis is a contributor (Figure 21.11). Mild brow ptosis is typically only a concern with respect to aesthetics. As the brow descends, it can become an issue with visual field disturbance. Patients may complain of frontal headaches and horizontal rhytids due to tonic contraction of the frontalis muscle to improve brow height.

DIFFERENTIAL DIAGNOSIS

Etiology of brow ptosis is most typically related to soft tissue laxity as the result of age and manifests laterally first. Other causes of a drooping brow must be ruled out prior to intervention. The frontalis muscle is the only brow elevator and thus loss of function can result in brow malposition. Neurologic causes related to decreased unilateral frontalis function include facial nerve paralysis associated with neuromas of cranial nerve VII or VIII, Bell's palsy, postsurgical deficits, other CNS or parotid tumors, or accidental trauma. Other neurologic disorders that may contribute to unilateral or bilateral deficits include myasthenia gravis, oculopharyngeal muscular dystrophy, and myotonic dystrophy. Primary skin neoplasms, metastatic lesions, or perineural invasion can cause a partial facial nerve weakness and brow ptosis by invading the upper branches of the facial nerve including the frontal branch. Muscular hyperfunction of the brow depressors such as the orbicularis oculi in patients with blepharospasm can pull the brow to a lower position by tonic contraction inferiorly.

PREOPERATIVE CONSIDERATIONS

Beginning your preoperative examination with a thorough ophthalmic examination is prudent in any periocular surgery. Visual acuity, extraocular muscle function, and pupillary examination should be recorded. Neurologic causes such as myasthenia gravis, myotonic and oculopharyngeal muscular dystrophy, or facial nerve impairment not previously described must be excluded or worked up prior to addressing brow ptosis. Asymmetries in brow position must

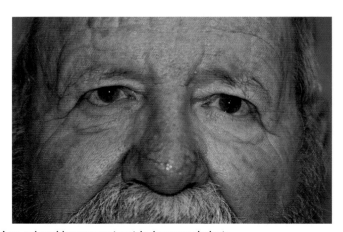

Figure 21.11 Age-related brow ptosis with dermatochalasis.

be noted preoperatively. Scars or a history of periocular trauma is important to recognize.

It is important for the patient to be in complete repose during evaluation. Often, patients with brow ptosis compensate by tonic contraction of the frontalis muscle. To achieve full repose, it may be beneficial to ask the patient to close their eyes, focus on relaxing the forehead, and gently open their eyes for a more precise analysis of brow position.

Men tend to have a heavier, thicker brow with little arc present that should lie approximately at the level of the superior orbital rim. The female brow is club shaped medially and tapers laterally with the medial border on a vertical line with the alar–facial crease. The lateral end of the brow lies on a line drawn from the alar–facial crease tangent to the lateral canthus. Of note, the medial and lateral brows are on the same horizontal plane.

The highest arch of a female brow is ideally at the lateral limbus or just lateral to this. Ideally, the brow in females should lie just above the superior orbital rim (Figure 21.12).[7]

Physical exam findings may deem a certain brow procedure more appropriate. Deep forehead rhytids or the level of the hairline may make one browlift technique more reasonable. The patient's overall health may also play a role in preoperative decisions. Unhealthy patients not suited for longer surgeries or general anesthesia may elect a less invasive approach. Botulinum toxin prior to browlifting may be helpful to eliminate the function of the brow depressors including the corrugator, procerus, and orbicularis oculi muscles.

The preoperative evaluation of brow ptosis is inextricably linked to the physical assessment prior to blepharoplasty surgery. This will be discussed in a separate chapter.

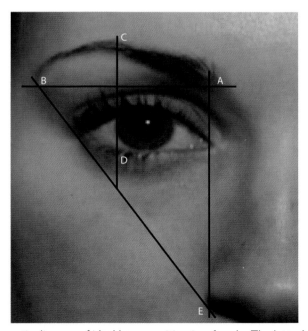

Figure 21.12 Schematic diagram of ideal brow position in a female. The lateral brow lies at or above the medial brow (A–B). The medial brow begins along a vertical line drawn from the nasal ala (A–E). The brow peaks at the lateral limbus of the iris (C–D). The lateral brow extends to a line drawn through the lateral canthus to the ala (B–E). (Modified from Gunter, JP and Antrobus, SD, *Plast. Reconstr. Surg.*, 99, 1808, 1997.)

TREATMENT

The main treatment for brow ptosis is surgical. There are multiple techniques used for browlifting that may be elected based on an individualized basis following complete examination and discussion of patient goals. The transblepharoplasty approach uses the upper eyelid crease, whereas the direct browlift uses an incision immediately along the upper border of the eyebrow. A mid-forehead browlift may be used in someone with deep forehead rhytids to camouflage the incision, especially within the male population. These three methods require less aggressive dissection and are ideal for patients with prevailing functional complaints or inability to tolerate a larger surgery or a general anesthetic.

The pretrichial approach is ideal for someone with a high hairline. The incision is placed just within the hairline in a trichophytic fashion. A coronal incision may also be used and is created just anterior to the vertex. This is an acceptable option if the patient has a lower hairline. The endoscopic approach is currently the most widely utilized within the aesthetic community. It requires 3–5 incisions posterior to the hairline that are well concealed and preserve scalp sensation. The endoscopic approach allows for earlier resolution of edema as well as minimal change in hairline position.

COMPLICATIONS

Complications vary with approach and incisions used. Poor scarring as well as scalp and forehead sensory deficits may occur. Sensation usually improves over the course of months. Alopecia may be related to incision creation or closure tension. Damage to the facial nerve can occur where it passes near the lateral brow. Brow asymmetry or inadequate elevation can frustrate surgeons as well. Adverse hairline alteration can hopefully be avoided with the appropriate choice of approach.

References

1. Niamtu J. 2014. Evaluation of the facelift patient. *Atlas of Oral and Maxillofacial Surgery Clinics of North America* 22(1):1–8.
2. Baker DC, Conley J. 1979. Avoiding facial nerve injuries in rhytidectomy. Anatomical variations and pitfalls. *Plastic and Reconstructive Surgery* 64(6):781–795.
3. Zimbler MS, Mashkevich G. 2009. Pearls in facelift management. *Facial Plastic Surgery Clinics of North America* 17(4):625–632.
4. Sadick NS. 2003. Update on non-ablative light therapy for rejuvenation: A review. *Lasers in Surgery and Medicine* 32:120–128.
5. Hassan KM, Benedetto, AV. 2013. Facial skin rejuvenation: Ablative laser resurfacing, chemical peels, or photodynamic therapy? Facts and controversies. *Clinics in Dermatology* 31:737–740.
6. Niamtu J. 2009. Complications in facelift surgery and their prevention. *Oral and Maxillofacial Surgery Clinics of North America* 21(1):59–80.
7. Gunter JP, Antrobus SD. 1997. Aesthetic analysis of the eyebrows. *Plastic and Reconstructive Surgery* 99:1808–1816.

Bibliography

American Academy of Facial Plastic and Reconstructive Surgery. 2012. Membership Study. Available at: http://www.aafprs.org/wp-content/themes/aafprs/pdf/AAFPRS-2012-REPORT.pdf (last accessed on June 2014).

Bassichis BA. 2007a. Cosmetic upper-lid blepharoplasty. *Operative Techniques in Otolaryngology* 18:203–208.

Bassichis BA. 2007b. Lower-lid blepharoplasty. *Operative Techniques in Otolaryngology* 18:209–216.

Berbos ZJ, Lipham WJ. 2010. Update on botulinum toxin and dermal fillers. *Current Opinion in Ophthalmology* 21(5):387–395.

Carruthers A, Kane MA, Flynn TC, Huang P, Kim SD, Solish N, Kaeuper G. 2013a. The convergence of medicine and neurotoxins: A focus on botulinum toxin type A and its application in aesthetic medicine—A global, evidence-based botulinum toxin consensus education initiative: Part I: Botulinum toxin in clinical and cosmetic practice. *Dermatologic Surgery* 39(3 Pt 2):493–509.

Carruthers J, Fagien S, Matarasso SL. 2004. Botox Consensus Group. Consensus recommendations on the use of botulinum toxin type a in facial aesthetics. *Plastic and Reconstructive Surgery* 114(Suppl. 6):1S–22S.

Carruthers J, Fournier N, Kerscher M et al. 2013b. The convergence of medicine and neurotoxins: A focus on botulinum toxin type A and its application in aesthetic medicine—A global, evidence-based botulinum toxin consensus education initiative: Part II: Incorporating botulinum toxin into aesthetic clinical practice. *Dermatologic Surgery* 39(3 Pt 2):510–525.

De Boulle K, Fagien S, Sommer B, Glogau R. 2010. Treating glabellar lines with botulinum toxin type A-hemagglutinin complex: A review of the science, the clinical data, and patient satisfaction. *Clinical Interventions in Aging* 26(5):101–118.

Fagien S, Raspaldo H. 2007. Facial rejuvenation with botulinum neurotoxin: An anatomical and experiential perspective. *Journal Cosmetic Laser Therapy* 9(Suppl. 1):23–31.

Flynn TC. 2012. Advances in the use of botulinum neurotoxins in facial esthetics. *Journal of Cosmetic Dermatology* 11(1):42–50.

Friedland JA, Lalonde DH, Rohrich RJ. 2010. An evidence based approach to blepharoplasty. *Plastic Reconstructive Surgery* 126(6):2222–2229.

Friedman O. 2005. Changes associated with the aging face. *Facial Plastic Surgery Clinics of North America* 13:371–380.

Fujinaga Y. 2010. Interaction of botulinum toxin with the epithelial barrier. *Journal of Biomedical Biotechnology* 2010:974943.

Kane M, Donofrio L, Ascher B, Hexsel D, Monheit G, Rzany B, Weiss R. 2010. Expanding the use of neurotoxins in facial aesthetics: A consensus panel's assessment and recommendations. *Journal of Drugs in Dermatology* 9(Suppl. 1):s7.

Klein AW, Carruthers A, Fagien S, Lowe NJ. 2008. Comparisons among botulinum toxins: An evidence-based review. *Plastic and Reconstructive Surgery* 121(6):413e–422e.

Lambros V. 2007. Observations on periorbital and midface aging. *Plastic and Reconstructive Surgery* 120(5):1367–1376.

Lelli GJ, Jr., Lisman RD. 2010. Blepharoplasty complications. *Plastic and Reconstructive Surgery* 125(3):1007–1017.

Naik MN, Honavar SG, Das S. 2009. Blepharoplasty: An overview. *Journal of Cutaneous and Aesthetic Surgery* 2(1):6–11.

Pepper JP, Moyer JS. 2013. Upper blepharoplasty: The aesthetic ideal. *Clinical Plastic Surgery* 40(1):133–138.

Stucker FJ, de Souza C, Kenyon GS, Lian TS, Draf W, Schick B (eds.). 2009a. Botox: Its use in facial lines and wrinkles. In: *Rhinology and Facial Plastic Surgery*. Berlin, Germany: Springer, pp. 839–852.

Stucker FJ, de Souza C, Kenyon GS, Lian TS, Draf W, Schick B (eds.). 2009b. Blepharoplasty. In: *Rhinology and Facial Plastic Surgery*. Berlin, Germany: Springer, pp. 877–887.

Suggested Reading

Bailey BJ, Johnson JT, Kohut RI et al. 2006. *Head and Neck Surgery-Otolaryngology*, 4th ed. Philadelphia, PA: Lippincott Williams & Wilkins, pp. 2761–2770.

Hetzler L, Sykes J. 2010. The brow and forehead in periocular rejuvenation. *Facial Plastic Surgery Clinics of North America* 18(3):375–384.

Lam S, Glasgold M, Glasgold R. 2007. *Complementary Fat Grafting*, 1st ed. Philadelphia, PA: Lippincott Williams & Wilkins.

Papel I. 2009. *Facial Plastic and Reconstructive Surgery*, 3rd ed. New York: Thieme Medical Publishers, Inc., pp. 227–242.

Skin: Refinement and Reconstruction

Devinder S. Mangat, Mark J. Been, Benjamin Marcus, Laura T. Hetzler, and Celeste Gary

Skin resurfacing with chemical peels

*Devinder S. Mangat
and Mark J. Been*

INTRODUCTION

The study and intervention of the aging face has become an increasingly popular field. Facial skin resurfacing has, in the last 50 years, undergone a transformation with a myriad of techniques and products available to the facial aesthetic surgeon. The most common techniques include chemical peels (chemexfoliation), laser resurfacing, and dermabrasion (mechanical exfoliation). Chemical peels, simply stated, involve the application of cytotoxic chemicals to the surface of the face. The goal is to create a controlled destruction of the epidermis and dermis in order to remove the unwanted superficial layers of the skin. Different depths of penetration and skin destruction can be achieved by altering the types and/ or concentrations of chemexfoliant applied to the skin.

Chemical peels represent a reliable technique for facial skin resurfacing. Advantages of this technique include highly predictable outcomes over large areas of the face with results equal or better than laser and dermabrasion. There is a relatively low incidence of pigmentation abnormalities for properly selected patients. The process of performing a chemical peel is fast and technically straightforward for the experienced practitioner. Additionally, the chemical agents involved are inexpensive to stock.

In the 1960s, the classic Baker–Gordon phenol-based chemical peel was described and became the gold standard in deep chemical peels.[1] Numerous other chemical agents are commercially available that demonstrate efficacy including trichloroacetic acid (TCA), Jessner's solution, alpha-hydroxy acids (e.g., glycolic acid), and, more recently, a modification of the Baker–Gordon formula described by Hetter that is based on the concentration of croton oil.[2] While the purpose of this chapter is not to delve into the variety of the chemical peels most commonly utilized, it is hoped that a greater understanding will be borne by students and clinicians alike regarding the factors involved in assessment and diagnosis of common aging face problems as well as preparation and execution of chemical peels.

WORKUP

The astute facial aesthetic surgeon must be able to perform critical facial analysis and recognize age-related changes that occur in the face. From a demographic standpoint, individuals with sequelae of chronic sun exposure or acne scarring may be most inclined to seek consultation for skin resurfacing (Figure 22.1). The following

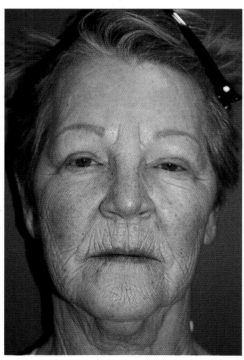

Figure 22.1 Preoperative photo of patient with diffuse facial rhytids and skin lentigenes.

are skin conditions commonly addressed with chemical peels:

1. Dyschromias, lentigines
2. Actinic skin damage
3. Facial rhytids
   a. Deep facial (forehead, glabella)
   b. Fine facial (periorbital, perioral)
4. Acne scars
5. Posttraumatic, surgical scars
6. Melasma

Not all individuals are candidates for chemical peels and one must discern favorable patient qualities prior to proposing the procedure. Based on skin character, the ideal patient is one with thin skin, fine rhytids, and Fitzpatrick skin types I or II (Table 22.1).[3] Individuals with darker skin, or higher Fitzpatrick skin types, carry increased risk of postoperative pigmentation complications. Other favorable factors include patients who are nonsmokers and those who are not opposed to wearing makeup during the healing process. The patient should be motivated and the practitioner must work to establish a good rapport with the patient. Patients must also diligently adhere to preoperative and postoperative regimens for optimal outcomes. Avoidance of significant sunlight exposure for 2–3 months postoperatively is paramount to reduce the likelihood of pigmentation anomalies.

Contraindications to performing chemical peels include the following conditions[4]:

1. Fitzpatrick skin types IV–VI
2. Active herpes outbreak
3. Immunosuppression
4. Recent isotretinoin treatment
5. Collagen disorders
   a. Scleroderma
   b. Ehlers–Danlos syndrome
6. Severe hepatic, renal, or cardiac dysfunction (phenol peels)
7. History of radiation to face or keloid formation
8. Telangiectasias
9. Unreliable patients

PREOPERATIVE ROUTINE

Preoperative measures may be performed to enhance the outcome of the chemical peel. Medications are started up to 6 weeks prior to performing the chemical peel.[5] Tretinoin (Retin-A) is a topical vitamin A derivative that is applied topically to the face. Tretinoin contributes to multiple favorable skin conditions including thinning of the stratum corneum, increased dermal collagen formation, and increased mitotic activity of follicular epithelium that allows for more rapid reepithelialization of the skin following the chemical peel.[6]

Hydroquinone and topical steroids are other medications applied topically to the face up to 6 weeks prior to the procedure.

Table 22.1 Fitzpatrick skin type classification

	Skin color	Tanning pattern	Burning pattern
Type I	Very white	Never tans	Always burns
Type II	White	Tans minimally	Usually burns
Type III	White to olive	Tans moderately	Sometimes burns
Type IV	Light brown	Tans readily	Rarely burns
Type V	Dark brown	Tans profusely	Very rarely burns
Type VI	Black	Tans profusely	Never burns

Hydroquinone inhibits the enzyme tyrosinase, which blocks the conversion of dopa to melanin. The clinical effects are suppression of melanocyte activity and reduction of potential pigmentation abnormalities. Topical steroids, such as hydrocortisone ointment, help reduce local inflammation. Antivirals, such as acyclovir or valacyclovir, are utilized perioperatively to prevent herpetic outbreaks.

TREATMENT

Chemical peels may be subdivided according to their depth of penetration into the skin. The peel agents create a keratocoagulation of surface proteins that prevents further penetration to deeper layers of the skin. Chemical peels are routinely divided into superficial, medium, and deep categories. Superficial chemical peels will cause full-thickness destruction of the epidermis. Medium-depth peels penetrate to the deep papillary dermis. Deep chemical peels typically penetrate to the superficial reticular dermis.

Chemical peels are routinely performed under monitored anesthesia with intravenous sedation and cardiac monitoring. A local anesthetic is used to perform nerve blocks and infiltrate the subcutaneous regions of the skin to be treated. The procedure may also be performed exclusively under local anesthesia if only treating limited areas with superficial-depth peel. In this instance, topical anesthetic products may be used to prevent the burning sensation that may be encountered after application of the peel agent.

After the patient is adequately anesthetized, the face is cleansed and degreased with acetone. Application of the peel agent is performed with cotton tip applicators or 4 × 4 gauze. The goal is to achieve a uniform frost in the treated area(s). The depth of penetration may be gauged intraoperatively by the color of the frost obtained. Light pink or whitish pink frost indicates penetration through the epidermis to the papillary dermis. Solid white frost indicates penetration through the papillary dermis to the upper reticular dermis and a whitish gray frost suggests deeper penetration to the mid-reticular dermis.

While performing the procedure, the face is divided into subunits. Intervals of 15 minutes are allowed between applications to the different subunits to decrease the risk of cardiac toxicity from any phenol-based peel. At the end of the procedure, the periphery of the peeled area is feathered with a superficial peel agent to blend the treated areas of the face with the surrounding skin.

General guidelines can be followed regarding the depth of chemical peel based on regions of the face. Considerations are dependent on the thickness of skin and associated condition(s) being treated. The lower eyelid, periorbital area, and nose should be limited to superficial chemical peels due to thin skin. On the eyelids, application of the peel may approach the ciliary margin. The upper eyelid is not routinely included in peels. Medium-depth peels may be performed on the cheeks and forehead; however, deeper peels may be necessary to address deep forehead and glabellar rhytids or acne-related scars. The perioral region and mentum have thicker skin and can tolerate medium to deep chemical peels. Application of the peeling agent may extend across the vermillion border without untoward effects. In general, chemical peels are not extended inferiorly below the submandibular region; however, in select cases, very superficial peels may be performed on the neck and upper chest.

POSTOPERATIVE CARE

Immediately following the procedure, the patient's skin will assume a light to deep red color depending on the depth of peel. The treated areas of the face are covered generously with topical emollient, and the patient is instructed to maintain adequate moisturization until the treated areas exfoliate and reepithelialization occurs. At this time, the patient's face resembles the erythematous

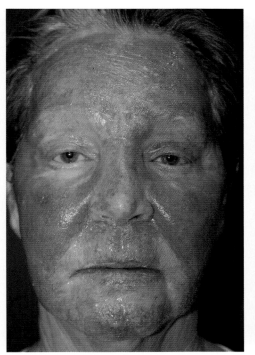

Figure 22.2 Postoperative day 6 following a medium-depth Hetter-based chemical peel.

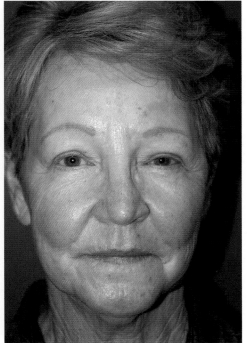

Figure 22.3 Six months following a medium-depth Hetter-based chemical peel.

nature of a sunburn (Figure 22.2). The time to reepithelialization is dependent on the depth of the chemical peel. The following outline may serve as a general guide for time to skin reepithelialization:

1. Superficial peel
   a. 5 days
2. Medium-depth peel
   a. 7–10 days
3. Deep peel
   a. 10–14 days

After reepithelialization occurs, the patient should continue to keep the skin moisturized. Application of topical steroids can help to decrease posttreatment inflammation of the skin. The final results are often apparent at 3–6 months following the procedure (Figure 22.3).

COMPLICATIONS

Listed in the following are potential complications associated with chemical peels:

1. Acne
2. Milia
3. Scarring
4. Prolonged erythema
5. Pigmentary
   a. Hypopigmentation
   b. Hyperpigmentation
6. Ectropion
7. Infectious
   a. Cellulitis
   b. Herpes outbreak

Complications are infrequent and almost always temporary in nature. Generally, posttreatment problems can be managed with conservative measures (e.g., skin cleansers, topical steroids). If complications persist, further medical and/or surgical intervention may be necessary.

CONCLUSION

Chemexfoliation is a safe and effective skin resurfacing technique to address a number of commonly encountered aging face problems. Chemical peels should be performed by experienced practitioners with detailed understanding of chemical peel agents to avoid possible complications.

Skin resurfacing with lasers

Benjamin Marcus

INTRODUCTION

Laser and light therapy for facial skin has become a mainstay of aesthetic practices. With the advent of newer technologies, we can offer patients treatments that span from minimal down time to major skin resurfacing—all with a high degree of safety and reliability.

BACKGROUND

The basic premise of laser and light therapy centers on the concept of the chromophore. Laser devices produce a singular frequency of light and that frequency is absorbed by particular color target or even water. With the correct chromophore and laser target pair, one can vaporize skin cells or gently target brown or red pigment (Figure 22.4).

Lasers can be classified into two main groups: ablative and nonablative lasers. Ablative lasers work by removing layers of skin cells. Nonablative lasers often target nonskin elements such as brown pigments or the red of blood vessels. Superficial or light ablative laser peels generally just ablate the outer surface (epithelium) of the skin. Medium-depth ablative laser peels penetrate into the upper (papillary) dermis. Deep ablative laser peels

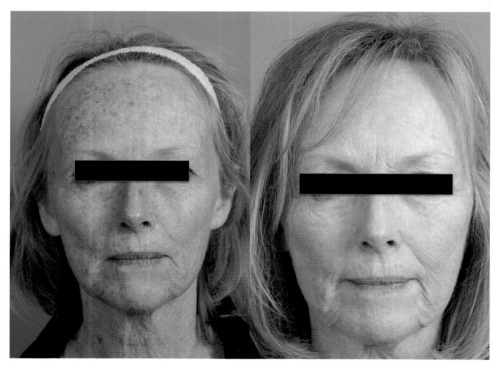

Figure 22.4 Patient before and after treatment with the noninvasive broad band light treatment.

are the most significant type of treatment and can reach into the upper reticular dermis. As with any wound, the closer one gets to the mid-reticular dermis, the greater the chance for scar or compromised wound healing.

Nonablative lasers generally bypass the epithelium and are absorbed by the deeper and pigmented elements of the skin. Examples include Nd:YAG lasers that target blood vessels or intense pulsed light that can target melanin.

INDICATIONS

Superficial ablative laser peels are indicated for patients who have very limited photoaging of the skin or for those patients who desire very minimal downtime. Patients can expect a mild improvement in their fine lines and minimal improvement in deeper rhytids. With repeated treatment, patients will note improvement in their skin pigmentation irregularities. Medium-depth and deep laser peels offer more significant ablation and therefore will have a more significant effect on fine lines and pigment variegation. At the deepest levels, the ablative laser peels can produce very significant skin results. A subcategory of ablative lasers is the fractional devices. These devices treat skin with microcolumns of ablative lasers that will create collagen and reduce wrinkles but trade a quicker recovery for a lesser overall result.

Conditions that are treated by nonablative lasers include photoaging of skin, solar lentigo, melasma, telangiectasias, and rosacea. Nonablative lasers can also be used for hair removal and other treatments but that is beyond the scope of this chapter. Laser and light therapies that target hemoglobin are suited to reduce telangiectasia and capillaries associated with photoaging or rosacea. Melanin is also removed with targeted light treatment from IPL or broadband light (BBL). The main advantage of nonablative treatments is their ability to improve skin appearance with little or no downtime (Figure 22.5).

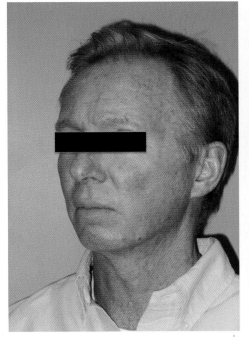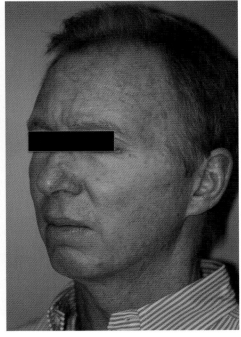

Figure 22.5 Patient after treatment with a Nd:YAG laser for reduction of capillaries.

TECHNICAL DETAILS

Nonablative laser treatments are almost always performed in the clinic setting and can be done with or without topical anesthesia. These can be performed by the physician or physician extender. Skin prep is performed with alcohol or acetone. Postprocedure care is centered on a gentle cleanser and moisturizer of choice. A limited skin peel may occur in 1–2 days followed by mild erythema. No viral prophylaxis is required.

Medium-depth and deep ablative treatments should be performed by the physician provider or by a physician extender under direct supervision. These procedures are usually performed in the clinic setting but may be combined with operative procedures. Skin prep is performed with alcohol or acetone. Postprocedure care is centered on an occlusive topical ointment such as Aquaphor or Vaseline. A full skin peel may occur in 2–3 days followed by moderate to significant erythema. Antiviral prophylaxis is required. Treatment endpoint for the deep peel is the upper reticular dermis. A full skin peel will occur in 2–3 days followed by significant erythema. Antiviral prophylaxis is required.

COMPLICATIONS

Complications associated with nonablative treatments are rare. Complications from ablative lasers include prolonged erythema, hypopigmentation, postinflammatory hyperpigmentation, and scar. Risk associated with superficial lasers is quite low with pigmentation changes and scarring at far less than 1%. As one moves into deeper peels, there is an increasing risk of pigmentation changes, especially hypopigmentation. This can reach as high as 15% with CO_2 lasers but is much lower with newer Er:YAG devices. For this reason, only experienced practitioners should perform deep laser resurfacing (Figure 22.6).

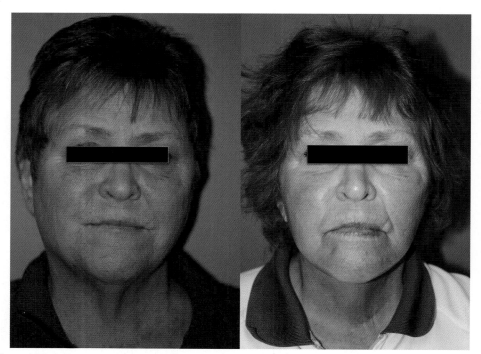

Figure 22.6 Patient before and after deep laser resurfacing. Photo is pre-procedure and 6 months post. Notice improvement in dyschromia and rhytids.

Advancement flaps

Laura T. Hetzler

DEFINITIONS AND CLINICAL FEATURES

Advancement flaps are local methods of tissue rearrangement that depend on the advancement of the surrounding tissue along a linear axis to close a defect. They may be unilateral, bilateral, or geometric in design to include V to Y or A to T closures (Figure 22.7). Classically, advancement flaps have a length-to-width ratio of 2:1 but can be designed at 3–4:1 within the head and neck secondary to its robust blood supply. With the increased length-to-width ratios, advancement flaps may create standing cutaneous deformities or "dog-ear" deformities. These deformities must also be addressed as part of the reconstructive plan.

UTILITY

Advancement flaps may be utilized following trauma or excision of benign and malignant lesions. Unilateral or bilateral advancement flaps are frequently used on the forehead or the upper lip where parallel limbs can fall within anatomic subunit lines, relaxed skin tension lines (RSTLs), or rhytids or if the vector of advancement will provide a favorable horizontal sling for support such as in eyelid reconstruction (Figure 22.8).

A to T closures are ideal when the defect abuts an anatomic border, such as the hairline, that is to remain mostly unmodified. V to Y advancement flaps recruit adjacent tissue that is pushed into the defect by closing the apex of the "V" primarily. These are best designed parallel to RSTLs.

WORKUP

Consideration of other reconstructive options need to be given in patients with poor overall health to include poorly controlled diabetes, smokers, or those with a history of bleeding disorders. Other deterrents to performing an advancement flap include those with concurrent local wound infection or those where tumor surveillance may be necessary or might be obscured by local flap creation.

EXECUTION

Advancement flaps are designed based on surrounding anatomy and subunit architecture.

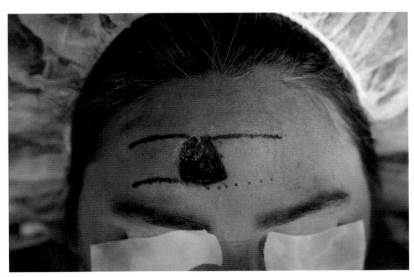

Figure 22.7 Designed bilateral advancement flaps.

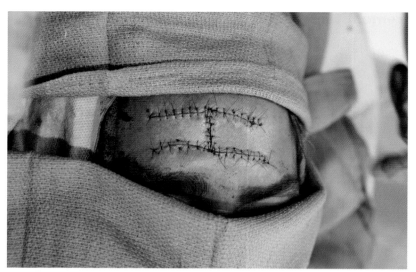

Figure 22.8 Closure of bilateral advancement flaps.

The flaps themselves are elevated deep to the dermis to preserve the subdermal plexus. Deep sutures of 4-0 or 5-0 Monocryl or Vicryl can be used in the deeper tissues for tension support. The skin itself may then be closed with 5-0 or 6-0 nylon or Prolene. Sutures are removed within 5–7 days and may be supported by taping at that time. Burow's triangles may be fashioned to improve the appearance of standing cutaneous or "dog-ear" deformities.

A to T flaps are designed to avoid distortion of a linear landmark such as the hairline or eyebrow. The defect is placed within the triangle of the "A" and the base of the triangle resting on the landmark to be preserved. Incisions are extended out from the base of the triangle and bilateral flaps are elevated within the subcutaneous plane (Figure 22.9). The bilateral flaps are advanced toward one another to create a "T"-shaped incision and scar (Figure 22.10).

V to Y advancement flaps are created by making a V-shaped incision involving the defect margin and advancing the broad base of the V into the defect

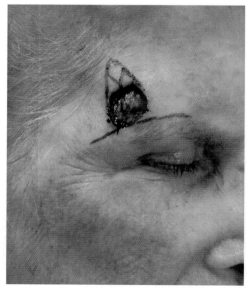

Figure 22.9 A to T flap designed superior to right brow with W-plasty superiorly to limit vertical extension of incisions.

leaving flap subcutaneously pedicled (Figures 22.11 through 22.13). The resulting defect is closed primarily resulting in a "Y" shape.

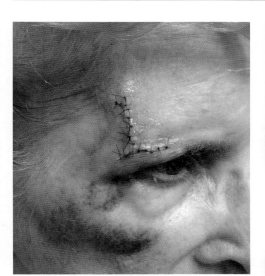

Figure 22.10 Closure of A to T flap.

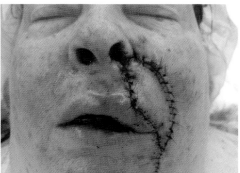

Figure 22.12 Closure with V to Y flap with subcutaneous pedicle.

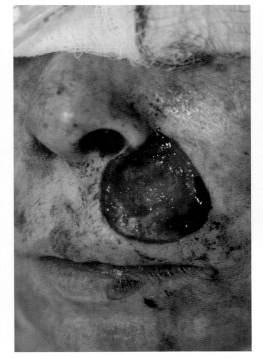

Figure 22.11 Large left upper lip and medial cheek defect.

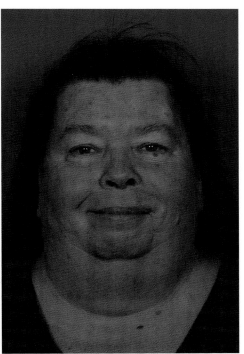

Figure 22.13 Four-month postoperative view.

COMPLICATIONS

Wound complications following advancement flaps include hematoma or infection. Poor scarring and wound dehiscence can be an issue when the closure is under tension. Ischemia and necrosis can occur with technical errors that include poor flap design and injury to the blood supply during dissection.

Transposition flaps

Laura T. Hetzler

DEFINITIONS AND CLINICAL FEATURES

Transposition flaps are local flaps harvested from an adjacent donor site and rotated over an incomplete bridge of skin to fill the proposed defect. Transposing tissue from a donor site leaves a secondary defect that must be closed primarily. Transposition flaps capitalize on adjacent skin laxity and redistribution of skin tension. The three classic transposition flap designs include the rhombic flap, bilobed flap, and Z-plasty. Resultant scars are geometric in shape and are ideally less conspicuous; however, the complex design of transposition flaps makes it difficult to create scars that will completely rest within RSTLs.

UTILITY

Transposition flaps may be utilized following trauma or excision of benign and malignant lesions as well as in scar revision. Rhomboid flaps have a wide range of utility to include reconstruction of the medial and lateral cheek, temple, chin, neck, lips, ears, and nose (Figure 22.14). Bilobed flaps are frequently elected with defects of the nasal tip and dorsum, temple, and cheek. A Z-plasty can be used in both reconstruction or more commonly to refine a preexisting scar when unsightly tethering or traction is occurring. Z-plasty principles allow reorientation of the scar to fall within RSTLs; lengthen a scar that is distorting an anatomic margin such as the eyelid, lip, or ala; and function in irregularization of a linear scar.

WORKUP

Consideration of other reconstructive options needs to be given in patients with poor overall health to include poorly

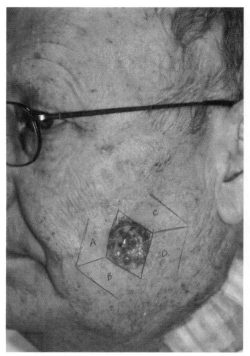

Figure 22.14 Left cheek defect, 3 cm × 3 cm, with a rhombus designed around the defect with angles of 60° and 120°. Two separate flaps can be extended from each 120° corner with the second limb drawn parallel to the adjacent side of the rhombus. The "D" flap was chosen as the optimal flap for reconstruction of this defect (see Figures 22.15 and 22.16).

controlled diabetes, smokers, or those with a history of bleeding disorders. Other deterrents to performing rotational flaps include those with concurrent local wound infection or those where tumor surveillance may be necessary or might be obscured by local flap creation. Patients on blood thinners or supplements that may act as anticoagulants are instructed to stop prior to their procedure.

EXECUTION

As in all local flaps, consideration must be given to adjacent areas of skin laxity and RSTLs; neighboring distortable landmarks such as the lid margin, ala, or lip; and nearby aesthetic subunits. The standard Limberg rhombic flap involves creating an equilateral parallelogram around a defect (Figure 22.15). The rhombus can be closed with one of four distinct flaps pending evaluation of the aforementioned considerations (Figure 22.16). Dufourmentel and the Webster modifications of the rhombic flap were designed to decrease angels of rotation resulting in less redundancy and smaller-standing cone deformities (Figure 22.17).

The bilobed flap is a double transposition flap that raises a second flap to fill the initial donor defect (Figure 22.18). The second donor site is then closed primarily. In the Esser modification, the total arc of rotation is 90° that creates less tension on the closure and less chance for a standing cone deformity. The first flap is designed to be

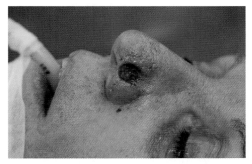

Figure 22.17 Left nasal alar and tip defect, 1.1 cm × 0.8 cm.

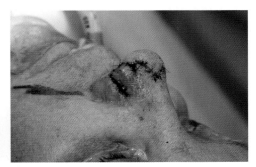

Figure 22.18 Transposed bilobed flap.

the size of the actual defect with the second flap being half of the initial flap. The donor site of the second flap is then closed primarily (Figure 22.19).

A Z-plasty is a double transposition flap used for scar revision. The central limb of the "Z" is based on the preexisting scar and the lateral limbs should be placed parallel to one another at equal angles from the central line. If the angles within the two transposition flaps are equal to 60°, a Z-plasty will lengthen a scar by 75%, while 45° and 30° designs lengthen scars by 50% and 25%, respectively. Deep sutures of 4-0 or 5-0 Monocryl or Vicryl can be used in the deeper tissues for tension support. The skin itself may then be closed with 5-0 or 6-0 nylon or Prolene. Sutures are removed within 5–7 days and may be supported by taping at that time.

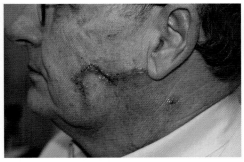

Figure 22.15 Closure of defect with rhombic transposition flap.

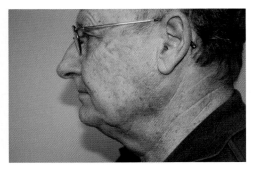

Figure 22.16 One-year postoperative view. Patient declined dermabrasion.

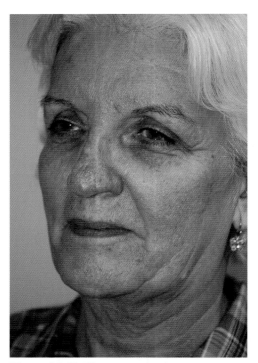

Figure 22.19 Three-month postoperative view.

COMPLICATIONS

Wound complications following advancement flaps include hematoma or infection. Poor scarring and wound dehiscence can be an issue when the closure is under tension. Ischemia and necrosis can occur with technical errors that include poor flap design and injury to the blood supply during dissection.

Rotation flaps

Laura T. Hetzler

DEFINITIONS AND CLINICAL FEATURES

Rotational flaps are named for the curved vector of motion around a fixed point or fulcrum into a defect. The flap is rotated along an arc that is ideally less than 30° toward the defect. The radius of the arc is approximately 2.5–3 times the diameter of the defect. The arc length is roughly four to five times the

width of the defect. It is rare to have a purely rotational flap without some component of advancement, and thus, these flaps are more appropriately labeled rotation/advancement flaps. The axis of rotation can be modified to increase or decrease the advancement contribution.

UTILITY

Rotation flaps may be utilized following trauma or excision of benign or malignant lesions (Figure 22.20). They allow reconstruction by mobilizing a large area of tissue with a wide vascularized base and rotating it into a theoretical triangular-shaped defect. Rotational flaps are used often in reconstruction of both the medial and lateral cheek. Double-rotation flaps, or the O to Z flap, may be used for scalp or facial reconstruction. For larger scalp defects, up to 50% triple rotation flaps can be used. Successful execution of rotational flaps bears the disadvantage of extensive undermining and dissection beyond the defect.

WORKUP

Consideration of other reconstructive options needs to be given in patients with poor overall health to include poorly controlled diabetes, smokers, or those with a history of bleeding disorders. Other deterrents to performing rotational flaps include those with concurrent local wound infection or those where tumor

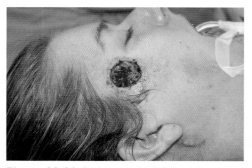

Figure 22.20 Right temple defect, 3.5 cm, post–melanoma excision.

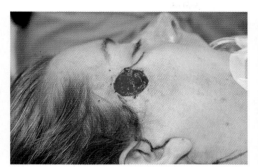

Figure 22.21 Proposed rotation advancement flap prior to reconstruction.

surveillance may be necessary or might be obscured by local flap creation.

EXECUTION
Rotational flaps are designed based on surrounding laxity of tissue and may have a variable component of advancement (Figure 22.21). The defect is best visualized as lying within a triangle though creation of a triangular-sized defect is not necessary. The flap itself is elevated deep to the dermis to preserve the subdermal plexus. The length of the flap is typically four to five times the diameter of the defect though may be less if there is significant tissue laxity or may be longer if more recruitment is needed. A Burow's triangle may be excised on the outer or longer limb of the arc to avoid bunching of the incision. Another standing cone deformity may occur in the region between the fulcrum and actual defect. Deep sutures of 4-0 or 5-0 Monocryl or Vicryl can be used in the deeper tissues for tension support. The skin itself may then be closed with 5-0 or 6-0 nylon or Prolene. Sutures are removed within 5–7 days and may be supported by taping at that time (Figure 22.22).

COMPLICATIONS
Wound complications following advancement flaps include hematoma or infection. Poor scarring and wound dehiscence can be an issue when the closure is under tension.

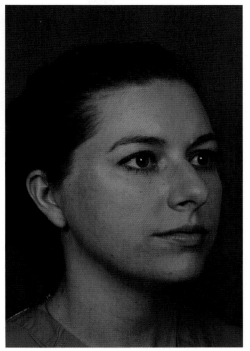

Figure 22.22 Ten-month postoperative result.

Ischemia and necrosis can occur with technical errors that include poor flap design and injury to the blood supply during dissection.

Interpolated flaps

Laura T. Hetzler

DEFINITIONS AND CLINICAL FEATURES
An interpolated flap is an example of a local flap that crosses over or under intervening tissue remaining attached to its blood supply by a pedicle. The blood supply is often a named artery and vein; however, the flap can be based off of a region of vessel confluence allowing the pedicle to have a robust blood supply for the distal flap. These so-called axial patterned flaps have a more generous blood supply and can therefore be designed longer than their random blood supply local flap counterparts. Pedicled flaps are typically two-stage flaps that require division and

inset at a later date once external blood supply has been established from surrounding tissue. In comparison to the transposition flap, whose base is adjacent to the defect to be repaired, an interpolated flap is harvested when surrounding tissue has poor mobility or is insufficient for reconstruction. The classic axial patterned facial interpolated flap is the paramedian forehead flap based off of the supratrochlear artery. An interpolated cheek flap (melolabial flap), loosely based off of branches of the facial artery, is an interpolated flap that is not uniformly described as having axial blood supply. The pedicle may include epidermis or be based off of the subcutaneous tissue.

UTILITY

Pedicle flaps may be utilized following trauma or excision of benign and malignant lesions. The paramedian forehead flap is frequently used to repair extensive defects of the nasal dorsum, nasal tip, ala, or full-thickness columella (Figure 22.23). The forehead flap may also be used as internal nasal lining either by reflecting the skin paddle internally or by creating a longer

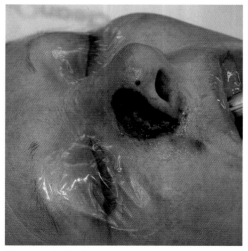

Figure 22.23 Preoperative right nasal ala and nasal sidewall defect.

flap folded at the alar rim, as described by Menick, to recreate vestibular lining.

The interpolated melolabial flap is used commonly for alar reconstruction when the entire alar subunit is missing. It has been used successfully in columellar reconstruction and may be used to recreate nasal lining as well.

WORKUP

Consideration of other reconstructive options needs to be given in patients with poor overall health to include poorly controlled diabetes, smokers, or those with a history of bleeding disorders. Patients that are smokers may have minimal initial flap manipulation and thinning and may undergo intermediate stages of refinement prior to pedicle division. Pedicle division may also be delayed in smokers or in patients that have been previously radiated.

Other deterrents to performing an interpolated flap include those with concurrent local wound infection or those where tumor surveillance may be necessary or might be obscured by local flap creation. Given the staged nature of an interpolated flap, expedient division and inset need to be planned if postoperative radiation therapy is needed. Patients that are unable to perform wound care related to the pedicle or are deemed unreliable to have an open wound for a period of time should not have a pedicled reconstruction.

EXECUTION

Interpolated flaps are elected based on inadequate adjacent tissue or improved aesthetic outcomes related to the skin thickness and texture afforded by the pedicled tissue. In nasal defects greater than 1.5 cm, the paramedian forehead flap offers large quantities of tissue coverage that closely matches the thickness, texture, and sebaceous quality of the native nasal skin. The paramedian forehead flap is designed based off of the supratrochlear artery. The neurovascular bundle is located between 1.7 and 2.2 cm from the midline glabella at the medial edge of the eyebrow. The nasal defect is then measured and a template is created. If greater than 50% of the nasal subunit is affected, the remaining portion of the subunit is often completely excised for improved aesthetic outcomes. The template is then reflected to the forehead and outlined superior to the neurovascular bundle. A 1.3–1.5 cm pedicle is designed centered on the supratrochlear neurovascular bundle (Figure 22.24). Elevation of the flap is performed in the subgaleal plane for the distal portions of the flap. The subperiosteal layer may be entered approximately 2 cm superior to the neurovascular bundle to protect axial blood supply. The distal flap may be thinned down

to the subdermal plexus and reflected inferiorly to the nasal defect. Securing the flap to the surrounding defect skin can be performed with 6-0 nylon or Prolene. If the flap is extending down to the vestibular lining, 5-0 chromic may be used.

The recommended period of 2–4 weeks should be allowed prior to division and inset (Figures 22.25 and 22.26). Patients that are smokers typically wait 4 weeks and may undergo an intermediate thinning stage prior to pedicle division.

The interpolated melolabial flap is designed based off of the alar facial crease in the region of the facial artery at the takeoff of the angular artery. It can be used for reconstruction of the alar subunit as well as the columella. The nasal defect is again

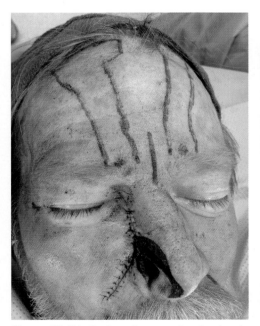

Figure 22.24 Design of paramedian forehead flap with single dot overlying the vascular pedicle 1.8 cm away from midline and a 1.5 cm pedicle. The patient is a heavy smoker and has already undergone advancement of the right cheek with bony fixation to the maxilla. Two paramedian forehead flaps are planned for intranasal lining and external skin coverage.

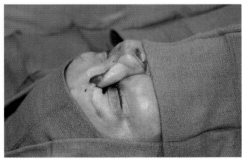

Figure 22.25 Right-sided paramedian forehead flap with pedicle in place.

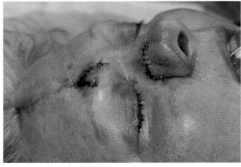

Figure 22.26 Right-sided paramedian forehead flap.

measured and a template created. The template should be placed with its medial edge at the nasolabial crease. The flap is designed with either a cutaneous or subcutaneous pedicle and sutured into the defect with 6-0 nylon to the nasal skin and 5-0 chromic for the nasal lining. The time period between the division and inset is similar to that of the paramedian forehead flap.

COMPLICATIONS

Wound complications following interpolated flaps are less common than are seen in random flaps as there is a more robust blood supply. Ischemia and necrosis can still occur with technical errors that include poor flap design and injury to the blood supply during dissection. Hematoma, infection, poor scarring, and wound dehiscence can occur as well.

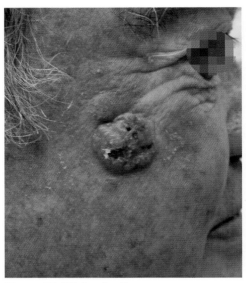

Figure 22.27 Basal cell carcinoma.

Skin cancer and Mohs micrographic surgery

Celeste Gary and Laura T. Hetzler

DEFINITIONS AND CLINICAL FEATURES

Skin cancer is the most common cancer in humans. While cancer can arise from all cell types that compose the skin, the most common forms of cutaneous malignancies involve cancers of the epidermis:

1. Basal cell carcinoma from epidermal precursor cells (Figure 22.27)
2. Squamous cell carcinoma from differentiated epidermal cells (Figure 22.28)
3. Melanoma from melanocytes (Figure 22.29)

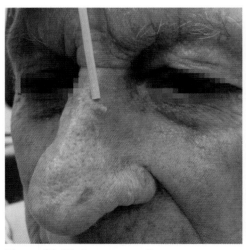

Figure 22.28 Squamous cell carcinoma.

Other skin malignancies include Merkel cell carcinoma from neuroendocrine cells, sebaceous carcinoma from sebaceous glands, eccrine carcinoma from eccrine glands, microcystic adnexal carcinoma from eccrine glands, extramammary Paget's disease from apocrine glands, dermatofibrosarcoma protuberans from fibroblasts, atypical fibroxanthoma from fibroblasts, malignant fibrous histiocytoma from fibroblasts, angiosarcoma from endothelial cells, and leiomyosarcoma from smooth muscle.

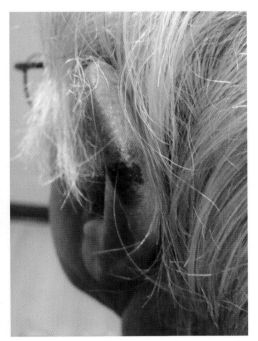

Figure 22.29 Melanoma. (Photo courtesy of Chad Prather.)

DIFFERENTIAL DIAGNOSIS

There are a wide variety of benign skin lesions that can appear concerning for skin cancer. Special consideration should also be given to premalignant lesions including actinic keratoses, Bowen's disease, and keratoacanthoma.

WORKUP

Individuals with fair skin and light eyes are more prone to skin cancers. The patient should be questioned about sun exposure history and history of prior skin cancers. Tanning bed usage has become a significant risk factor for melanoma in younger populations. A family history of melanoma should also be elucidated.

Principles of self-examination and public screening are often referred to as the A, B, C, D, and Es of melanoma: A = asymmetry, B = irregular borders, C = color variations, D = diameter > 6 mm, and E = evolving over time (Figure 22.29).

A thorough examination of the skin of the scalp, ears, face, and neck should be performed. Irregular areas that appear discolored, painful, ulcerated, raised, or otherwise abnormal should be biopsied.

Biopsy methods include

1. Shave biopsy
2. Punch biopsy
3. Incisional biopsy
4. Excisional biopsy

Diagnosis is determined by permanent pathology of the specimen.

Shave biopsy should be avoided in hyperpigmented lesions concerning for melanoma. If the lesion is small enough for excisional biopsy with primary closure, this may be performed with a 2 mm margin. In larger lesions that are not amenable to excision with simple closure, punch biopsy through the thickest portion of the hyperpigmented area is recommended.

TREATMENT

The mainstay of skin cancer treatment is wide local excision. The goal of surgery is complete removal of the skin cancer with clear margins.

This can be accomplished in two ways:

1. Excision with measured marked margins:
   a. Goal margins for skin cancer by type (margins may be modified to accommodate individual anatomic or functional considerations):
      i. Basal cell carcinoma < 2 cm: 4 mm
      ii. Basal cell carcinoma > 2 cm: >4 mm
      iii. Squamous cell carcinoma < 2 cm: 4–6 mm
      iv. Squamous cell carcinoma > 2 cm: 9 mm
      v. Melanoma in situ: 1.0 cm

      vi. Melanoma $\leq$ 1.0 mm: 1.0 cm

     vii. Melanoma 1.01–2.0 mm: 1–2 cm

   viii. Melanoma > 2.01: 2.0 cm

2. Mohs excision that provides complete margin examination

    a. Advantages include a high rate of complete excision and skin cancer cure and narrower initial surgical margins that is advantageous for lesions next to complex structures of the head and neck, for example, the eye, lip, and nasal valve.

Techniques such as cryotherapy, CO_2 laser ablation, and radiation therapy also have roles in the treatment of skin cancer.

Scar revision

Laura T. Hetzler

DEFINITIONS AND CLINICAL FEATURES
Scar revision is performed to improve upon the appearance or position of a scar. It may also be necessary to resolve a scar's distorting effects on nearby structures. Scar revision may include reorientation of the existing scar to fall within RSTLs or alter the scar to more closely approximate a nearby facial subunit border. Irregularization procedures such as running W-plasty or geometric broken line closure can be performed to camouflage a previously linear scar that is more easily recognized by the human eye. Distortion of free facial margins such as the lip, eyelid, or alar rim by suboptimal scars can be released by Z-plasty techniques that provide scar lengthening, reorientation, and irregularization (Figure 22.30).

DIFFERENTIAL DIAGNOSIS
Scar revision may be considered in any setting of suboptimal healing following accidental trauma, surgery, or prior reconstruction. Scars may be considered

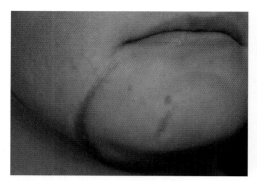

Figure 22.30 Preoperative suboptimal scar following dog bite 14 months prior.

unfavorable because of their relationship to facial anatomic units or RSTLs. Risk factors for poor scarring include unfavorable incision angle, depth, and mechanism of injury, wounds that are subject to persistent contractile forces, or pathologic healing process such as infection or poor wound care. Contributing factors include suboptimal repair technique such as inadequate closure, traumatic closure with poor tissue handling, or excessive cautery. Consideration to underlying soft tissue contraction must be considered as well before a cutaneous refinement is attempted.

WORKUP
Facial and skin analysis must be addressed prior to scar revision. Expectations must be managed preoperatively by explaining that any scar revision is simply replacing one scar with another that is anticipated to be more aesthetically acceptable.

The timing of scar revision does require some understanding of wound healing. Scars mature or remodel over 12–18 months with the strength attained being only 80% of the native tissue preinjury. A patient's ability to heal must be assessed as well. Diabetics, smokers, or patients on prolonged systemic steroids or with poor nutritional status and impaired microvascular circulation need to be informed of the limitations in their aptitude to heal. Attention should be paid to patients with a history of poor scar formation such as those with a tendency to hypertrophic or keloid scarring.

TREATMENT

Goals of intervention: (1) reorientation of the scar in the direction of RSTLs or aligning it more optimally with an anatomic landmark or subunit, (2) interruption of the length of the scar making it less visible, (3) release of a contracted scar by lengthening, and (4) optimization of the relationship of the superficial scar to the deeper scar.

MEDICAL MANAGEMENT

Nonsurgical treatment includes cosmetics for camouflage. Further prevention of poor scar formation may be possible with application of pressure dressings, silicone, or polyurethane sheeting.

Less invasive measures include dermabrasion, laser resurfacing, or steroid injections. Triamcinolone acetate 10 mg/mL can be used for intralesional injections at bimonthly intervals to prevent further thickening or promote softening of a forming scar. Nonsurgical treatment of keloid scars may involve intralesional injection of triamcinolone acetate 40 mg/1 mL approximately every 4 weeks. Recent support of injections of 5-FU for preexisting keloids has been described.

SURGICAL MANAGEMENT

Simple excision is an option for shorter depressed keloid or hypertrophic scars. Serial excision of widened thicker scars or keloid scars may be necessary. Postexcision injection with triamcinolone acetate with or without the addition of 5FU is frequently recommended following keloid excision. Tension-free closure is paramount. Radiation therapy has been used in the past to avoid recurrence.

Irregularization is the act of turning a linear scar into an irregularly shaped scar in the hopes of being less perceptible. How this principle assists in scar camouflage

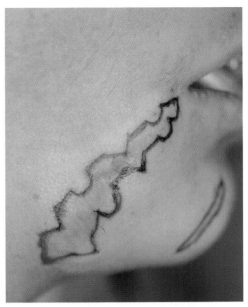

Figure 22.31 Intraoperative template for GBLC (Photo courtesy of Jonathan Sykes).

requires an understanding of wound and scar dynamics as well as how linearity is perceived by the human eye. Linear scars have a tendency to bowstring over surfaces. The original scar is excised within the new construct and care is taken to reapproximate the skin edges. GBLC, running W-plasty, and Z-plasty are all options of irregularization (Figure 22.31).

Z-PLASTY

Z-plasty is an irregularization and lengthening procedure. The classic Z-plasty has three limbs of equal length set at identical angles from one another. The amount of lengthening needed determines the angle used. For example, utilizing an angle of 60° will yield a 75% length increase; a 45° angle, a 50% length increase; and a 30° angle, a 25% length increase. The final result places the central limb (previous scar) perpendicular to its original orientation and lengthens the linear dimension. The lateral limbs need to be designed as parallel as possible to RSTLs. Z-plasty may also be performed in a serial fashion for longer contracture-type scars for additive lengthening and irregularization.

W-PLASTY

W-plasty is an irregularization procedure that allows the surgeon to interrupt the linear perception of a scar. This procedure consists of creating consecutive small triangular flaps on opposing sides of a scar to be excised. Typically, a triangle should not be taller than 6 mm with angles 90° or less. W-plasty is a great option for long curvilinear scars with larger triangular flaps designed on the outer curve of the wound. Precise angular excision must be performed with an 11 blade scalpel. Deep closure must be used to reduce epidermal tension.

GEOMETRIC BROKEN LINE CLOSURE

GBLC is an irregular irregularization procedure based on the same illusory principles as the W-plasty. The goal is to create an irregular linear scar that is less visible than those produced from a regular patterned configuration such as in the W-plasty. Similar to the W-plasty, GBLC does not lengthen the original scar. The design of GBLC utilizes a pattern of irregular geometric shapes on opposing sides of the scar to be excised. Use of angles shapes (squares, triangles) rather than curvilinear shapes (half circles) allows for more precise healing and approximation (Figure 22.32).

CONTRAINDICATIONS

Scar revision is to be avoided in patients with limited chances for a favorable or improved outcome. Often, a period of reassurance is needed as the new revised scar will be more noticeable in the acute setting than the previous chronic scar.

Avoid intervention in patients that are not psychologically prepared or have unrealistic expectations. Relative contraindications exist

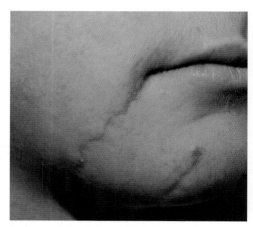

Figure 22.32 2.5-month follow-up from GBLC scar revision (Photo courtesy of Jonathan Sykes).

for those with a history of hypertrophic or keloid scarring.

References

1. Baker TJ, Gordon HL. 1961. The ablation of rhytids by chemical means: A preliminary report. *Journal of the Florida Medical Association* 48:451.
2. Hetter GP. 2000. An examination of the phenol-croton oil peel: Part IV. Face peel results with different concentrations of phenol and croton oil. *Plastic and Reconstructive Surgery* 105(3):1061–1083.
3. Fitzpatrick TB. 1988. The validity and practicality of sun-reactive skin types I–VI. *Archives of Dermatology* 124:869.
4. Brody HJ. 1989. Complications of chemical peeling. *Journal of Dermatologic Surgery* 15:1010.
5. Monheit GD. 1994. Advances in chemical peeling. *Facial Plastic Surgery Clinics of North America* 2(1):7.
6. Baldwin HE, Nighland M, Kendall C, Mays DA, Grossman R, Newburger J. 2013. 40 years of topical tretinoin use in review. *Journal of Drugs in Dermatology* 12(6):638–642.

Suggested reading

Bailey BJ, Johnson JT, Kohut RI et al. 2006a. *Head and Neck Surgery-Otolaryngology*, 4th ed. Philadelphia, PA: Lippincott Williams & Wilkins, pp. 2357–2368.

Bailey BJ, Johnson JT, Kohut RI et al. 2006b. *Head and Neck Surgery-Otolaryngology*, 4th ed. Philadelphia, PA: Lippincott Williams & Wilkins, pp. 2411–2420.

Bailey BJ, Johnson JT, Kohut RI et al. 2006c. *Head and Neck Surgery-Otolaryngology*, 4th ed. Philadelphia, PA: Lippincott Williams & Wilkins, pp. 2421–2452.

Bailey BJ, Johnson JT, Kohut RI et al. 2006d. *Head and Neck Surgery-Otolaryngology*, 4th ed. Philadelphia, PA: Lippincott Williams & Wilkins, pp. 1455–1468.

Baker S. 2007. *Local Flaps in Facial Reconstruction*, 2nd ed. Philadelphia, PA: Elsevier Inc.

Myers EN. 2008. *Operative Otolaryngology-Head and Neck Surgery*, 2nd ed. Philadelphia, PA: Elsevier, pp. 719–736.

National Comprehensive Cancer Network Version 2. 2014: Melanoma.

Papel I. 2009. *Facial Plastic and Reconstructive Surgery*, 3rd ed. New York: Thieme Medical Publishers, Inc., pp. 59–66.

Papel I. 2009. *Facial Plastic and Reconstructive Surgery*, 3rd ed. New York: Thieme Medical Publishers, Inc., pp. 41–58, 807–820.

Papel I. 2009. *Facial Plastic and Reconstructive Surgery*, 3rd ed. New York: Thieme Medical Publishers, Inc., pp. 721–744.

Patel K, Sykes J. 2011. Concepts in local flap design and classification. *Operative Techniques in Otolaryngology-Head and Neck Surgery* 22(1):12–23.

CHAPTER 23

Medical and Surgical Hair Restoration

Lane D. Squires and Jonathan Sykes

- **Definitions and clinical features**
- **Differential diagnosis**
- **Pertinent anatomy**
- **Clinical workup**
- **Treatment: Medical therapy**
- **Treatment: Surgical therapy**
- **Complications**
- **References**

Definitions and clinical features

A person's physical appearance conveys immediate information to the beholder and can dramatically affect social and cultural perceptions. Western society places high regard on the appearance of youthfulness and abundant hair is integral in projecting a youthful image. Early or significant loss of hair, or alopecia, may lead to diminished perceptions of one's attractiveness, assertiveness, or youthfulness.[1] While this process is biologically benign, appearance alterations that result from alopecia can negatively impact the individual's quality of life.[2]

There are multiple etiologies of alopecia, each with varied clinical and pathological findings. Two main categories exist: permanent versus temporary alopecias. Permanent alopecias caused by inflammatory infiltrates lead to scarring within the scalp, whereas the nonscarring permanent alopecias impair the hair follicle without signs of inflammation.[3] Otolaryngologists largely diagnose and treat the latter type, with the most common form being androgenic alopecia (AGA). AGA was formally known as male pattern baldness; however, since AGA can affect adult females in a similar pattern, the term "male pattern baldness" is no longer used. Alopecia areata is another common form of nonscarring permanent alopecia seen by otolaryngologists. The patchy diffuse hair loss seen in alopecia areata is caused by an unknown autoimmune phenomenon.

Differential diagnosis

Alopecia may result from a vast number of endocrine disorders, including hypopituitarism, hypothyroidism, hypoparathyroidism, diabetes mellitus, hyperprolactinemia, polycystic ovary syndrome, and Cushing syndrome.[4] Additional associations have been shown with dyslipidemia and cardiovascular disease.[5] Other etiologies should be considered, such as fungal infections, medication-induced hair loss (chemotherapeutics, oral contraceptives, anabolic steroids), poor nutrition, or prior trauma. It is important that the clinician consider and diagnose any treatable medical conditions prior to initiating definitive treatment for hair loss.

Pertinent anatomy

Human hair follicles all share a common, basic structure and growth pattern (Figure 23.1) despite varying dramatically in their size and shape, based on their location or exposure to androgen.[6] The dermally based hair bulb is responsible for housing the rapidly proliferating matrix cells that manufacture the hair shaft. Hair pigment is produced by melanocytes within the matrix

of the bulb. The dermal papilla is at the base of every hair bulb and helps regulate the timing of proliferation for each hair follicle. Each human is born with a limited number of follicles. Of the approximately 5 million total hair follicles, 150,000 are located in the scalp.[6] Hair follicles are continuously regenerating in a cyclical process. The stages of a follicle's morphogenesis are known as anagen (growth), catagen (involution), and telogen (quiescence). Though each hair follicle is constantly recycling, no new follicles develop after birth.[6]

Despite its many limitations, the current standard used by most clinicians for categorizing male pattern hair loss is the Norwood–Hamilton classification system.[8,9] This system includes seven categories, accounting for the hair loss along the anterior hairline and the vertex of the scalp (Figure 23.2).[10] Typically, bitemporal recession occurs first, followed by balding of the vertex, with subsequent unification of both hair loss areas across the entire frontoparietal region, sparing only the inferior occipital and temporal scalp. While females can also be categorized using this system, the Ludwig classification system may best reflect actual female pattern loss, especially loss seen with AGA (Figure 23.3).[11]

Clinical workup

A thorough history and physical examination should be performed on every patient focusing on the timing and pattern of hair loss, rapidity of progression, prior attempted therapies, and coexisting medical conditions. A thorough review of the patient's family history should be performed, focusing on direct ancestors with early hair loss and the presence of metabolic or endocrine disorders.

Quantifying the degree of hair loss can be accomplished by several methods, depending on the level of invasiveness.[12] Noninvasive measures include clinical inspection,

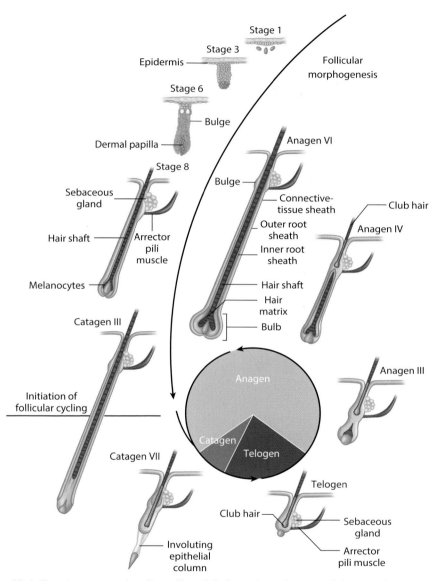

Figure 23.1 Development and cycling of hair follicles: selected stages of the morphogenesis of hair follicles and the three stages of follicular cycling (anagen, catagen, and telogen) are shown. The roman numerals indicate morphologic substages of anagen and catagen. The pie chart shows the proportion of time the hair follicle spends in each stage. (From Paus, R and Cotsarelis, G, *N. Engl. J. Med.*, 341, 491, 1999.)

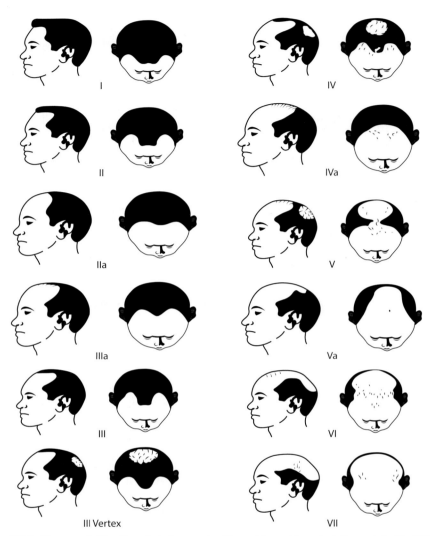

Figure 23.2 Norwood–Hamilton hair loss scale. (From Hong, H et al., *J. Dermatol.*, 40, 102, 2013.)

trichoscopy, self-assessment questionnaires, daily hair counts, standardized wash testing, or global photographs. A trichogram, or direct sampling of 50–100 hairs via plucking from the frontal and occipital scalp, is a semi-invasive method to assess the degree of loss. However, use of the trichogram has fallen out of favor due to its increased invasiveness and resulting pain.

Finally, a scalp biopsy can be considered to help determine the cause of alopecia; however, this too is often deferred for noninvasive measures. Unfortunately, no single diagnostic method has been shown to be preferable over others. The clinician is thus left to determine their most preferred route to measure hair loss in their patient population.

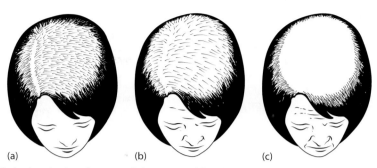

Figure 23.3 Ludwig's classification of the types of female-type androgenetic alopecia. (a) Perceptible thinning of the hair on the crown. (b) Pronounced thinning of the hair on the crown. (c) Full baldness of the hair on the crown. (From Ludwig, E, *Br. J. Dermatol.*, 97, 247, 1977.)

Treatment: Medical therapy

Patients who seek medical or surgical therapies for hair restoration will have likely experienced unwelcomed attention due to their alopecia. Practitioners should approach these patients with individualized treatment strategies, as each patient's motivation for seeking medical assistance and anticipated outcomes of their therapy will vary dramatically. Taking an individualized approach will increase the likelihood of establishing realistic expectations and improve the chance of satisfying the patient.

Prior to seeking medical therapies, some patients will try the use of hair prosthetics (hair pieces, wigs, toupees) to temporarily ameliorate appearance changes associated with alopecia.[13] Two main medical therapies exist for treatment of alopecia. Topical minoxidil is often the first-line medical therapy attempted. Minoxidil is a potent vasodilator that influences hair follicle growth via the increased blood flow to the remaining dermal papillae. Its use is encouraged once to twice daily and should be used indefinitely to ensure continued vascular nourishment to existing follicles. For patients with AGA, finasteride may be used as first-line therapy. Finasteride, or its counterpart, dutasteride, is an orally administered 5-alpha reductase inhibitor. Patients with AGA have been shown to have increased 5-alpha reductase

activity, which increases the local production of dihydrotestosterone. This hormonal change leads to the loss of hair follicles by an unknown mechanism. Blocking this hormonal effect can lead to cessation of hair follicle loss and improve hair strength for up to 86% of patients.[14] Unfortunately, the effects of 5-alpha reductase inhibitors are maintained only as long as a patient uses the medication.

Treatment: Surgical therapy

Traditional hair transplantation techniques, such as plug grafts, scalp reductions, and rotational flaps, have been replaced with follicular unit transplantation. Follicular units are naturally occurring groups of one to four terminal hairs. A midoccipital donor strip of scalp is excised (approximately 1 cm in width by 10–30 cm in length) at a level just below the hair follicles within the subcutaneous fat layer.[15] Using a magnification, hair technicians separate the donor scalp into vertical graft segments consisting of one to four hairs. Superficial stab incisions are made into the recipient hairline in a grid pattern and grafts are inserted with proper orientation, angulation, and great care so as not to crush the follicle itself. Generally, the appropriate thickness can be achieved when transplanting 20–40 follicular units per square centimeter; however, patients should be counseled that two to four grafting sessions may be required to recreate a substantial anterior hairline and an increase in overall hair density. Postoperatively, antibiotics, pain medication, and moistening sprays with saline are used until that patient is allowed to shower and shampoo gently after 72 hours.

Complications

While relatively uncommon, there are a few complications from follicular unit transplantation that every clinician should review with their patients prior to the procedure. In general, scarring is insignificant; however, repeated donor harvests may lead to a more noticeable midoccipital scar over time. The transplantation itself may induce temporary hair loss (telogen effluvium) in both the donor and the recipient areas as a result of the surgical manipulation of the adjacent hairs. This hair loss may last up to 3 months, but patients are to be reassured that hair regrowth will occur. Temporary decreased sensation along the scalp above the donor site may occur. Ingrown hairs or epidermal cysts may develop in a delayed fashion, weeks after the original procedure.

References

1. Muscarella F, Cunningham MR. 1996. The evolutionary significance and social perception of male pattern baldness and facial hair. *Ethology and Sociobiology* 17:99–117.
2. Cash TF. 1999. The psychological consequences of androgenic alopecia: A review of the research literature. *British Journal of Dermatology* 141:398–405.
3. Olsen EA, Bergfeld WF, Cotsarelis G et al. 2003. Summary of North American Hair Research Society (NAHRS)-sponsored Workshop on Cicatricial Alopecia, Duke University Medical Center, February 10 and 11, 2001. *Journal of the American Academy of Dermatology* 48:103–110.
4. Wiwanitkit S, Wiwanitkit V. 2013. Alopecia due to common metabolic diseases. *Diabetes Metabolic Syndrome* 7:116–117.
5. Arias-Santiago S, Gutiérrez-Salmerón MT, Buendía-Eisman A, Girón-Prieto MS, Naranjo-Sintes R. 2010. A comparative study of dyslipidemia in men and woman with androgenic alopecia. *Acta Dermato-Venereologica* 90:485–487.
6. Whiting DA. 2004. *The Structure of the Human Hair Follicle: Light Microscopy of Vertical and Horizontal sections of Scalp Biopsies.* Fairfield, NJ: Canfield Publishing.
7. Paus R, Cotsarelis G. 1999. The biology of hair follicles. *New England Journal of Medicine* 341:491–497.
8. Hamilton JB. 1951. Patterned loss of hair in men: Types and incidence. *Annals of the New York Academy of Science* 53:708–728.
9. Norwood OT, Shiell RC. 1984. *Hair Transplant Surgery.* Springfield, IL: Charles C Thomas.
10. Hong H, Ji JH, Lee Y, Kang H, Choi GS, Lee WS. 2013. Reliability of the pattern hair loss classifications: A comparison of the basic and specific and Norwood–Hamilton classifications. *Journal of Dermatology* 40:102–106.
11. Ludwig E. 1977. Classification of the types of androgenetic alopecia (common baldness) occurring in the female sex. *British Journal of Dermatology* 97:247–254.
12. Dhurat R, Saraogi P. 2009. Hair evaluation methods: Merits and demerits. *International Journal of Trichology* 1:108–119.
13. Tsuboi R, Itami S, Inui S, Ueki R, Katsuoka K, Kurata S, Kono T, Saito N, Manabe M, Yamazaki M. 2012. Guidelines for the management of androgenetic alopecia (2010). *Journal of Dermatology* 39:113–120.
14. Rossi A, Cantisani C, Scarnò M, Trucchia A, Fortuna MC, Calvieri S. 2011. Finasteride, 1 mg daily administration on male androgenetic alopecia in different age groups: 10-year follow-up. *Dermatology and Therapy* 24:455–461.
15. Bernstein RM, Rassman WR. 1999. The logic of follicular unit transplantation. *Dermatologic Clinics* 17:277–295.

Trauma

Sean Weiss, Laura T. Hetzler, Christopher Tran, Celeste Gary, Neal M. Jackson, and Daniel W. Nuss

- **Mandible fractures**
- **Le Fort fractures**
- **Orbital floor fractures**
- **Zygomatic fractures**
- **Nasal trauma**
- **Frontal sinus trauma**
- **Facial reanimation**
- **References**
- **Bibliography**
- **Suggested reading**

Mandible fractures

Sean Weiss and Laura T. Hetzler

DEFINITION AND CLINICAL FEATURES

Mandible fractures are typically caused by blunt trauma and are most often associated with sports injury, vehicle accidents, assaults, and falls. The prominent nature of the adult human mandible makes it particularly susceptible to injury, as it is frequently the initial point of contact for trauma.

The mandible has an interesting anatomy and relationship with its surrounding structures. The bone has an outer and inner cortex with a cancellous inner layer. The anatomic components of the mandible include the condyle, the coronoid process, ramus, angle, body, parasymphysis, symphysis, and alveolus (Figure 24.1). The most common areas of fracture are the parasymphyseal region, the angle, and the subcondylar region.[1]

The mandible has 16 teeth associated with it, and their occlusal relationship with the teeth of the maxilla is important to consider when addressing mandible fractures. Angle's classification of dental occlusion uses the mesiobuccal cusp of the maxillary

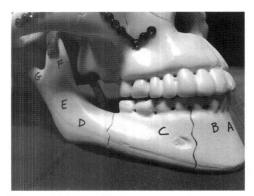

Figure 24.1 Mandibular anatomy: A—symphysis, B—parasymphysis (canine to canine), C—body, D—angle, E—ramus, F—coronoid process, G—condyle.

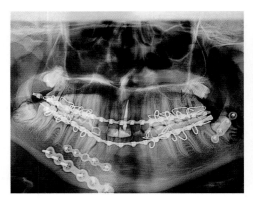

Figure 24.2 Panorex showing right parasymphyseal and left angle fractures postrepair with open reduction internal fixation methods and intermaxillary fixation with arch bars.

first molar as a point of reference to classify various types of dental occlusion.

It is important also to have knowledge of the relationship of the mandible and the various muscles of mastication. These muscles impose forces on the mandible that can either displace fractured segments of bone or hold fractured segments in a reduced position. When the segments are distracted from one another, it is considered to be an unfavorable fracture, and when the segments are pulled toward the reduced position, it is considered to be favorable.

PHYSICAL EXAM

A detailed physical exam is usually sufficient for diagnosing a mandibular fracture. Common findings include intraoral bleeding, pain, swelling, trismus, malocclusion, and deviation of the jaw upon opening. Other findings may include a palpable step-off at the fracture site, ecchymosis of the cheek, skin, or mucosa, and the ability to elicit pain with manipulation of the mandible or with biting. The fracture may also involve one or more teeth with bleeding, loose, or missing teeth.

IMAGING

Panoramic radiographs of the jaw or panorex provides the most information at the least expense (Figure 24.2). While the panorex

will detect mandible fractures more accurately, if the patient is not cooperative, a mandibular series is indicated.[2] This would include lateral oblique views, posterior–anterior view, and Towne's view. Computed tomography (CT) scans can provide more detailed information of fractures; however, they are costly and typically not necessary (Figure 24.3). The panorex should be the imaging modality of choice.

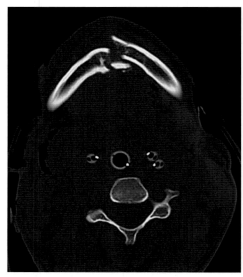

Figure 24.3 Comminuted symphyseal fracture.

TREATMENT

The basic principles of managing mandible fractures require establishment of preinjury dental occlusion, reduction of the fracture, and stabilization until the bone has healed. Stabilization can be achieved by either semi-rigid or rigid fixation.

Semirigid fixation allows for some movement at the fracture line and is acceptable for minimally displaced, favorable fractures. Semirigid fixation can be accomplished through techniques such as placement of arch bars with interdental wiring, Ivy loops, external fixation devices, and four-screw intermaxillary fixation. The mandible is held in preinjury dental occlusion by heavy elastic bands or wire. Fixation is maintained for 2–6 weeks. Traditionally, longer periods of fixation have been used; however, satisfactory healing occurs with fixation for only 2 weeks and allows for quicker recovery of maximal mouth opening, better oral hygiene, and less weight loss in appropriately selected patients.[3]

Rigid fixation involves the use of plates and/or screws for fracture fixation and immobilization of the fracture segments. The most common material used is titanium. After reduction has been accomplished, in most cases a plate is positioned over the fracture line and secured using screws placed into healthy bone on either side of the fracture. Care is taken when selecting the plate to ensure that it is strong enough to withstand the normal loads encountered with mastication and speech.

As described by Champy in the 1970s, under normal circumstances, bringing the teeth into occlusion results in tension on the alveolar surface of the mandible while compression forces are encountered along the inferior border. These varying forces are due to the complex nature of the muscles exerting force on different portions of the bone. When a fracture is present, these forces can displace the bone, and oftentimes a tension band is needed to support stabilization.

The purpose of the tension band is to overcome distracting forces at the alveolar portion of the mandible. A tension band can be created using an arch bar or wires. In addition, miniplates across the fracture line secured with monocortical screws can provide stabilization while avoiding injury to the tooth roots.

Compression plates are form of fixation device used in mandible fractures with decreasing frequency. These plates are designed with two holes on either side of the fracture line, which have a beveled surface that allows a screw being threaded through the hole to slide toward the medial aspect of the plate. The screw, being driven into the bone, will move the bone medially toward the fracture line as well. When both screws have been placed on opposite sides of the fracture, the opposing surfaces are compressed against one another producing an axial preload force within the fracture line and increased friction, which facilitates stabilization.

Lag screws are another way of achieving compression. These screws are placed by drilling an oversized hole in the outer cortex of one segment and an appropriately sized tap, which matches the size of the screw on the other side of the fracture line. The screw is passed through the overdrilled hole and the threads are allowed to engage the bone of the opposite side of the fracture. When the screw is tightened, the two fragments are drawn toward each other and compression is achieved at the fracture line. Lag screws are most often for fractures at the symphysis; however, they can also be used for oblique fractures of the body, angle, and subcondylar region if there is adequate overlap of the fragments.

MANAGEMENT OF TEETH

Teeth that are fractured at the root or pulp chamber or those with carious decay or abscess should be removed prior to reduction and fixation. Teeth in the fracture line can result in higher rates of infection.[4]

COMPLICATIONS

The complication rate has been reported to be 40% or greater in the literature, with infection, nonunion, malunion, tooth loss, anesthesia, facial nerve injury, trismus, and malocclusion being among some of those reported.[5]

Le Fort fractures

Christopher Tran and Laura T. Hetzler

DIFFERENTIAL DIAGNOSIS

A major contributor to differential diagnosis of facial fractures is determination of the mechanism of injury. The type of weapon and direction of force can implicate common fracture patterns or involvement of different bony structures. Facial fractures can seldom be classified purely as Le Fort I, II, or III (Figure 24.4). Nevertheless,

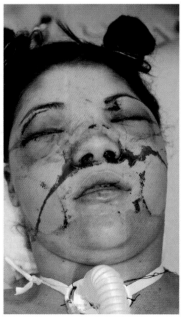

Figure 24.4 Facial distortion related to extensive facial trauma resulting in Le Fort III and naso-orbito-ethmoid fractures.

understanding the Le Fort classification can aid in the description of facial fractures within the medical record and among caretakers. Other common fracture patterns often seen in facial trauma can be closely associated with Le Fort–type fractures (Table 24.1).

Naso-orbital-ethmoidal fractures carry the potential for injuries to the ethmoidal roof, lacrimal system, medial canthal tendons, cribriform plate, and nasal vasculature. Potential signs and symptoms include cerebrospinal fluid (CSF) rhinorrhea, epistaxis, anosmia, epiphora, and telecanthus. Nasofrontal duct injury can lead to mucocele development.

Zygoma fractures can be implicated by a V-shaped depression of the cheek, the result of zygomatic arch fractures occurring at the ends and center of the zygoma. The infamous zygomaticomaxillary "tripod fracture" usually involves articulation(s) of the zygoma, frontal bone, temporal bone, sphenoid bone, and maxilla. Extension to the orbital floor is often encountered, as this type of fracture can be associated with force directed at the cheek and/or eye.

In pediatric facial trauma, a special consideration is due to the higher cartilaginous content of the nose. With increased flexibility of the nose, children are more likely to have more evenly distributed force across the midface, leading to more complex and less predictable fracture patterns and massive facial edema.

EXAM

Evaluation of the airway is of paramount importance in the workup of facial trauma. After the primary trauma survey is complete, physical examination in the setting of facial trauma consists of evaluation of neurologic function and structural integrity. Neurologic exam should include overall neurologic status (i.e., level of consciousness, cognition) and cranial nerve function if possible. Paresthesia below the eye indicates infraorbital nerve involvement from orbital

Table 24.1 Le Fort fracture classification

	Le Fort I	Le Fort II	Le Fort III
Fracture outline			

	Le Fort I	Le Fort II	Le Fort III
Name	"Horizontal maxillary"	"Pyramidal maxillary"	"Craniofacial dysjunction"
Classification key element	Maxilla fracture only	Infraorbital rim involved	Zygomatic arch involved
Structures involved	Piriform aperture	Nasal dorsum	Nasal dorsum
	Lateral maxillary or nasal wall	Medial orbital wall	Ethmoid bone
	Pterygoid plate	Posterior to lacrimal bone	Medial orbital wall
		Infraorbital rim	Orbit
		Below ZM buttress[a]	Lateral orbital wall
		Pterygoid plate	ZF buttress[a]
			Sphenoid skull base
			Zygomatic arch
			Pterygoid plate
Physical exam clues	Misalignment of teeth	Mobility of central face	Massive facial edema/ elongation
		Infraorbital paresthesia	

Source: Richardson, ML, Department of Radiology, University of Washington, Seattle, WA, www.rad.washinton.edu/ mskbook/facialfx.html. With permission.

[a] ZM, zygomaticomaxillary; ZF, zygomaticofrontal.

floor or inferior orbital rim fractures. Bony prominences should be palpated for bony step-offs or defects. Hematoma, bruising, or edema indicates underlying injury. Impaired ocular movements could indicate entrapment of the orbital tissues within an orbital floor fracture.

Le Fort fractures classically demonstrate mobility of the maxilla on physical exam. This finding is elucidated by grasping the maxilla firmly between the thumb and forefinger and performing a gentle rocking motion to evaluate for stability. Oral exam includes removal of dentures, evaluation of teeth and alveolar mobility, occlusion, and presence of foreign bodies or lacerations. Alveolar fractures are suspected with loose teeth and bruised or bleeding gingiva. Trismus can result with bony impingement from the zygomatic arch on the temporalis or masseter muscle or mandibular involvement. Any active hemorrhage or clear rhinorrhea or otorrhea should be evaluated appropriately as this could indicate ethmoid fracture or posterior table of the frontal sinus (FS) fracture.

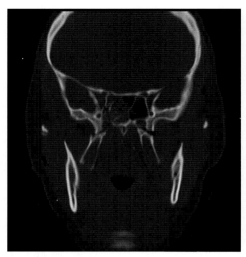

Figure 24.5 Fracture of bilateral pterygoid plates.

IMAGING

Le Fort fractures all characteristically involve fractures of the pterygoid plates (Figure 24.5). Radiographic evaluation of Le Fort fractures consists of the standard imaging protocols for any facial fracture. Namely, CT scans specialized for maxillofacial or sinus protocols are useful for detailed delineation of fracture lines. A CT head scan without contrast may be indicated to evaluate for cranial and skull base defects as well as intracerebral hemorrhage that may be associated with head trauma. Oftentimes, 3D reconstruction technology is helpful to visualize complex or comminuted fracture(s) globally (Figure 24.6).

TREATMENT

Optimal timing for reduction and fixation of facial fractures depends upon several factors. Significant edema distorts anatomy;

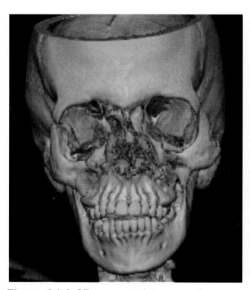

Figure 24.6 3D computed tomography reconstruction of true craniofacial dysjunction or Le Fort III.

thus, definitive treatment of fractures is often delayed until swelling has improved. However, it is generally optimal to treat facial fractures within 1 week of onset to avoid healing in a nonreduced state.

Observation may be indicated for nondisplaced or minimally displaced fractures without malocclusion or if the patient has comorbidities that impart great surgical risk.

Fractures that may require more urgent surgical intervention are those that include the orbital apex or entrapment of extraocular muscles, causing vision loss and/or diplopia.

Treatment to include open reduction with internal fixation of Le Fort I fractures is often performed via a sublabial incision for plating of the lower maxilla. Maxillomandibular fixation is often performed. If palatal instability is present, a splint may be fashioned and secured into place. Le Fort II fractures necessitating open reduction and internal fixation (ORIF) may require sublabial incisions as well as periocular incisions to address the orbital rim, orbital floor, or medial wall and occasionally a coronal approach for nasofrontal fractures. Le Fort III fractures, or true craniofacial disjunction, may require all of the aforementioned approaches and is frequently associated with severe cranial injury and other fracture patterns of the craniofacial skeleton such as naso-orbito-ethmoid (NOE) fractures and zygoma or "tripod" fractures.

Orbital floor fractures

Celeste Gary and Laura T. Hetzler

DEFINITIONS AND CLINICAL FEATURES
Most fractures involving the bones of the orbit are a consequence of blunt trauma to the face. Isolated orbital floor fractures are often the result of low-velocity blunt injury to the midface with higher velocity injuries often involving fractures of other facial bones. While some orbital fractures involve the orbital rim, true "blowout" fractures of the orbit involve fractures of the orbital floor, medial wall, or orbital roof without a rim fracture. Orbital floor fractures involve the inferior portion of the orbit (the roof of the maxillary sinus) without involvement of the rim.

DIFFERENTIAL DIAGNOSIS
Orbital floor fractures can often be associated with other facial fractures.

WORKUP
Since most orbital floor fractures are obtained during trauma, initial evaluation of the patient should be focused on the trauma algorithm including establishment of the airway, breathing, and circulation. Facial trauma should be investigated during the secondary survey of the patient. Assessment of all facial bones should be conducted.

When available, an examination of the globe and orbit by an ophthalmologist is ideal prior to surgical repair of an orbital trauma. Examination of all aspects of the orbit should be conducted including

1. Pupil size, shape, reactivity
2. Hyphema
3. Conjunctival injection, hemorrhage, chemosis, laceration
4. Periorbital edema, ecchymosis, laceration
5. Proptosis or enophthalmos
6. Visual acuity
7. Presence or absence of diplopia on all gazes
8. Extraocular movements
9. Palpation of the bony rim of the orbit

The classic triad of orbital blowout fractures includes enophthalmos, hypesthesia of the cheek, and deficiency of upgaze (Figure 24.7).

Maxillofacial CT without contrast is used to evaluate the extent of facial fractures (Figure 24.8).

Determination of the need for repair is based on the size of the injury, injury to other adjacent structures, associated symptoms, and characteristics of the patient.

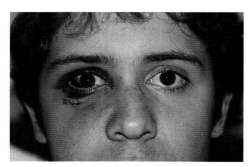

Figure 24.7 Young patient postinjury with repaired laceration, relative enophthalmos, and ecchymosis.

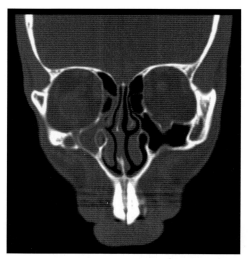

Figure 24.8 Left orbital blowout fracture with entrapment of the inferior rectus.

TREATMENT

Orbital floor fractures with entrapment of extraocular muscles, most commonly the inferior rectus, require urgent repair, ideally within 24 hours, to prevent fibrosis of the involved muscle and permanent diplopia.

Presence of oculocardiac reflex occurs more often in the pediatric population and is considered an indication for imminent repair.

Enophthalmos and diplopia serve as clinical indicators for the need for repair. In general, fractures involving more than 50% of the orbital floor are likely to cause later enophthalmos. Fractures, which are 1 cm^2 in size, will produce approximately 1 mm of enophthalmos. Enophthalmos of the eye up to 2 mm is often unnoticeable aesthetically.

Repair of orbital floor fractures without entrapment that qualify for intervention can be delayed up to 7–10 days.

Surgical repair involves access to the floor using a preexisting laceration, a transconjunctival approach, a subciliary approach, a mideyelid or subtarsal approach, or a rim incision approach. The medial, lateral, and posterior extents of the fracture should be exposed. Once the orbital contents are retracted back into the orbit, an implant is used to recreate the orbital floor. Many options are available including pliable absorbable materials, pliable nonabsorbable materials, titanium plates, and coated plates. Fixation of these materials can be performed with small self-drilling titanium screws but is not mandated (Figure 24.9).

The postoperative goal is resolution of diplopia and prevention of enophthalmos.

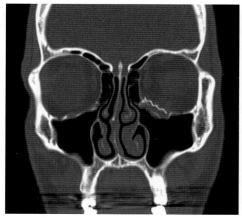

Figure 24.9 Left orbital blowout fracture following repair.

Zygomatic fractures

Sean Weiss and Laura T. Hetzler

DEFINITIONS AND CLINICAL FEATURES

The zygomatic bone is a major structural component for both anterior and lateral projection of the midface. It has direct associations with the temporal bone, the frontal bone, the maxillary bone, and the sphenoid bone, forming distinct buttresses, which support the position of the malar eminence. The zygomatic bone has superficial relationships with the frontal, temporal, and maxillary bones, and it has deep projections associating it with the sphenoid bone, along the lateral orbital wall, and the maxilla, along the lateral aspect of the orbital floor.

Fractures of the zygomaticomaxillary complex (aka zygomaticomalar complex [ZMC]) involve injury to the zygomatic bone at all four buttresses and displacement of the malar eminence. There are variations on the severity and complexity of ZMC fractures, which have been classified by several authors. The Zingg classification system of ZMC fractures organizes fractures according to anatomic structures injured and the severity of the injury.[6] Because the zygomatic bone contributes to both horizontal and vertical arcs of contour, repair of such fractures can involve unique complexities for repositioning of the anterior and lateral projection of the cheek and the vertical height of the malar eminence.

DIFFERENTIAL DIAGNOSIS

Assessment of facial fractures must include evaluation of the airway, cervical spine, hemodynamic stability, and in severe trauma, assessment for intracranial pathology. Once these have been addressed, focus can be turned to assessment of the facial skeletal exam and evaluation of the remainder of the head and neck. Oftentimes, ZMC fractures can be associated with other head and neck injuries and a thorough evaluation for these injuries is needed. Of particular importance is assessment of injuries to the eye and orbital adnexa. The potential for impairment of visual function mandates an ophthalmologic assessment in cases involving violation of the bony orbit prior to any surgical intervention. In these circumstances, additional consideration should be made for injury to the skull base and possible compression of the superior orbital fissure due to hematoma or bony malposition.

WORKUP

Assessment should include history of details surrounding the mechanism of injury and the setting in which the injury took place. Clues to the severity of the injury can be obtained with focused attention to the symptoms associated with the injury such as trismus, diplopia, facial numbness, and headache, for example.

The physical exam must be detailed and complete in order to guide decisions for further diagnostic and therapeutic interventions. This should include palpation of the facial skeleton to assess for any bony step-offs or point tenderness. A visual acuity exam and extraocular muscle evaluation can help to identify possible entrapment or a more concerning ophthalmologic process. Attention to the oral cavity should include assessment for trismus, which may indicate temporalis compression by a depressed zygomatic arch, and it should assess for proper dental occlusion. In addition, a complete cranial nerve exam should be performed. It is particularly important to elicit any numbness over the cheek region, which may indicate compression of the infraorbital neurovascular bundle. More importantly, the cranial nerve exam can help detect signs of optic neuropathy, which could result from direct injury to the optic nerve or globe but is more commonly the result of an indirect injury such as edema or hematoma (Figure 24.10).[7]

In today's modern age, a CT scan is preferred over plain films for evaluation of facial fractures (Figure 24.11). With plain

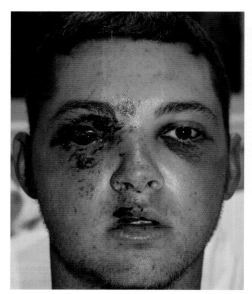

Figure 24.10 Preoperative image of patient with severely comminuted right zygomatico-maxillary complex fracture. Note flattening of malar bridge and enophthalmos.

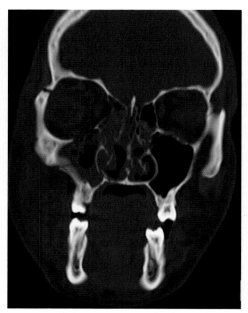

Figure 24.11 Coronal bone window computed tomography demonstrating fractures of the right zygomatic arch, lateral buttress and orbital rim (zygoma to maxilla), and zygomaticofrontal region.

film radiographs for zygomaticomaxillary fractures, historically, Water's view gave some indication that a fracture was present; however, plain films are not adequate for a complete evaluation.[8,9]

CT imaging is the imaging modality of choice for ZMC fractures and fractures that may involve the bony orbit. Axial images provide the best view of the zygomatic arch, vertical orbital walls, and maxillary sinus, and coronal cuts demonstrate the zygomaticofrontal suture line along with the lateral and inferior orbital rim (Figure 24.12).

TREATMENT

Early management of facial fractures can avoid difficulty due to scar contracture and collapse of skeletal support. The goal should be to reestablish the horizontal and vertical buttresses through proper repositioning of the zygoma to restore the horizontal width of the midface and height of the malar eminence.

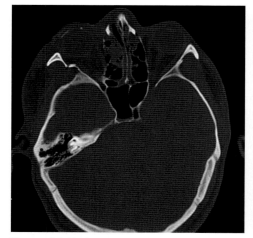

Figure 24.12 Axial bone window computed tomography showing comminution of the zygomaticosphenoid region.

In rare cases where there is minimal displacement of the fractures and there is no comminution, closed techniques or simple observation may suffice. However, more complex fractures require an open procedure with reduction and fixation of the fracture sites for stabilization needed for healing in proper alignment. Multiple approaches may be needed to access all of the fractured components depending on the severity of the injury. The zygomaticofrontal suture can be approached through an extended upper lid blepharoplasty incision or a lateral brow incision. The orbital rim can be accessed through a transconjunctival incision or through a subciliary incision. A gingivobuccal sulcus incision is used to access the anterior face of the maxilla and zygomaticomaxillary buttress. Extended dissection in this area can give access to the zygomatic arch. In addition, the arch can be approached by way of a coronal incision, and this approach should be used if there is questionable exposure or ability to reduce the fracture at the zygomatic arch or if there is severe comminution. The entire extent of all fracture lines should be exposed and evaluated to ensure proper alignment and reduction.

Internal fixation is accomplished well using craniofacial miniadaptation plates secured via transosseous screws. These plates maintain the reduction while bone healing takes place. A variety of plating systems exist, and there are plates designed for specific fracture patterns as well as plates that can be shaped to fit the surgeons' need (Figure 24.13).

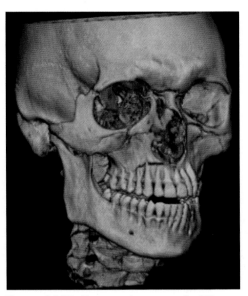

Figure 24.13 Computed tomography 3D reconstruction demonstrating mobility of zygoma-given fractures of the zygomatic arch, zygomaticofrontal region, zygomaticosphenoid region, and orbital rim and lateral buttress where the zygoma articulates with the maxilla.

COMPLICATIONS

Complications associated with treatment of the ZMC fractures include injury to the eyelid resulting in lid malposition, implant visibility, and possible implant extrusion, malunion, ocular damage including vision loss and enophthalmos, and facial asymmetry related to failure to reestablish the proper positioning of the malar eminence.

Nasal trauma

*Neal M. Jackson and
Laura T. Hetzler*

BACKGROUND

The nasal bones are the most commonly fractured bones in the body and are involved in approximately 40% of all maxillofacial trauma.

The nasal bones are at higher risk of injury because of their prominence on the face and their relative thinness compared to other facial bones.

Because the nose is visibly prominent and acts to warm, humidify, and deliver inspired air to the lower airway, proper management of nasal trauma addresses both cosmetic and functional concerns.

The most commonly involved demographic is young males in the second and third decades of life. For this group, most injuries are caused by assaults, sports injuries, falls, and motor vehicle collisions.

For geriatric and pediatric populations, falls and motor vehicle collisions are the main causes.

NASAL ANATOMY

The nose is a pyramid-shaped structure composed of bone, cartilage, and soft tissue. Its superior portion is composed of the paired nasal bones that articulate with the maxillary and frontal bones. The lower portion is composed of the paired upper lateral and lower lateral cartilages that contribute to nasal airway patency and nasal tip projection, respectively.

The nasal septum is a vertical segment separating the left and right nasal cavities that is composed of four parts: quadrangular cartilage anteriorly, perpendicular plate of the ethmoid bone posterosuperiorly, vomer posteroinferiorly, and the maxillary crest inferiorly.

Epistaxis, bleeding from inside the nasal cavity, is a common occurrence with nasal trauma due to the rich vascular supply of the nasal mucosa.

PRINCIPLES OF NASAL TRAUMA EVALUATION

Patients suffering from nasal trauma should be evaluated acutely.

In the acute setting, epistaxis control is important to enable adequate physical examination of the nasal cavity and to prevent significant blood loss.

A mucosal laceration may indicate a fracture of the underlying bones or cartilage.

The nasal septum should be examined to rule out a nasal septal hematoma.

DIAGNOSIS

History and complete head and neck physical exam alone are typically sufficient to diagnose a nasal fracture or soft tissue injury.

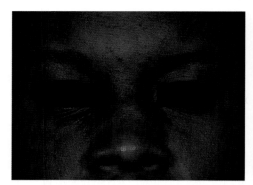

Figure 24.14 Preoperative image demonstrating right facial laceration and fullness of left nasal sidewall consistent with outward displacement of the left nasal bone and inward collapse of the right nasal bone.

A history should include mechanism of injury, time since injury, any previous deforming trauma and/or surgery, and any previous sinonasal problems such as rhinitis, sinusitis, or polyps.

Physical exam should begin with a preinjury photograph of the patient's face for comparison with the postinjury appearance.

The external nose may show a skin laceration, obvious bony step-off, crepitus, or tenderness to palpation (Figure 24.14).

The internal nose should be suctioned clean of any blood and then can be examined before and after administration of topical decongestant. Findings may include nasal septal deviation, septal hematoma, or an obvious source of hemorrhage.

Any clear drainage should alert the physician to the possibility of a CSF leak from the skull base, possibly from fracture of the cribriform plate.

IMAGING

Plain x-rays may show a fracture or dislocation of the bony nose but offer limited information about soft tissue defects. As a general consideration, any patient with known or suspected maxillofacial trauma should receive a CT scan of the maxillofacial

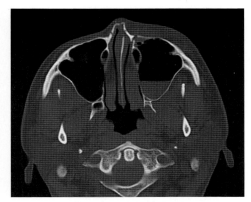

Figure 24.15 Comminution of the left nasal bone and ascending maxilla.

region to investigate for midface, orbital, skull base, and frontocranial fractures (Figure 24.15).

MANAGEMENT PRINCIPLES

The primary goal is to restore premorbid function and cosmesis of the nose.

If a patient still complains of nasal airway obstruction and deformity after allowing 3–5 days for posttraumatic swelling to subside, surgical correction may be indicated.

The decision to surgically correct an acquired nasal deformity is based on both appropriate patient expectations and surgeon experience. Factors include premorbid deficits, remaining intact structures, presence of chronic sinonasal disease, and overall surgical candidacy. There are many successful techniques for a wide variety of acquired deformities.

Depending on the extent of functional and cosmetic deficits, the surgical spectrum includes observation, closed reduction, septoplasty, rhinoplasty, and septorhinoplasty.

The timing of fracture treatment may vary depending on the degree of fracture and surgeon preference. Many surgeons often delay significant intervention, such as septoplasty or rhinoplasty until months have passed and healing and swelling are complete.

For an isolated closed nasal bone fracture occurring within 24–48 hours, a closed reduction to reduce the fracture within 7–10 days of the injury under local or general anesthesia depending on patient and surgeon preference requires no external incisions and simply reduces the nasal bones or nasal septum into a premorbid position.

Isolated closed nasal bone fractures occurring over 2 weeks ago may require osteotomies as bones may have healed together in poor alignment.

Isolated nasal mucosa lacerations can be reapproximated with 5-0 chromic.

Nasal septal hematomas need to be treated immediately with incision and drainage or 18-gauge needle aspiration. Nasal packs should be inserted to apply pressure against septum and prevent reaccumulation. Prophylactic antibiotics should be prescribed while packs are in place. Failure to recognize nasal septal hematomas can lead to septal necrosis and subsequent nasal collapse.

COMPLICATIONS

Each method of surgical correction has its inherent risks.

Bruising and pain are common in the acute postoperative period.

Delayed complications such as chronic nasal airway obstruction or poor cosmetic outcome may present weeks to months later as the healing process occurs and the operative structures settle into permanent positions. Risks, benefits, and alternatives discussed should include the limitations of closed reduction. Closed nasal fracture reduction improves alignment of the nose in a frontal view. It cannot alter the likelihood of callus formation or bony hump. Closed reduction does not absolutely decrease the risk of nasal obstruction as related to subluxation of upper lateral cartilages beneath the nasal bones and later collapse of the internal nasal valve.

Frontal sinus trauma

Neal M. Jackson and Laura T. Hetzler

BACKGROUND

The FS is the air-filled, mucosa-lined paranasal sinus cavity located superior to the orbit and anterior to the frontal lobe of the brain.

The development and anatomy of the FS is quite varied. It is a paired sinus, with the left and right parts that are usually not symmetric and approximately 15% of patients have only one unilateral FS. It is the last sinus to develop, beginning in first 3 years of life as extension of air cells from the ethmoid sinuses. It reaches adult aeration and size by the end of the second decade of life. About 1 in 25 patients does not develop FSs at all.

The FS is described as having two bony walls or "tables" as well as a floor. The anterior table is behind the skin and soft tissue of the forehead, and with a width of 2–12 mm, it can be one of the thickest bones in the body. The posterior table, which separates the sinus cavity from the dura of the frontal lobe, is relatively thin, measuring 0.1–5 mm (Figure 24.16). The floor overlies the orbits laterally and the ethmoid air cells medially.

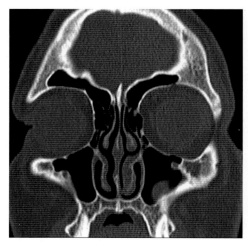

Figure 24.17 Normal patent frontal sinus outflow tract.

The FS drains into the middle meatus of the nasal cavity through the frontal sinus outflow tract (FSOT), which is an hourglass-shaped drainage avenue normally 2–10 mm in diameter (Figure 24.17). From superior to inferior, the FSOT includes the FS infundibulum, the FS ostium, and then the frontal recess. Partial or complete obstruction at any of these passageways can lead to chronic sinusitis, mucocele, and/or infection.

FRACTURES OF FRONTAL SINUS

Of the facial bones, the frontal bone has the highest tolerance of direct trauma. Between 800 and 2200 lb of pressure can be required to fracture the FS. The thick anterior table is more resistant to fracture than the thin posterior table. The degree of soft tissue injury does not accurately predict the extent of FS injury.

FS fractures account for 5%–12% of all facial fractures. FS trauma can range from isolated nondisplaced fracture of the anterior table to concomitant anterior and posterior comminuted fractures with exposure of intracranial contents. Because the force needed to fracture the FS is high, the presence of an FS fracture suggests other

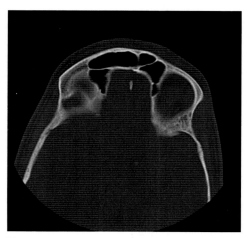

Figure 24.16 Normal septate frontal sinus.

wounds exist such as lacerations and/or fractures of the orbit, NOE complex, and maxilla. Approximately two-thirds of FS fractures occur with other craniofacial fractures.

Injury to the brain in the form of cerebral contusion, epidural hematoma, subdural hematoma, subarachnoid hemorrhage, intracerebral hemorrhage, or CSF peak may occur in up to 18%–38% of FS fractures. Incidence of ophthalmic injuries such as ruptured globe, optic nerve injury, extraocular muscle injury, or lens subluxation may be up to 25%. Patients with severe, comminuted fractures often have associated intracranial or ophthalmic injuries. Combined anterior and posterior table fractures are most commonly caused by motor vehicle collisions.

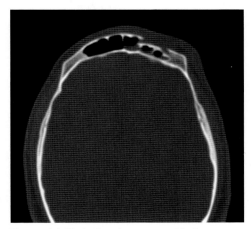

Figure 24.18 Isolated anterior table fracture with posterior displacement of fractured segment.

EPIDEMIOLOGY

The most common causes of FS trauma are motor vehicle collisions (~50%), gunshot wounds and physical altercations (~25%), and falls and recreational injuries (10%–15%).

Males in the third decade of life are by far the most commonly affected demographic group.

The use of seat belts and airbags has been thought to explain the decrease in the overall incidence of FS trauma.

DIAGNOSIS

The history of FS trauma is often straightforward and typically includes an acutely traumatic event. Any patient with a suspected FS trauma should receive a full trauma assessment. Physical exam findings suggest that FS trauma include forehead lacerations or abrasions, palpable step-offs, and hematoma.

The gold standard is a CT scan with thin 1.0–1.5 mm axial cuts with sagittal, coronal, and 3D reconstruction views. Axial views best show anterior and posterior table involvement (Figure 24.18); coronal images depict orbital roof/FS floor injury. Sagittal views are best for assessing frontal recess patency; 3D views help to view the external contour deformity. CT also allows study of soft tissue and intracranial injury.

If the patient reports watery drainage through the nose or salty tasting postnasal drip, the clinician should suspect a CSF leak. A bedside "halo test" can be done, though testing the fluid for beta-2 transferrin is the definitive test for CSF leak. Beware that this test can take 5–7 days for results to return, so diagnosis is often confirmed after treatment has begun. CSF leaks may occur in up to one-third of patients with FS trauma.

CLASSIFICATION OF FRONTAL SINUS FRACTURES

Many classification systems have been developed to classify FS fractures. Newer schemes have focused on more pertinent characteristics (isolated anterior vs. combined anterior and posterior wall fractures, dural tear with CSF leak, etc.).

Five general categories exist: isolated anterior table fracture, isolated posterior tablet fracture, combined anterior and posterior table involvement, any fracture that impedes flow through FSOT, and any fracture that leads to dural tear.

Injury to the frontonasal outflow tract is suspected if the fracture involves the supraorbital rim, nasoethmoid complex, or floor of FS.

MANAGEMENT PRINCIPLES

Multiple management algorithms exist. Five main interests that guide management include anterior table displacement, posterior table injury, FSOT impairment, CSF leak, and comminution of involved bone or extent of cosmetic defects.

While some clinicians believe that antibiotics may be used prophylactically to prevent sinusitis as well as intracranial contamination, they are not clearly indicated. If antimicrobials are used, third generation cephalosporins with high CSF penetration and anaerobic coverage are recommended.

In general, all patients should receive extended follow-up as complications have been known to present years later.

CSF leaks can be managed conservatively with bed rest, elevation of head of bed, and possibly placement of a lumbar drain. Any CSF leak persisting for greater than 5 days may be surgically treated, usually with cranialization of the FS and direct repair of the dural tear.

TREATMENT OPTIONS

The most conservative option is observation with close and long-term follow-up, as well as nasal decongestants and possibly antimicrobials. This can be utilized in patients with isolated anterior table injuries with minimal displacement.

Endoscopic transnasal sinus surgery to correct isolated FSOT injury is typically performed months after injury when serial imaging demonstrates maintained secretions or mucocele in the injured FS indicating inadequate drainage.

For visibly displaced anterior table fractures, ORIF of fractured bone utilizes miniplates, mesh, or other biomaterials via a bicoronal, subbrow, supraorbital brow, or other approaches. Use of any existing soft tissue lacerations and the endoscope may reduce invasiveness.

For comminuted fractures, microplates can be placed to reform the bony fragments.

In fractures that compromise the FSOT, in the past sinus obliteration has been performed. Obliteration is a procedure that removes all sinus mucosa and a thin layer of inner cortex of the sinus wall; this includes obliteration of the frontonasal outflow tract as well. The remaining cavity is then filled with a biomaterial, most often autogenous fat graft, temporalis fascia, pericranium, or cancellous bone from the pelvis. Alloplastic materials such as hydroxyapatite bone cement and calcium phosphate bone cement are alternatives. This has become less favored in recent years due to concerns over infected grafts and mucoceles as well as the ease at which endoscopic sinus procedures may be performed to reopen the obstructed outflow tract.

In fractures that result in defects of the posterior table and CSF leaks, FS cranialization involves removal of the posterior table and all FS mucosa, leaving the anterior sinus wall exposed to anterior cranial contents (dura and frontal lobe). The FS outflow tract must be obliterated to avoid intracranial contamination from the nasal cavity.

COMPLICATIONS

Complications may occur with any extent of FS trauma and can be categorized as sinus related, intracranial, or cosmetic.

The most common sinus problems include persistent headache, chronic sinusitis, and mucocele development, which are related to retained mucus due to outflow tract obstruction. Mucoceles are well known to present months to decades (average = 7.5 years) after the injurious event, which makes long-term follow-up imperative.

Major intracranial complications are subarachnoid hemorrhage, intracerebral hemorrhage, CSF leak, cerebral contusion, and infection in the form of brain abscess, epidural abscess, or meningitis.

Common cosmetic concerns are scar or soft tissue changes, sensory deficits in the injured areas, and a palpable step-off or visible depression of the forehead.

Facial reanimation

Laura T. Hetzler and Daniel W. Nuss

CLINICAL FEATURES AND DEFINITIONS

Facial paralysis can be devastating both emotionally and functionally. The direst functional loss related to impaired facial nerve function relates to ocular protection. Loss of orbicularis oculi function, and therefore inability to close the eye, results in a lack of tear film distribution and lubrication that may result in desiccation and corneal ulceration. Loss of frontalis muscle function can lead to brow ptosis and vision impairment. Loss of buccal branch function can result in nasal obstruction as well as loss of upper lip and oral commissure excursion resulting in smile impairment. Impairment of buccinator function disturbs the formation of an adequate food bolus and allows food trapping within the cheek during mastication. Paralysis of the lip depressors via the marginal mandibular nerve can result in asymmetry of the mouth when speaking and opening of the oral aperture as well as oral incompetence. Loss of function to orbicularis oris can result in poor articulation and contributes to oral incompetence (Figures 24.19 and 24.20).

DIFFERENTIAL DIAGNOSIS

The differential diagnosis of facial paralysis is extensive and includes trauma, infection, congenital, metabolic, neoplastic, toxic, or iatrogenic etiologies.

Infectious etiologies such as Lyme disease, Guillain–Barre syndrome, herpes simplex, herpes zoster, middle ear infections, meningitis, temporal bone osteomyelitis, and many others must be considered. Inflammatory conditions including autoimmune and connective tissue disorders can affect facial nerve function.

Tumors anywhere along the length of the facial nerve can be responsible for paralysis. Intracranial lesions such as acoustic neuromas, meningiomas, and others can affect

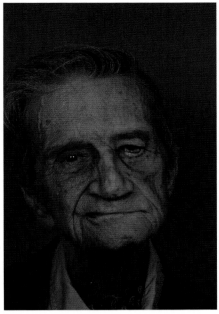

Figure 24.19 Facial paralysis patient in repose demonstrating brow ptosis, lower lid ectropion, and facial droop.

the facial nerve as well as cranial nerves VIII and V. *Intratemporal* facial nerve tumors to include neuromas, hemangiomas, or primary tumors of the middle ear and skull base must be considered. *Extratemporal* tumors involving primary and metastatic malignancies of the parotid may also cause facial paralysis.

Penetrating and blunt trauma causing temporal bone fractures or direct injury to facial nerve anywhere along its length is possible. In this setting, facial nerve status needs to be assessed in the initial evaluation. Iatrogenic injuries to the facial nerve following tumor ablation are unfortunately sometimes unavoidable in head and neck surgery.

WORKUP

A complete history and head and neck examination are critical. A diagnosis of Bell's palsy should not be accepted unless other plausible diagnoses have been

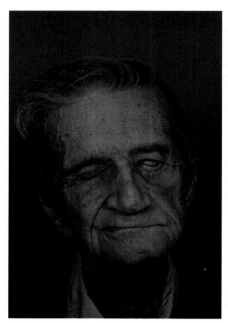

Figure 24.20 Facial paralysis patient with attempted eye closure demonstrating lagophthalmos, lower lid ectropion, and Bell's phenomenon.

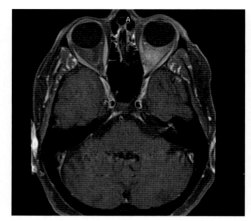

Figure 24.21 Facial nerve enhancement on T1 MRI with gadolinium supporting a diagnosis of Bell's palsy.

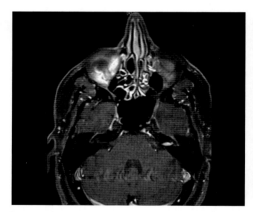

Figure 24.22 Facial neuroma in the internal auditory canal on T1 MRI with gadolinium.

thoroughly investigated. Prior incisions and integrity of other cranial nerves must be noted. Age, comorbidities, and life expectancy may contribute to decision-making in facial reanimation. Interestingly, radiation therapy, whether planned or past, has minimal influence in reconstructive planning. Imaging to evaluate the course of the facial nerve to include an MRI or CT may be helpful (Figures 24.21 and 24.22).

The availability of proximal and distal facial nerve must be assessed. The viability of facial musculature and motor end plates is key in reconstructive planning and is often the hindrance in longer-term facial paralysis patients. For patients in whom questionable continuity or viability is an issue, electrical testing may be in order. Electroneuronography is of value between 3 days and 3 weeks of onset to evaluate facial nerve function. Greater than 90%

degeneration as compared to the functioning facial nerve bears a poor prognosis of functional recovery. Electromyography is used starting 2–3 weeks after onset to predict recovery. Fibrillations indicate a poorer prognosis.

The mechanism of injury and time since injury are key when designing a reconstructive plan. Complete or partial facial motion impairment should be noted to include whether weakness or complete paralysis in some or all of the branches is present.

The House–Brackmann scale is the most commonly utilized facial nerve grading scale because of its reproducibility and ease of use, but is insufficient and was not intended for precise assessment of different branches or regions of the face, and therefore, explicit analysis and documentation is also needed.

Independent assessment of the upper, middle, and lower face is imperative. Facial tone must be noted. A complete nasal exam is necessary to describe alar and columellar position, septal position, and valve collapse related to poor nasal sidewall support. Ocular status of lagophthalmos, ectropion or laxity, conjunctival injection or irritation, lacrimal punctal position and epiphora, Bell's phenomenon, and brow position must be noted. Corneal ulceration may expedite intervention. Oral examination to identify cheek biting, difficulty with mastication, lip position, and oral incompetence must be noted.

Finally, patient expectations must be managed to prepare for incomplete recovery even in the best of reconstructive efforts. In cases during which the loss of neural continuity is expected, recovery may at best provide complete eye closure with persistent asymmetries present during motion.

TREATMENT
Medical management
Preventing vision loss and injury to the ocular surface is the most important initial goal. Conservative measures include artificial tears and ointment, application of moisture chambers, contact lenses, and taping. A simple eye patch is to be avoided.

Steroids with or without antivirals can be used as medical therapy in patients with Bell's palsy or trauma. Observation and conservative treatment is appropriate when recovery is anticipated and the integrity of the nerve is felt to be preserved.

Adjunct procedures such as botulinum toxin can be used to improve facial symmetry.

Surgical management
Surgical interventions are categorized as static and dynamic procedures.

STATIC PROCEDURES: UPPER FACE
Brow ptosis can be repaired with a brow lift utilizing multiple techniques including direct, midforehead, and endoscopic approaches.

Lagophthalmos is most often rehabilitated with upper lid loading with either a gold or platinum weight ranging from 0.6 to 1.8 g. Upper lid springs are successfully used as well; however, they are more technically challenging than upper lid weight insertion. Lagophthalmos correction and improved eye closure promotes tear distribution and corneal health.

Lower lid laxity is treated with both medial and lateral canthopexy techniques. Lateral canthal tightening can be performed with wedge excisions as well as lateral tarsal strip procedures (Figures 24.23 and 24.24). In the face of corneal ulceration a tarsorrhaphy, temporary or permanent, may be necessary to allow the corneal surface time to heal. Some patients with cranial nerve V deficits may require permanent tarsorrhaphy given the lack of sensory input that is needed to protect the eye.

Periocular static reanimation may be performed even if recovery is anticipated. Aggressive ocular intervention is promoted

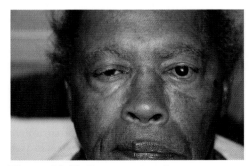

Figure 24.23 Preoperative photo demonstrating ocular asymmetry related to facial paralysis.

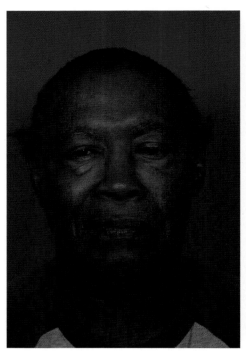

Figure 24.24 Postoperative photo with correction of asymmetry and lagophthalmos with platinum weight insertion and lateral tarsal strip of the left eye.

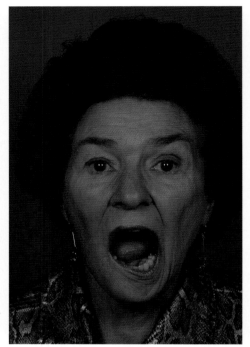

Figure 24.25 Preoperative right-sided isolated marginal branch weakness demonstrating distortion of lower lip to contralateral side and asymmetry related to DAO and DLI paralysis.

given the risk of permanent injury and vision loss in the unprotected eye.

STATIC PROCEDURES: MIDFACE

Static slings are employed in patients unfit for larger dynamic operations, patients who have a poor prognosis, or patients who do not desire extensive intervention for facial reanimation. Materials used for slings range from autologous fascia lata to allografts including acellular human dermis (Alloderm) and polytetrafluoroethylene (Gore-Tex). Rhytidectomy or midface lifts are a useful adjunct in patients who have extensive hemifacial ptosis related to facial paralysis.

STATIC PROCEDURES: LOWER FACE

Paralysis of the marginal mandibular branch of the facial nerve results in loss of lower lip support and pull of the midline lower lip to the contralateral side. The lower lip and oral commissure can be supported with static slings. Lower lip wedge excision can be performed to shorten the affected lip giving the appearance of improved muscular support as would be present with a functioning depressor anguli oris (Figures 24.25 and 24.26). Cheiloplasty recreates the function of the depressor labii inferioris by causing an outward roll of the affected lower lip. Platysma or digastric transpositions can be performed to rehabilitate marginal nerve weakness.

DYNAMIC PROCEDURES

Dynamic facial reanimation techniques follow an order of preference for optimal results. If the nerve has been transected and can be repaired without tension, primary

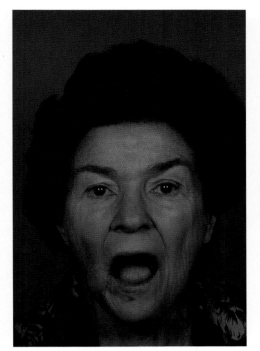

Figure 24.26 Three weeks postoperative photo following botox to contralateral lip depressors and ipsilateral lower lip wedge on right.

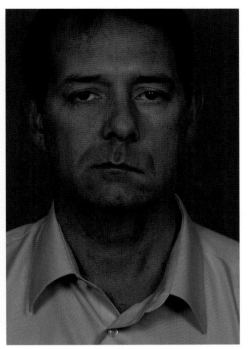

Figure 24.27 Preoperative left flaccid facial paralysis.

neurorrhaphy is ideal. If an intervening segment of nerve is lost and tension-free repair is not possible, interposition grafts between the two facial nerve ends are appropriate. If the facial nerve is not available or primary or cable grafting methods are not possible, nerve transposition, muscle transposition, and free tissue transfer may be warranted.

NERVE TRANSPOSITION

Nerve transposition is considered when there is a lack of proximal facial nerve segment with an intact distal segment and viable facial musculature. Donor nerves used include the hypoglossal nerve, spinal accessory nerve, nerve to the masseter (branch of V3), and the contralateral facial nerve.

The hypoglossal nerve is the most frequently used of all nerve transpositions and commonly used in the setting of acoustic neuroma resections. Its use is promoted for the recovery of facial tone yet unreliable for movement (Figures 24.27 through 24.29). The facial nerve may be divided at its exit from the temporal bone, or if more length is needed, it can be exposed within the mastoid and divided proximally at the second genu and reflected inferiorly to reach the hypoglossal nerve. Distal dissection of the facial nerve into the parotid gland with removal of the gland inferiorly may allow for increased mobilization and negate the need for an interposition graft. Upon isolation of the hypoglossal nerve distal to the ansa cervicalis, only 1/3 of the hypoglossal nerve is transected to minimize hemiglossal atrophy. The facial nerve is then approximated to the proximal neurotomy of the hypoglossal nerve (Figure 24.30). If the facial nerve is too short, an interposition graft may be used between the stump of the facial

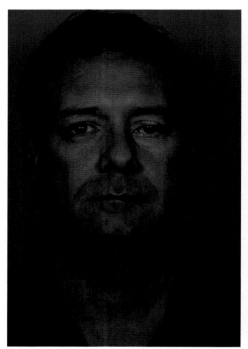

Figure 24.28 Six months post XII–VII neuror-rhaphy in repose showing improved tone.

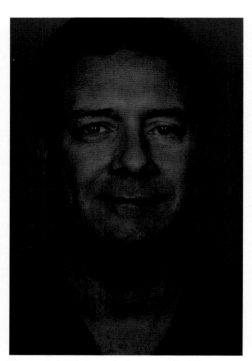

Figure 24.29 Six months post XII–VII neurorrhaphy with gentle smile demonstrating oral commissure excursion with smiling.

nerve and the hypoglossal nerve. Recovery of function will continue to improve over the course of 2 years.

MUSCLE TRANSPOSITION

Muscle transposition techniques are used when there has been long-standing facial paralysis of greater than 2–3 years or when other cranial nerves have been sacrificed, and therefore, transposition techniques are not suitable. If the trigeminal nerve is intact, the masseter muscle and temporalis muscle are most frequently used for dynamic facial reanimation. These two muscles can be used simultaneously for upper and lower face reanimation.

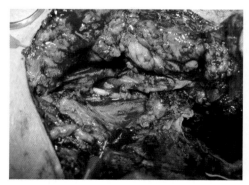

Figure 24.30 Intraoperative photo demonstrating the "split" facial nerve to hypoglossal nerve neurorrhaphy.

The temporalis muscle can be used for both periocular and perioral reanimation. Anterior strips of the temporalis muscle have been used for improvement of palpebral position and eye closure. The main body of the temporalis muscle may be reflected over the zygomatic arch or tunneled beneath it and has an ideal vector for oral commissure and midface reconstruction. Orthodromic temporalis tendon transfer has been described as releasing the temporalis tendon from the coronoid process and securing it to the modiolus of the orbicularis.

The masseter muscle may be used for perioral dynamic reanimation. The vector of pull is more horizontal than the temporalis muscle and therefore less ideal.

FREE TISSUE TRANSFER

Free tissue transfer is the preferred method of facial reanimation in patients suffering from congenital facial paralysis. This technique is also applicable in patients who have undergone resections of the facial nerve and its distal branches or who have long-standing facial paralysis. Muscle flaps that have been used include the gracilis, serratus anterior, latissimus dorsi, pectoralis minor, and extensor digitorum brevis.

Autologous free muscle transfer is often performed in two stages. The initial stage includes a nerve graft, commonly the sural nerve, attached to a distal branch of the facial nerve of the contralateral normal face and tunneled to the paralyzed side. A second stage is performed 6–9 months later, with free muscle transfer and neurorrhaphy between the cross facial nerve graft and the nerve of the free tissue complex.

Single-stage procedures may be performed when utilizing free muscle transfer with a donor nerve long enough to reach the contralateral facial nerve. Single-stage free tissue transfers have also been performed employing the ipsilateral proximal facial nerve remnant or the masseteric branch of the trigeminal nerve to power the free muscle.

References

1. Olson RA, Fonseca RJ, Zeitler DJ et al. 1982. Fractures of the mandible: A review of 580 cases. *Journal of Oral and Maxillofacial Surgery* 40:23.
2. Chayra GA, Meador LR, Laskin DM. 1986. Comparison of panoramic and standard radiographs for the diagnosis of mandibular fractures. *Journal of Oral and Maxillofacial Surgery* 44(9):677–679.
3. Bailey BJ, Johnson JT. 2006. *Head & Neck Surgery—Otolaryngology*. Philadelphia, PA: Lippincott Williams & Wilkins.
4. Ellis E, Sinn DP. 1993. Treatment of mandibular angle fractures using two 2.4-mm dynamic compression plates. *Journal of Oral and Maxillofacial Surgery* 51:969–973.
5. Fonseca RJ. 2000. Mandible fractures. In: Spina, AM and Marciani, RD (eds.), *Oral and Maxillofacial Surgery*, 1st ed. Philadelphia, PA: WB Saunders Company, Vol. 3.
6. Warner JE. 1995. Traumatic optic neuropathy. *International Ophthalmology Clinics* 35:57.
7. Kassel EE, Noyek AM, Cooper PW. 1983. CT in facial trauma. *Journal of Otolaryngology* 12:2.
8. Zilkha A. 1982. Computed tomography in facial trauma. *Radiology* 144:545.
9. Zingg M, Laedrach K, Chen J et al. 1992. Classification and treatment of zygomatic fractures: A review of 1,025 cases. *Journal of Oral and Maxillofacial Surgery* 50:778–790.

Bibliography

Bailey BJ, Johnson JT, Kohut RI et al. 2006. *Head and Neck Surgery—Otolaryngology*, 4th ed. Philadelphia, PA: Lippincott Williams & Wilkins, pp. 973–993.

Bell RB. 2009. Management of frontal sinus fractures. *Oral and Maxillofacial Surgery Clinics of North America* 21(2):227–242.

Brown DJ, Jaffe JE, Henson JK. 2007. Advanced laceration management. *Emergency Medicine Clinics of North America* 25(1):83–99.

Chadha NK, Repanos C, Carswell AJ. 2009. Local anaesthesia for manipulation of nasal fractures: Systematic review. *The Journal of Laryngology and Otology* 123(8):830–836.

Donald P. 2005. *Frontal Sinus and Nasofrontoethmoidal Complex Fractures*, Self Instructional Package. Alexandria, VA: American Academy of Otolaryngology—Head and Neck Surgery Foundation.

Doonquah L, Brown P. 2012. Management of frontal sinus fractures. *Oral and Maxillofacial Surgery Clinics of North America* 24(2):265–274.

Duvall AJ, Porto DP, Lyons D et al. 1987. Frontal sinus fractures. Analysis of treatment results. *Archieves of Otolaryngology Head and Neck Surgery* 113(9):933–935.

Escada P, Penha RS. 1999. Fracture of the anterior nasal spine. *Rhinology* 37(1):40–42.

Fischer C, Bertelle V, Hohlfeld J, Forcada-Guex M, Stadelmann-Diaw C, Tolsa JF. 2010. Nasal trauma due to continuous positive airway pressure in neonates. *Archives of Disease in Childhood—Fetal and Neonatal Edition* 95(6):F447–F451.

Frodel JL. 2012. Revision of severe nasal trauma. *Facial Plastic Surgery* 28(4):454–464.

Garr JI, McDonald WS. 2004. Zygoma fractures. In: Thaler, SR and McDonald, WS (eds.), *Facial Trauma*. New York: Marcel Dekker Inc., pp. 367–368.

Higuera S, Lee EI, Cole P, Hollier LH, Stal S. 2007. Nasal trauma and the deviated nose. *Plastic and Reconstructive Surgery* 120(7 Suppl. 2):64S–75S.

Jung SN, Shin JW, Kwon H, Yim YM. 2009. Fibrolipoma of the tip of the nose. *The Journal of Craniofacial Surgery* 20(2):555–556.

Kalavrezos N. 2004. Current trends in the management of frontal sinus fractures. *International Journal of Care of the Injured* 35:340–346.

Koento T. 2012. Current advances in sinus preservation for the management of frontal sinus fractures. *Current Opinion in Otolaryngology and Head and Neck Surgery* 20(4):274–279.

Lauder A, Jalisi S, Spiegel J, Stram J, Devaiah A. 2010. Antibiotic prophylaxis in the management of complex midface and frontal sinus trauma. *Laryngoscope* 120(10):1940–1945.

Litschel R, Tasman AJ. 2009. Current controversies in the treatment of frontal sinus fractures. *Laryngorhinootologie* 88(9):577–581.

Mondin V, Rinaldo A, Ferlito A. 2005. Management of nasal bone fractures. *American Journal of Otolaryngology* 26(3):181–185.

Moskovitz JB, Sabatino F. 2013. Regional nerve blocks of the face. *Emergency Medicine Clinics of North America* 31(2):517–527.

Myers EN. 2008. *Operative Otolaryngology—Head and Neck Surgery*, 2nd ed. Philadelphia, PA: Elsevier, pp. 935–945.

Papel ID. 2009. *Facial Plastic and Reconstructive Surgery*, 3rd ed. New York: Thieme Medical Publishers, Inc.

Rohrich RJ, Adams WP. 2000. Nasal fracture management: Minimizing secondary nasal deformities. *Plastic and Reconstructive Surgery* 106(2):266–273.

Rontal ML. 2008. State of the art in craniomaxillofacial trauma: Frontal sinus. *Current Opinion in Otolaryngology & Head and Neck Surgery* 16:381–386.

Sabatino F, Moskovitz JB. 2013. Facial wound management. *Emergency Medicine Clinics of North America* 31(2):529–538.

Tiwari P, Higuera S, Thornton J et al. 2005 The management of frontal sinus fractures. *Journal of Oral and Maxillofacial Surgery* 63(9):1354–1360.

Wright RJ, Murakami CS, Ambro BT. 2011. Pediatric nasal injuries and management. *Facial Plastic Surgery* 27(5):483–490.

Ziccardi VB, Braidy H. 2009. Management of nasal fractures. *Oral and Maxillofacial Surgery Clinics of North America* 21(2):203–208, vi.

Zingg M, Laedrach K, Chen J et al. 1992. Classification and treatment of zygomatic fractures: A review of 1025 caswes. *Journal of Oral and maxillofacial Surgery* 50:778–790.

Suggested reading

Bailey BJ, Johnson JT, Kohut RI et al. 2006a. *Head and Neck Surgery—Otolaryngology*, 4th ed. Philadelphia, PA: Lippincott Williams & Wilkins, pp. 2467–2480.

Bailey BJ, Johnson JT, Kohut RI et al. 2006b. *Head and Neck Surgery—Otolaryngology*, 4th ed. Philadelphia, PA: Lippincott Williams & Wilkins, pp. 919–934, 1027–1046.

Papel I. 2009. *Facial Plastic and Reconstructive Surgery*, 3rd ed. New York: Thieme Medical Publishers, Inc., pp. 869–896.

Papel I. 2009. *Facial Plastic and Reconstructive Surgery*, 3rd ed. New York: Thieme Medical Publishers, Inc., pp. 991–1000.

SECTION 6

PEDIATRICS

CHAPTER 25

Ear Disease

Oliver Adunka

- **External ear**
- **Auricular malformations**
- **Inner ear**

External ear

PREAURICULAR PIT/CYST
Definition and clinical features
It is characterized as sinus tracts or cysts that are present under the skin near the ear cartilage and lined by squamous epithelium that can occasionally sequester to form cysts that can become infected. Caused by duplication of the external auditory canal (EAC), these are divided into two types:

1. Type 1 pits/cysts are formed from duplication of the external auditory canal, run parallel to it, and are lined by skin. They are found in the preauricular or postauricular areas.
2. Type 2 pits/cysts are true congenital duplications of the external auditory canal and are comprised of skin and cartilage. Both sinuses and cysts have an intimate association with the perichondrium of the ear. Many are asymptomatic but can become infected and present with cellulitis of the skin or purulent drainage (Figures 25.1 and 25.2).

Differential diagnosis
First branchial cleft cyst, cellulitis, and trauma.

Workup
Due to the association between preauricular pits/cysts and congenital syndromes, a formal audiogram must be performed. In addition, some children with multiple abnormalities may benefit from a renal ultrasound. Associations include branchiootorenal syndrome, Beckwith–Wiedemann syndrome, and mandibulofacial dysostosis.

Treatment
While most are asymptomatic throughout life, it can present with fever, cellulitis around the ear, or purulent drainage or as an enlarging mass, which should be acutely managed with antibiotics and possible incision and drainage. Once acute episode has resolved, surgical removal of the pit/cyst should be considered. Surgery is typically limited to lesions that cause recurrent infections. Due to the intimate association with the perichondrium of the auricle, surgical

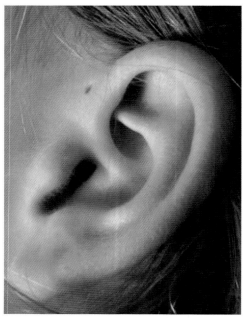

Figure 25.1 Type 1 preauricular pit.

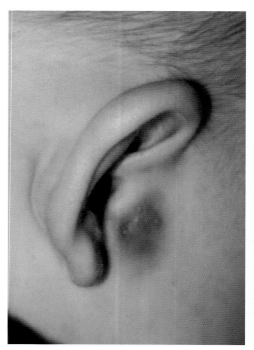

Figure 25.2 Type 2 preauricular cyst that has become infected.

excision must typically include the perichondrium at the base of the lesion to prevent recurrence.

PREAURICULAR TAG/APPENDAGE
Definition and clinical features

Commonly found in asymptomatic infants, tags are characterized as one or multiple fleshy epithelial mounds found near the ear. Nontender and similar to the surrounding skin, these lesions may be located behind the ear, on the lobule, in front of the auricle, or within the ear. They are most commonly found around the tragus in the preauricular region. They are caused by supernumerary hillocks that remain from embryonic development. In comparison to preauricular pits, these lesions have cartilaginous or bony components and are not associated with the ear canal or middle ear (Figure 25.3).

Workup

The lesions, especially those near the tragus, are sometimes associated with syndromes including Goldenhar syndrome, hemifacial microsomia, first and second branchial arch syndrome, and malformations in the facio-auriculo-vertebral spectrum. Therefore, children noted to have these lesions should have

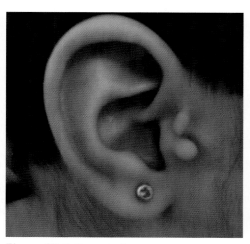

Figure 25.3 Preauricular tag.

a formal audiometric assessment to check for unilateral versus bilateral hearing loss.

Differential diagnosis
These lesions are usually fairly easy to recognize, but other skin or cartilaginous lesions, such as epidermal inclusion cysts, dermoid cysts, or other growths, are possible.

Treatment
While these lesions are completely asymptomatic, many infants will present for evaluation for removal due to cosmetic concerns. When these lesions are noted to have a very narrow base, they may occasionally be tied at their base with suture in clinic. For large or broad-based lesions, complete excision with proper closure must take place in the operating room. This is typically deferred until anesthesia is considered safe for the child.

Auricular malformations

LOP EAR
Definition and clinical features
It is characterized as a normal-size auricle found in proper position with significant protrusion from the side of the head. This is caused by incomplete formation of the antihelical fold. While cosmetic concerns are common, this typically does not have any functional consequences. It may be associated with syndromes including Ehlers–Danlos syndrome and Towns–Brocks syndrome (Figure 25.4).

Workup
A complete otolaryngologic examination is advisable including audiometric testing.

Treatment
While no treatment is required due to lack of functional impairment, parents or patients themselves will seek correction due to cosmetic concerns. Otoplasty may be performed when the child is 4–6 years old.

Various surgical techniques have been described. Most commonly, the procedure

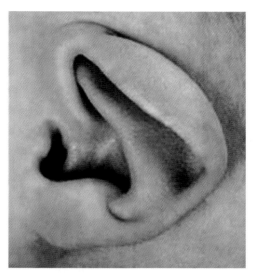

Figure 25.4 Lop ear.

includes four steps: excision of the conchal cartilage, formation of an antihelical fold, placement of a mastoid suture, and addressing the lobule of the auricle. Nonabsorbable sutures should be used to maintain a permanent result. The difficulty of the procedure is to shape the anterior side of the auricular cartilage framework from a posterior incision. The superior aspect of the auricle should not protrude for more than 2 cm. Care should be taken not to overcorrect the concha mastoid angle and hence to produce an unnatural cosmetic appearance.

MICROTIA
Definition and clinical features
These are abnormalities leading to small, deformed, or absent ears caused by variable levels of incomplete development of the pinna. These abnormalities can be categorized on a spectrum into three types based on the severity of the deformity:

- Grade 1 describes mild malformations. Specifically, grade 1 microtic auricles are generally well formed but are perceptibly smaller.

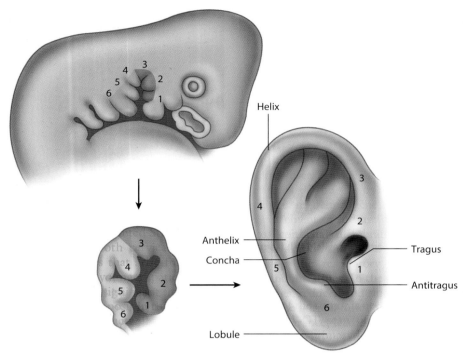

Figure 25.5 Development of the auricle from the 6 hillocks of His.

- Grade 2 characterizes more severe abnormalities associated with malformation of the auricle, which is at least 50% smaller than the contralateral side.
- Grade 3 describes the most severe deformities as patients have no identifiable auricle but have only a peanut-shaped collection of tissue (remnant of the hillocks of His) (Figure 25.5).
- Grade 4 is the complete absence of an auricle.

This group of abnormalities is typically seen more commonly in boys, children of diabetic mothers, increasing altitude, and increasing birth order. It is more commonly unilateral affecting the right more than the left. It can be associated with prenatal exposures to alcohol, isotretinoin, mycophenolate, and thalidomide. Patients may have microtia as an isolated defect or in association with other malformations. Two-thirds of these deformities are associated with sporadic genetic abnormalities (Figure 25.6).

Differential diagnosis

Preauricular skin tags, familial ear shape. Syndromic associations include Crouzon disease, CHARGE association, Duane syndrome, Franceschetti syndrome, Goldenhar syndrome, hemifacial microsomia, oculo-auriculo-vertebral dysplasia, Pierre Robin syndrome, retinoic acid embryopathy, rubella infection, Treacher Collins syndrome, trisomy 21, and VATER complex.

Workup

Each patient should receive a formal otolaryngologic examination. Other potentially associated anomalies should be identified and properly diagnosed. A visit with the

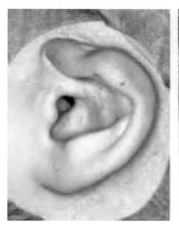 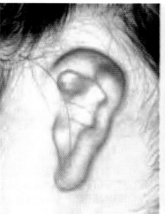 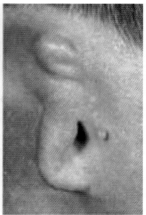

Figure 25.6 Grades of microtia. Grade 1 on the left. Grade 2 in the middle. Grade 3 on the right.

craniofacial team should be planned especially with bilateral anomalies. Genetic testing can be offered.

Many cases of microtia are associated with atresia of the external auditory canal. In these cases, especially with bilateral appearance, hearing concerns and subsequent speech and language development are probably more important than the cosmetic issues. In any case, a thorough audiometric examination should be carried out often including a bone conduction auditory brainstem response (ABR) assessment.

Treatment

Due to the association of microtia, either unilateral or bilateral, with a variety of syndromes, complete evaluation precedes repair. Surgical repair is typically not considered until children reach the ages of 4–6. Therefore, children with significant hearing loss must have this addressed prior to reconstruction. Reconstruction is done primarily for cosmetic reasons. It requires several stages in which a cartilaginous framework is developed from the costal cartilage that is transferred to the mastoid area. Should this multistage reconstruction be too risky for certain patients, a prosthetic auricle with osseointegrated pegs may also serve as an option.

MACROTIA

Definition and clinical features

It is characterized as ears that are well shaped but larger than normal based on their relationship to the rest of the face. This typically describes ears with a large auricle in which the exaggerated portion is the scaphoid fossa. This is typically bilateral and symmetric and associated occasionally with autosomal dominant inheritance, therefore running in families (Figure 25.7).

Differential diagnosis

Lop ear, familial ear shape.

Workup

Audiogram and genetic testing; syndromic associations include Marfan syndrome, cerebro-oculo-facial skeletal syndrome, fragile X syndrome, and Cornelia de Lange type 2 syndrome.

Treatment

No treatment required; however, cosmetic procedures may be performed to decrease size. In addition, management of hearing loss and syndromic malformations may be necessary.

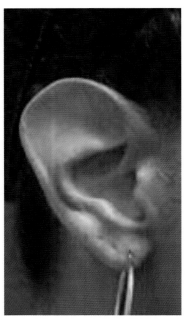

Figure 25.7 Macrotia with exaggerated scaphoid fossa.

SYNOTIA
Definition and clinical features
It is characterized as ears that are close together in the midline due to abnormalities in embryonic development and is typically associated with other significant craniofacial abnormalities.

Workup
Audiogram and genetic testing.

Differential diagnosis
Syndromic associations include trisomy 18, Noonan syndrome, and Pena Shokeir phenotype.

Treatment
Management of global craniofacial abnormalities.

ATRESIA
Definition and clinical features
Atresia is characterized as absent or stenotic external ear canal due to failure of complete invagination of external auditory canal during embryonic development. This failure of recanalization leads to improper formation of the tympanic membrane as well. The ossicles are formed from the first and second branchial clefts; therefore, atresia causes abnormalities of the ossicles as well, as they may be fused. While children may have significant abnormalities of the outer ear, the middle ear can be normal. Therefore, they can present with acute otitis media (AOM) like normal children. Children with bilateral atresia have an associated maximal conductive hearing loss (60 dB) and require early bone conduction hearing aids early in life in order to promote normal speech and language development. Children are also at risk for cholesteatoma; therefore, close monitoring should be performed (Figures 25.8 and 25.9).

Workup
Audiometric testing, high-resolution computed tomography (HRCT) of the temporal bones, and possible MRI of the brain.

Clinical staging
Jahrsdoerfer devised a clinical staging system mainly based on CT morphologic presence of certain structures. Based on this assessment, surgical candidacy for microtia repair can be further assessed (Tables 25.1 and 25.2; Figure 25.10).

Treatment
Children who are born with unilateral atresia should undergo proper audiometric assessment to evaluate hearing in the contralateral ear and to document sensorineural function on the affected side. Should the child have normal hearing in the contralateral ear, surgical repair is typically not required. In addition, bone conduction hearing aids to the affected ear are not helpful in that they do not help with localization of sound. Should the contralateral ear have some degree of hearing loss, amplification is important to assist with proper speech and language development.

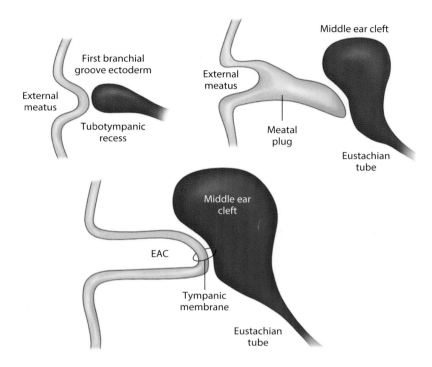

Figure 25.8 Development of the external auditory canal.

Children may also suffer from episodes of acute otitis media, presenting with fevers and ear pain. They should be treated with antibiotics in the same fashion as their counterparts.

The timing of imaging has been a controversial topic. It is important, however, to keep in mind that children with aural atresia are at risk for cholesteatoma development. Thus, a CT scan within the first few years of life may be advisable. At the same time, surgical candidacy can be assessed via the Jahrsdoerfer grading scheme and parents can be counseled adequately (Figure 25.11).

The consultation should include a thorough discussion of the surgical risks and the potential timeframe especially in cases of combined microtia and aural atresia. Specifically, the family's goals for repair and hearing care should be carefully discussed until expectations are at a realistic level.

Typically, microtia repair should precede surgery for aural atresia since scarring of the periauricular soft tissues from atresia repair will interfere with the cosmetic procedures from microtia surgery. In any case, a team approach is advisable where the otologist or pediatric otolaryngologist works in tandem with a facial plastic surgeon specializing on this kind of procedure (Figure 25.12).

Without any concerns from combined procedures, surgery to repair the atresia is typically performed at the end of the first decade of life. By this age, the mastoid has become more pneumatized, making the procedure easier. Surgery includes creation of a new ear canal with skin lining and creation of a new tympanic membrane. In addition, should ossicular abnormalities be present, mobilizing or repositioning of the ossicles must occur to allow for normal transmission of sound (Figure 25.13).

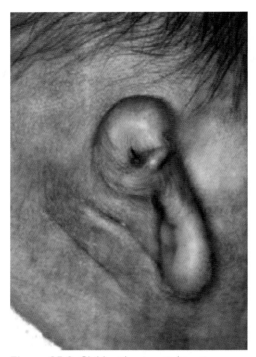

Figure 25.9 Child with microtia/atresia.

Table 25.1 Parameters assessed for the Jahrsdoerfer grading scheme

Parameter points	Points
Stapes present	2
Oval window open	1
Middle ear space	1
Facial nerve	1
Malleus/incus complex	1
Mastoid pneumatized	1
Incus–stapes connection	1
Round window	1
Appearance external ear	1
Total available points	**10**

If atresia repair is not advisable, a bone-anchored hearing appliance or similar bone conduction technologies have been recently utilized to provide hearing to patients with (bilateral) atresia, who have an unfavorable

Table 25.2 Grades of external auditory canal stenosis or atresia

Rating	Type of candidate
10	Excellent
9	Very good
8	Good
7	Fair
6	Marginal
5 or less	Poor

morphologic situation. Newer techniques include placement of active middle ear implants on the round or oval windows if these remain surgically accessible. These indications remain under clinical investigation and are not yet FDA approved.

CONGENITAL CHOLESTEATOMA
Definition and clinical features
A congenital cholesteatoma is similar to an acquired cholesteatoma in its composition of squamous epithelial lining and desquamated debris accumulating in the center of the expansile cyst. A congenital cholesteatoma arises in the middle ear space (or the more medial aspects of the temporal bone) from embryonic ectodermal remnants most commonly at the geniculate ganglion medial to the malleus. Typically, a congenital cholesteatoma is identified in the anterior superior mesotympanum with an intact tympanic membrane and no history of otitis media or middle ear disease. On otoscopy, a congenital cholesteatoma is often evident as a well-demarcated anterior mesotympanic mass with an intact tympanic membrane (Figure 25.14).

Differential diagnosis
Cholesteatoma, paraganglioma (glomus tympanicum, glomus jugulare), benign adenoma, sarcoma, endolymphatic sac tumor, and vascular (high-riding jugular bulb, persistent stapedial artery, aberrant internal carotid artery).

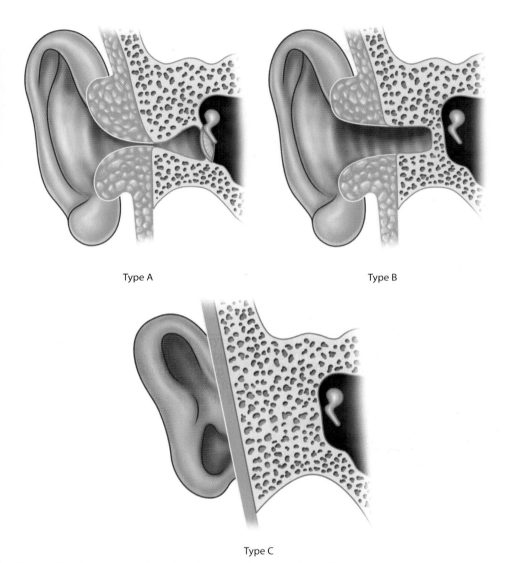

Type A   Type B

Type C

Figure 25.10 Interpretation of the Jahrsdoerfer anatomic grading system to assess microtia repair candidacy.

Workup

Although it is not necessarily recommended in the clinical evaluation of cholesteatoma in children, HRCT of the temporal bone can assist in determining both the site and the extent of a congenital cholesteatoma. In particular, this may allow the clinician to obtain a greater understanding of ossicular chain and otic capsule involvement.

Treatment

Surgical treatment is the definitive therapy for congenital cholesteatoma. Relative contraindications for operative management would

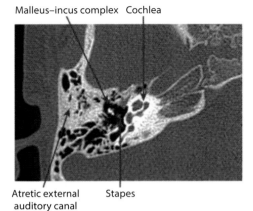

Malleus–incus complex Cochlea

Atretic external Stapes
auditory canal

Figure 25.11 CT morphologic example of a favorable case of aural atresia. Please note the good mastoid pneumatization as well as the present stapes.

include poor surgical candidacy or disease within the only hearing ear. Patients should be counseled that multiple procedures may be necessary including ossicular chain reconstruction and that depending on the location of the cholesteatoma, there is a risk that surgical treatment could worsen hearing.

ACUTE AND CHRONIC OTITIS MEDIA (REQUIRING VENTILATORY TREATMENT)
Definition and clinical features
When a child suffers from recurrent acute otitis media, persistent effusion for greater than 3 months, or a 20 dB HL conductive hearing loss, the indicated treatment is myringotomy with tympanostomy tube placement. Tympanostomy tubes (or pressure equalization [PE] tubes) allow for a consistent aeration of the middle ear space via the tympanic membrane opening. This, of course, provides an alternative route in the setting of the childhood Eustachian tube dysfunction. Specifically, the pediatric Eustachian tube assumes a more horizontal alignment when compared to the adult configuration. Once midfacial development proceeds, the Eustachian tube assumes a more vertical trajectory since the level of the palate moves inferiorly relative to the position of the middle ear. Also, hypertrophic adenoids have been postulated as being part of the pathogenesis via blocking the pharyngeal Eustachian tube ostium (Figures 25.15 through 25.17).

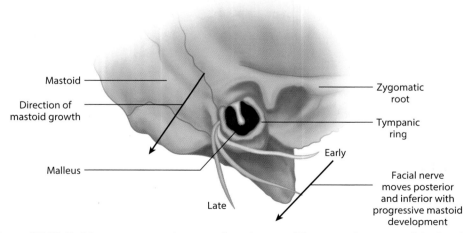

Mastoid

Direction of
mastoid growth

Malleus

Late

Early

Zygomatic
root

Tympanic
ring

Facial nerve
moves posterior
and inferior with
progressive mastoid
development

Figure 25.12 Facial nerve anatomy in cases of aural atresia. The mastoid segment of the facial nerve is moved inferiorly during the process of mastoid development.

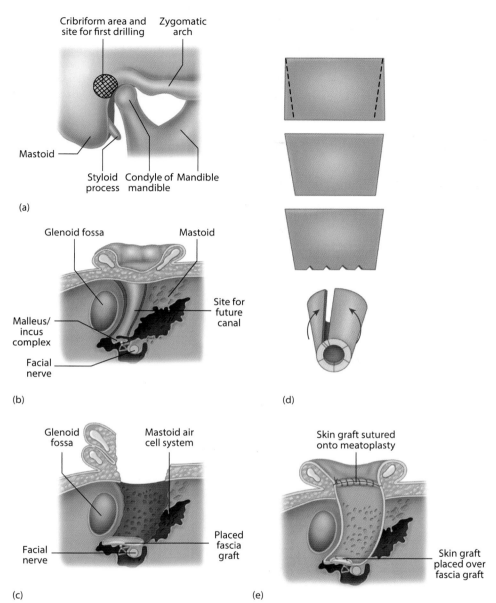

Figure 25.13 Surgical steps for aural atresia repair. (a) Cribriform are where ear canal drilling should be started. (b) Illustration of the atresia plate with the fused incus and malleus. Also, the bony attachment of the neck of the malleus with the atresia plate is a common finding. (c) Placement of the fascia graft after ear canal drilling has been completed. The mastoid air cell system should remain unopened. (d) Preparation of the split-thickness skin graft to conform to the newly drilled external auditory canal. (e) Placement of the split-thickness skin graft over the fascia graft in the position of the tympanic membrane.

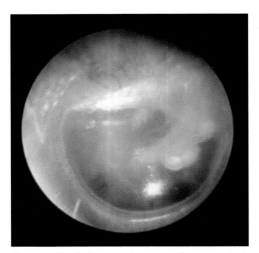

Figure 25.14 Otoscopic image of a congenital cholesteatoma presenting behind an intact eardrum in an ear with a white mass located in the anterior superior quadrant.

It appears that Eustachian tube functionality should assume an adult level at around age 7. At this point, the child's anatomic configuration has matured enough. Also, the immune system has developed and the adenoid cushion has retracted to provide ample ventilation of the tympanomastoid compartment (Figures 25.18 through 25.20).

Workup

Otoscopy, tympanometry, audiometric testing, and good patient history are all that are typically necessary to determine the need for tympanostomy tubes. If chronic infection persists, oftentimes, a sample of the middle ear effusion can be obtained for culture and sensitivity in order to tailor antibiotic therapy.

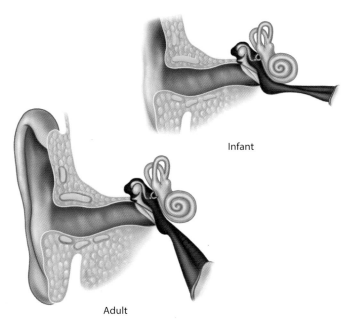

Infant

Adult

Figure 25.15 Adult and pediatric Eustachian tube configuration.

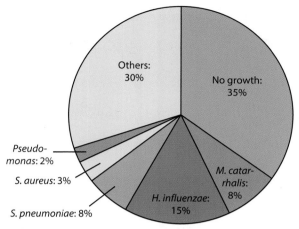

Figure 25.16 Common pathogens in chronic otitis media with effusion.

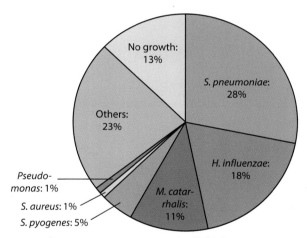

Figure 25.17 Common pathogens in acute otitis media (AOM).

Treatment

There are a variety of types of tympanostomy tubes that can be placed based on disease process, patient age, and surgeon preference:

Popular types of tubes include

1. Armstrong grommets
2. T-tubes (flexible flange)
3. Collar button tubes
4. Titanium tube

The indication for tympanostomy tube placement is chronic otitis media with effusion. As such, a child should have bilateral effusions for more than 3 months, which do not respond to antibiotic treatment. With unilateral effusions, a more conservative approach can be attempted. However, close clinical follow-up is mandatory (Figures 25.21 and 25.22).

Also, tympanostomy tubes are indicated with (imminent) complications from

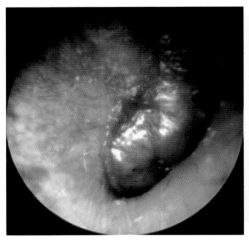

Figure 25.18 Otoscopic image of a bulging tympanic membrane observed in the clinical setting of acute purulent otitis media.

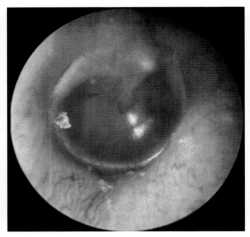

Figure 25.19 Chronic otitis media with effusion. The tympanic membrane is radially injected.

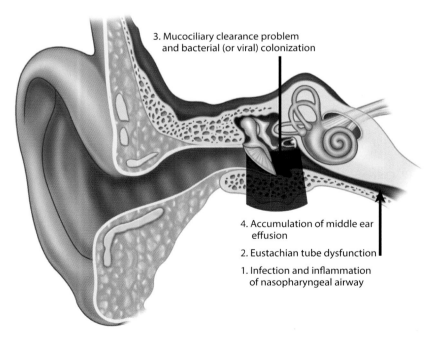

3. Mucociliary clearance problem and bacterial (or viral) colonization

4. Accumulation of middle ear effusion

2. Eustachian tube dysfunction

1. Infection and inflammation of nasopharyngeal airway

Figure 25.20 Typical pathophysiological pathway in the development of otitis media.

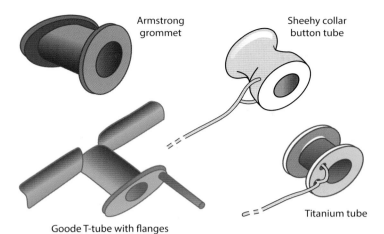

Armstrong grommet

Sheehy collar button tube

Titanium tube

Goode T-tube with flanges

Figure 25.21 Types of tympanostomy tubes.

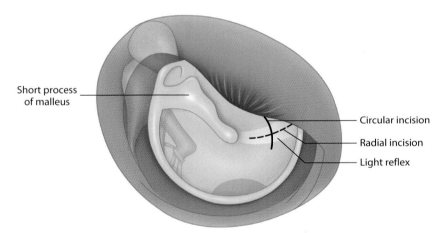

Short process of malleus

Circular incision

Radial incision

Light reflex

Figure 25.22 Placement of a myringotomy incision in the anterior inferior quadrant.

otitis media. Sometimes, emergent PE tube placement has to be contemplated especially with CNS complications. Due to the mostly symmetric functional impairment of the Eustachian tube, tympanostomy tubes should be placed in both ears even in the setting of a unilateral effusion. Exemptions to this rule exist, however. In older children with new-onset effusions, nasopharyngeal pathology must be excluded (Figure 25.23; Table 25.3).

COMPLICATIONS OF ACUTE OTITIS MEDIA/MASTOIDITIS
Definitions
Mastoiditis and the complications of acute and chronic otitis media have fortunately become rare events. Bacteria can enter the tympanomastoid compartment either via the middle ear in AOM or originating from the mastoid cavity in chronic otitis media (COM). The complications of otitis media are then divided between intra- and

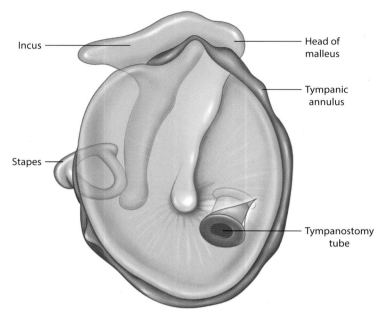

Incus — — Head of malleus

— Tympanic annulus

Stapes —

— Tympanostomy tube

Figure 25.23 Correct PE tube placement within the anterior inferior quadrant of the tympanic membrane.

extracranial categories. The most common complication of AOM is a postauricular, subperiosteal abscess. In the evaluation of potential mastoiditis or complications of otitis media, a detailed history with an exact timeline of events is critical. Specifically, complications are typically the result of an initially successful antibiotic treatment of otitis media with a recurrence about 10 days into the course. This is typically caused by bacterial strains not covered by the initial antibiotic treatment (Figure 25.24).

Differential diagnosis
Cranial/intratemporal complications
Mastoiditis (coalescent, chronic)

1. Ossicular erosion (conductive hearing loss)
2. Tympanic membrane perforation
3. Cholesteatoma formation

Table 25.3 Complications of tympanostomy tubes

Tube otorrhea (~25% of cases) result of water contamination, otitis media, hypersensitivity to tube material, biofilm formation on tube surface (removal typically required) less frequent after myringotomy only

Permanent perforation (~5%–10%) depending on length of intubation, tube size, otorrhea

Premature tube extrusion in rare cases, monolayer vs. bilayer, tympanic membrane

Retention of tube rarely, a tube can migrate into the middle ear space and remain in the middle ear

Tube migration

Cholesteatoma formation rare, typically extending from tube site in anterior inferior quadrant

a. Epidural abscess
b. Cerebellar abscess
c. Temporal lobe abscess
3. Sigmoid sinus thrombosis
4. Lateral sinus thrombosis
5. Subdural empyema
6. Otitic hydrocephalus

Workup

A complete neurological examination, audiometric testing, as well as laboratory studies and imaging studies are critical. Specifically, a contrasted CT scan of the temporal bones should be completed. With suspected intracranial complications, an MRI should be ordered to delineate potential CNS involvement. Often, these studies have to be obtained in a timely fashion (Figure 25.25).

TREATMENT

All patients with these complications will typically benefit from at least tympanostomy tube placement and culture-directed antibiotics with or without cortical mastoidectomy. A Bezold or subperiosteal abscess will require incision and drainage. Petrous apicitis (Gradenigo syndrome) requires prolonged IV antibiotic therapy, mastoid decompression with a PE tube, and/or cortical mastoidectomy and, in rare cases, surgical decompression of the petrous apex. Intracranial abscess will require drainage in conjunction with neurosurgical services. Systemic steroids should be considered (Figures 25.26 through 25.28).

CONGENITAL CONDUCTIVE HEARING LOSS

Definition and clinical features

The most common form of congenital ossicular anomaly with stapes footplate fixation is seen without evidence of otosclerotic bone changes. These patients present with conductive hearing loss that is nonprogressive, and there is no history

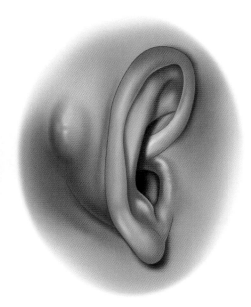

Figure 25.24 Postauricular abscess formation (subperiosteal abscess) typically seen in mastoiditis.

4. Labyrinthitis (serous, suppurative)—progression of infection into labyrinth through round or oval window
5. Bezold abscess—erosion of mastoid tip with infection of soft tissues of neck
6. Soft tissue/subperiosteal abscess—postauricular incision and drainage
7. Petrous apicitis—inflammation of petrous apex (Gradenigo syndrome—petrous apicitis with trigeminal neuralgia, abducens palsy, otorrhea)
8. Labyrinthine fistula
9. Facial nerve complications
10. Encephalocele and cerebrospinal fluid leakage

Intracranial/extratemporal complications

1. Meningitis
2. Intracranial abscess

Enlarged bony aperture of ELS
Mastoid effusion
Incomplete cochlear partitioning

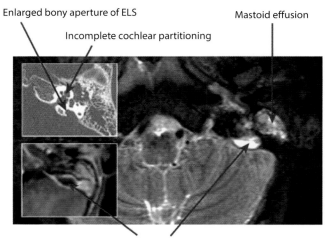

Abscess formation within an ELS

Figure 25.25 Axial CT and MRI of an endolymphatic sac abscess within the left temporal bone. The patient had a previously undiagnosed Mondini malformation (enlarged vestibular aqueduct and incomplete cochlear partitioning). ELS, endolymphatic sac.

Abscess formation of the sigmoid sinus

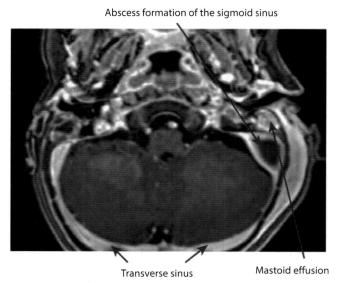

Transverse sinus   Mastoid effusion

Figure 25.26 Abscess formation of the left sigmoid sinus as a complication of otitis media.

of trauma or infection. Children will present with normal otoscopic examination, without changes to the eardrum. Abnormalities to the stapes footplate are typically isolated from other ossicular anomalies secondary to different embryologic origin. It is caused by fixation between the peripheral lamina stapedialis and the annular ligament and is typically bilateral.

Petrous apex inflammation

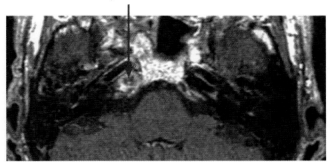

Figure 25.27 Gradenigo syndrome caused by right petrous apicitis. The patient complained of retroorbital pain, CN VI palsy, and otitis media.

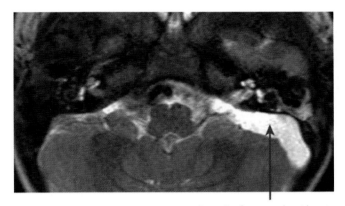

Posterior fossa arachnoid cyst

Figure 25.28 Postinfectious development of a posterior fossa (laterocerebellar) arachnoid cyst. The patient had a sigmoid sinus abscess.

Differential diagnosis

Congenital malleus head fixation, other ossicular chain fixation, congenital cholesteatoma, incompleted external aural atresia, posttraumatic ossicular chain fixation, and oval or round window atresia.

Workup

Audiogram and HRCT of the temporal bones. It is critical to obtain stapedius reflex testing since children with a third window pathology such as an enlarged vestibular aqueduct can present with (pseudo)conductive hearing loss. Surgical management of these cases will likely result in a profound sensorineural hearing loss on the affected ear. Thus, children presenting with a conductive hearing loss with a present stapedius reflex should be further evaluated using a CT of the temporal bones.

Treatment

In general, children with congenital conductive hearing loss can be managed both surgically and nonsurgically. The latter involves conventional amplification via a hearing aid. Unilateral versus bilateral involvement as well as the child's educational situation should be considered. Thus, a team approach working with audiologists, speech and language pathologists, and educators seems critical in making the correct decision.

Surgical management typically involves a middle ear exploration with subsequent ossiculoplasty. In case of true stapes fixation, a stapedotomy/stapedectomy can be performed. Care must be taken intraoperatively to evaluate the ear in a comprehensive fashion. With present reflexes and a conductive hearing loss, imaging studies should be obtained to rule out a third window pathology and thus a pseudoconductive involvement.

Inner ear

PEDIATRIC SENSORINEURAL HEARING LOSS
Definition and clinical features
About 3–4 children in 1000 live births are born with a significant hearing impairment with 25% ultimately being diagnosed with severe-to-profound sensorineural hearing loss, thus being considered for cochlear implantation. Early intervention remains critical since central auditory developments depend on appropriate acoustic stimulation. Hence, a hearing decision has to be made prior to the onset or speech and language (or the lack thereof) (Figure 25.29; Table 25.4).

Differential diagnosis
There are nongenetic (25%), genetic (50%), and idiopathic (25%) causes. Genetic causes can be nonsyndromic (70%) or syndomic (30%). Common autosomal dominant syndromic causes of hearing loss include Waardenburg, branchio-oto-renal, and Treacher Collins syndromes. Common autosomal recessive syndromic causes of hearing loss include Usher, Pendred, and Jervell and Lange-Nielson syndromes (Figure 25.30).

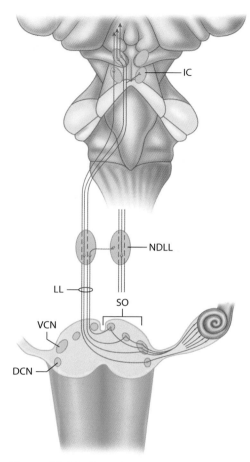

Figure 25.29 Central auditory pathway to the inferior colliculus.

Workup
Most developed countries have hearing screening programs available. These are based either on automated ABR algorithms or on otoacoustic emissions (OAEs). The latter method only measures hair cell function and will thus not likely pick up hearing loss due to auditory neuropathy spectrum disorder (ANSD). The newborn screening rate in North Carolina, for example, is 99.7%. As with many screening tests, newborn infant hearing screening features a high sensitivity and low specificity (Figure 25.31).

Table 25.4 Common genetic causes of sensorineural hearing loss (DFN: gene loci for DeaFNess) .

DFN	Gene	Onset	Type and degree
DFNB1	*GJB2 GJB6*	Prelingual	Usually unstable
DFNB2	*MYO7A*	Prelingual, postlingual	Unspecified
DFNB3	*MYO15*	Prelingual	Stable
DFNB4	*SLC26A4*	Prelingual, postlingual	Stable or progressive
DFNB6	*TM1E*	Prelingual	Stable
DFNB7/11	*TMC1*	Prelingual	Stable
DFNB8/10	*TMPRSS3*	Postlingual/prelingual	Progressive or stable
DFNB9	*OTOF*		
DFNB12	*CDH23*		
DFNB16	*STRC*		
DFNB18	*USH1C*		Stable
DFNB21	*TECTA*		Stable
DFNB22	*OTOA*	Prelingual	
DFNB29	*CLDN14*		
DFNB30	*MYO3A*		
DFNB31	*DFN31*		—
DFNB36	*ESPN*		—
DFNB37	*MYO6*		
DFNA1	*DIAPH1*	Postlingual/first	Low frequency progressive
DFNA2	*GJB3 KCNQ4*	Postlingual/second	High frequency progressive
DFNA3	*GJB2 GJB6*	Prelingual	
DFNA4	*MYH14*	Postlingual	Flat/gently downsloping
DFNA5	*DFNA5*	Postlingual/first	High frequency progressive
DFNA6/14/38	*WFS1*	Prelingual	Low frequency progressive
DFNA8/12	*TECTA*	Prelingual	Midfrequency loss
DFNA9	*COCA*	Postlingual/second	High frequency progressive
DFNA10	*EYA4*	Postlingual/third, fourth	Flat, gently downsloping
DFNA11	*MYO7A*	Postlingual/first	Flat, gently downsloping
DFNA13	*COL11A2*	Postlingual/second	Midfrequency loss
DFNA15	*POU4F3*		
DFNA17	*MYH9*		High frequency progressive
DFNA20/26	*ACTG1*		High frequency progressive
DFNA22	*MYO6*	Postlingual	
DFNA28	*TFCP2L3*	Postlingual	Flat, gently downsloping
DFNA36	*TMC1*		Flat, gently downsloping
DFNA39	*DSPP*		High frequency progressive
DFNA48	*MYO1A*		
DFN3	*POU3F4*		Variable, often progresses to profound

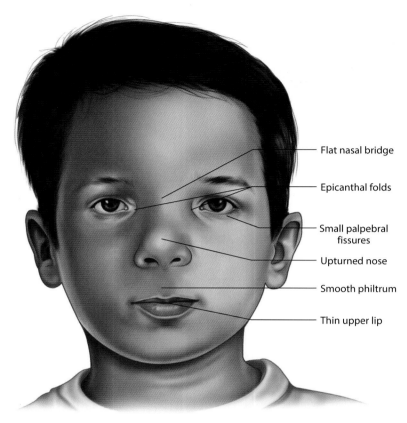

Flat nasal bridge

Epicanthal folds

Small palpebral fissures

Upturned nose

Smooth philtrum

Thin upper lip

Figure 25.30 Facial features typically observed in Waardenburg syndrome.

With a failed screening test, children are typically referred to an otolaryngologist and a pediatric audiologist within the first few months. In fact, it is advisable to perform a diagnostic ABR before the child has reached 2 months of age since most of these tests can be done under natural sleep. With older children, however, a sedated ABR should be scheduled. The results of the ABR are typically utilized to estimate ear-specific pure-tone thresholds and fit hearing aids. A medical evaluation process can be initiated at this point. This typically consists of an imaging study (we recommend an MRI) to assess both labyrinthine and central nervous system pathologies. An EKG should be obtained to rule out Jervell and Lange-Nielsen syndrome since the cardiac conduction deficit can typically be managed to avoid sudden death (Figures 25.32 and 25.33).

Also, genetic testing can be offered either via a direct blood draw or with blood obtained from a Guthrie card. Similarly, a Guthrie card can be used to test for perinatal CMV infection, a not uncommon cause for hearing loss.

With about 7–8 months of age, many children can be conditioned for visual response audiometry (VRA), a test used to confirm the thresholds previously obtained via the ABR. With lack of progress from conventional amplification, thresholds in

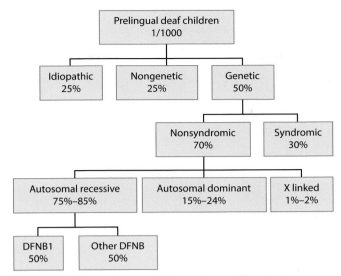

Figure 25.31 Common etiologies of congenital sensorineural hearing loss.

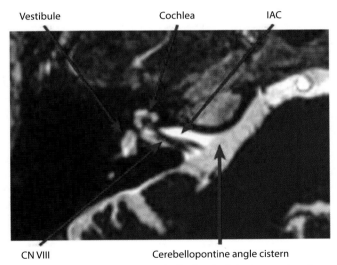

Figure 25.32 Axial CISS-sequence MRI through the level of the internal auditory canal (IAC) demonstrating normal morphology.

the severe-to-profound range, and no obvious contraindications, a cochlear implant should be considered. Implantation should be performed around the first birthday to facilitate proper speech and language development.

Some children demonstrate a progressive sensorineural hearing loss and should be followed closely. With proper speech and language development until a certain point, cochlear implantation remains a great tool for hearing rehabilitation. Late implantation

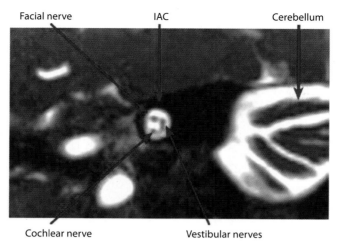

Figure 25.33 Normal contents of the internal auditory canal (IAC) as evidenced via this oblique parasagittal MRI (CISS sequence) to illustrate all four nerves within the lateral end (fundus) of the canal.

in profoundly hearing impaired children without proper speech and language development has been shown to lead to variable results and there appears to be a clear dependency of speech outcomes and age at implantation (Figure 25.34).

A team approach including multiple specialties appears to be critical when dealing with pediatric sensorineural hearing loss. The otolaryngologist should work closely with pediatric audiologists, educators, speech and language pathologists, and other specialties to improve outcomes and to provide adequate multidisciplinary care.

LABYRINTHINE MALFORMATIONS
Definitions
About 20% of pediatric sensorineural hearing losses are due to dysplasia of the bony labyrinth. Normal inner ear development can be arrested at various stages. Thus, a spectrum of labyrinthine malformations has been described. Arrested development of the otic placode, for example, results in a Michel deformity with the complete absence of the vestibulocochlear structures. Arrest at later stages of development can lead to either a common cavity deformity with rudimentary neuroepithelium or other cystic anomalies. After this stage, the cochlea or individual vestibular canals can be hypoplastic, a condition often encountered with syndromic involvement. The most common labyrinthine malformation is an enlargement of the vestibular aqueduct. This describes an abnormally large connection between the utricle and the endolymphatic sac. The large sac can be observed on T2-weighted MRI, whereas the CT scan can show the enlarged bony aperture of the endolymphatic duct. This malformation is often accompanied by a large vestibule and an incompletely partitioned cochlea. Children are sometimes born with residual hearing, but they typically also show a progressive loss of auditory function (Figure 25.35).

Absence of semicircular canals has been associated with cochlear nerve deficiency and syndromic cases are mostly due to CHARGE association.

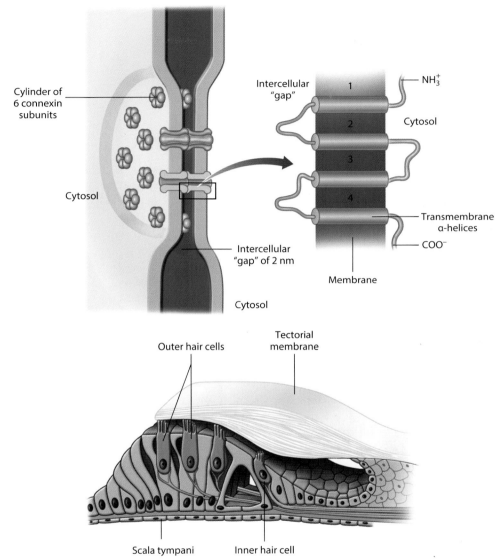

Cylinder of
6 connexin
subunits

Cytosol

Intercellular
"gap"

NH_3^+

Cytosol

1

2

3

4

Transmembrane
α-helices

COO^-

Intercellular
"gap" of 2 nm

Membrane

Cytosol

Tectorial
membrane

Outer hair cells

Scala tympani

Inner hair cell

Figure 25.34 Intracochlear distribution of Connexin 26, a gap junction protein responsible for potassium recirculation in the stria vascularis. It is the most common cause for nonsyndromic, autosomal recessive sensorineural hearing loss (GJB2).

Differential diagnosis

Michel deformity, common cavity deformity, hypoplasia of the cochlear of vestibular canals, enlarged vestibular aqueduct, and cochlear nerve deficiency. The labyrinthine malformation may be the only problem or part of a syndrome.

WORKUP

MRI and/or CT.

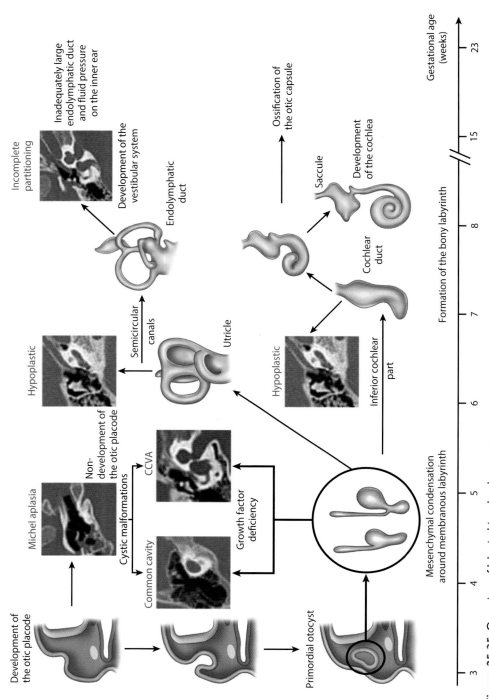

Figure 25.35 Overview of labyrinthine development.

TREATMENT

Cochlear implantation can be quite successful, even in the setting of a malformed inner ear. In fact, children with malformations of the incomplete cochlear portioning spectrum typically are excellent cochlear implant candidates. Children with cystic malformations typically do not perform well with cochlear implants and Michel deformities are considered contraindications to implantation (Figures 25.36 and 25.37).

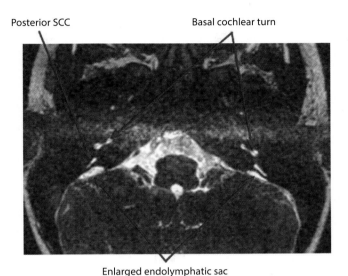

Figure 25.36 Axial MRI (CISS sequence) demonstrating bilaterally enlarged vestibular aqueducts.

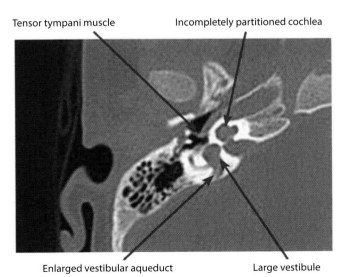

Figure 25.37 Axial high-resolution computed tomography (HRCT) demonstrating a Mondini malformation (enlarged vestibular aqueduct, large vestibule, incomplete cochlear partitioning).

AUDITORY NEUROPATHY SPECTRUM DISORDER

ANSDs have recently been recognized as a cause for sensorineural hearing loss. In fact, it is estimated that about 10%–15% of pediatric sensorineural hearing loss are caused by ANSD. The electrophysiological pattern describes a working cochlea with a neuropathic cochlear nerve. In some cases, the nerve can be anatomically absent or hypoplastic (termed cochlear nerve deficiency). In most cases, however, the nerve is physically present, but it is unable to conduct the electrical information to the cochlear nucleus (Table 25.5).

Various risk factors have been described. Prematurity, high bilirubin levels, and an extensive stay in the NICU have been discussed. The electrophysiological patterns observed are quite consistent, however. Specifically, affected children show a lack of central auditory activation (no ABR waves) with a present cochlear microphonic potential. This potential is a hair cell potential that follows the polarity of the stimulus. Thus, with sound stimuli alternating polarity during the ABR, the cochlear microphonics of both phases will cancel each other and thus be not present. Thus, a single polarity ABR should be obtained to conclude the proper diagnosis (Figure 25.38).

Affected children have variable thresholds and speech perception issues beyond what would be expected for the specific level of hearing impairment. Since ABRs typically do not demonstrate distal waves that could be utilized to estimate hearing levels, threshold estimation has to wait until children are able to be conditioned to VRA testing. This occurs around ages 7–8 months. Thus, early intervention in terms of early amplification is delayed until these data are available (Figures 25.39 and 25.40).

Cochlear implantation has been performed with variable success in these children. Also, a subset of children performs well with conventional amplification. With cochlear nerve deficiency, especially with bilateral involvement, auditory brainstem implantation might be a reasonable option in the future (Figures 25.41 and 25.42).

Table 25.5 Clinical characteristics of auditory neuropathy spectrum disorder (ANSD)

Pure-tone threshold: variable; can be normal

Speech recognition in quiet: variable, typically poor in noise

Otoacoustic emissions: normal or absent

Middle ear muscle reflexes: absent

Cochlear microphonic (CM): present (inverts with stimulus polarity reversal)

ABR: CM and absent distal waveform

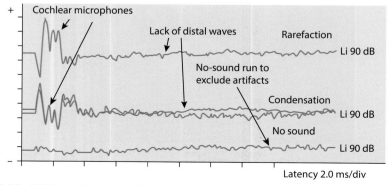

Figure 25.38 ABR in a child with auditory neuropathy spectrum disorder (ANSD).

Intracochlear part of electrode array   Receiver/stimulator

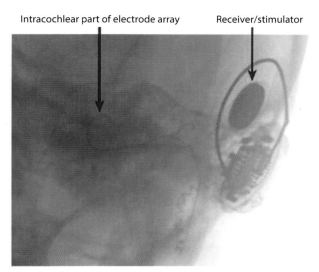

Figure 25.39 Transorbital projection obtained intraoperatively demonstrating appropriate positioning of a cochlear implant within the cochlea.

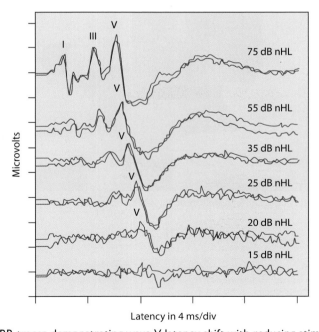

Figure 25.40 ABR traces demonstrating wave V latency shift with reducing stimulus intensities.

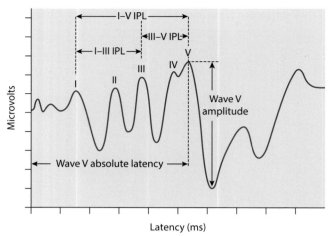

Figure 25.41 Normal ABR waveform.

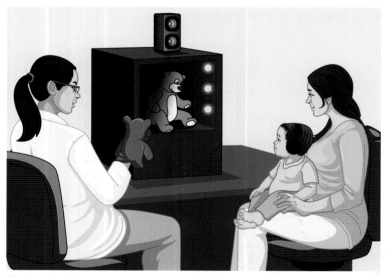

Figure 25.42 Visual reinforcement audiometry (VRA).

Sinonasal Disease

Austin S. Rose

- **Normal pediatric airway**
- **Adenoid hypertrophy**
- **Arhinia**
- **Choanal atresia**
- **Congenital nasolacrimal duct cyst**
- **Cystic fibrosis**
- **Nasal dermoid sinus cyst**
- **Nasal glioma and encephalocele**
- **Nasopharyngeal hairy polyp**
- **References**

Normal pediatric airway

Children can have many of the same causes of nasal pathology as an adult, including allergic rhinitis, nasal polyposis, chronic sinusitis, and benign or malignant tumors. However, this chapter focuses on pathologies that are likely to present in childhood. Many congenital lesions appear early in childhood. The neonate is an obligate nasal breather. As such, congenital lesions of the nose may result in life-threatening airway obstruction and/or difficulty with feeding during this period. Additional symptoms include "cyclical cyanosis," characterized by awake periods of agitation or crying during which the neonate may mouth breath and appear stable but followed by periods of calm or sleep where nasal breathing is not possible and apnea and cyanosis occur. Congenital lesions with less severe obstruction can often present later in childhood.

Adenoid hypertrophy

DEFINITION AND CLINICAL FEATURES
Adenoid hypertrophy is one of the most common causes of nasal obstruction in children. Lymphoid hyperplasia occurs by the same pathophysiology as tonsil hypertrophy. Adenoid often regresses in late childhood; however, hypertrophy is common in young children and may cause nasal obstruction. Symptoms may include snoring, chronic mouth breathing, dental problems, and hyponasal speech.

DIFFERENTIAL DIAGNOSIS
Antrochoanal polyp, turbinate hypertrophy, choanal atresia, deviated septum, and foreign body.

WORKUP
There is a limited role for further workup of adenoid hypertrophy in children beyond the history and physical examination as radiographs are unlikely to impact clinical decision making. However, if another etiology of nasal obstruction is suspected, the differential diagnosis may warrant imaging, flexible nasopharyngoscopy, or both.

TREATMENT
Intranasal steroids are an option for treatment in children with allergic rhinitis. Indications for adenoidectomy include adenoid hypertrophy resulting in nasal obstruction in addition to sinusitis, recurrent otitis media, and sleep-disordered breathing. Velopharyngeal insufficiency is a potential complication, occurring in about 1/1,500 adenoidectomies (Figure 26.1).

Arhinia

DEFINITION AND CLINICAL FEATURES
Arhinia, or congenital absence of the nose and nasal airway, is an extremely rare anomaly with less than 20 reported cases in the literature. This condition includes absence

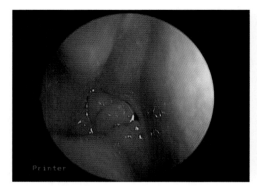

Figure 26.1 Adenoid tissue filling the nasal airway as seen on sinonasal endoscopy through the right side of the nose.

of the external nose and nasal airways, hypoplasia of the maxilla, a small high-arched palate, and hypertelorism. In most cases, there is a lack of the olfactory nerves and bulbs. In addition, there may be other associated anomalies including encephalocele, absence of paranasal sinuses, midface anomalies including cleft palate, low set ears, and various eye anomalies. Any associated ocular abnormalities are usually minor as the eye begins to form at an earlier stage of embryologic development. The occurrence of arhinia is thought to be sporadic and no specific maternal risk factors or associated chromosomal abnormalities have been identified. The immediate complications are severe airway impairment, due to the dependence of neonates on their nasal airway, and difficulties in feeding (Figure 26.2).

DIFFERENTIAL DIAGNOSIS
Other congenital nasal anomalies and choanal atresia.

WORKUP
Because infants are obligate nasal breathers, failure to recognize the implications of total nasal obstruction can result in hypoxia and death immediately after birth. The first priority in newborn patients with arhinia,

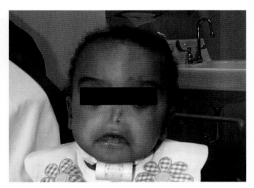

Figure 26.2 Neonate with arhinia status post tracheostomy tube placement.

therefore, is to establish a safe airway. An oral airway can be helpful initially and a McGovern nipple may be used for training an infant to breathe through the mouth and for feeding. Endotracheal intubation is necessary in some cases, and for those newborns unable to be extubated, tracheotomy is appropriate. Due to feeding difficulties, many infants with arhinia also require a gastric feeding tube for nutrition. Once the primary issues of airway and feeding have been addressed, the child with arhinia should be carefully evaluated for other congenital anomalies. A CT scan and MRI of the head and face should be obtained to rule out associated anomalies and to plan future efforts at reconstruction (Figure 26.3).

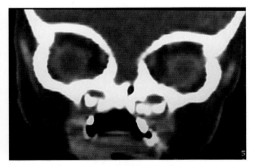

Figure 26.3 Coronal CT scan demonstrating the absence of nasal passages and cribriform plate.

TREATMENT

The goals of surgical treatment in patients with arhinia are to establish a patent nasal airway and to correct the external cosmetic defect. The recommended timing of initial surgical intervention varies from 4 weeks[1,2] to preschool age when facial development is more complete.[3] As a child with arhinia approaches school age, psychological issues relating to his or her cosmetic appearance become a more pressing issue. Currently, there is no consensus on surgical treatment or technique. While some authors have performed simultaneous reconstruction of the internal and external nose, others describe the creation of internal nasal passages with delayed external reconstruction.[2] In one report, an external nasal reconstruction was performed without the creation of internal nasal cavities.[4] In some cases, children have been managed solely with a prosthetic external nose.

Choanal atresia

DEFINITION AND CLINICAL FEATURES

Choanal atresia is the congenital absence of the normal pathway between the posterior nasal cavity and the remainder of the upper aerodigestive tract. Occurring approximately once in every 8000 births, it is seen twice as often in females as in males.[5] The obstruction between the nasal cavity and nasopharynx is usually composed of bone, though in some cases may be described as primarily membranous or mixed in nature. Choanal atresia is most commonly unilateral, though when it occurs bilaterally it is a neonatal emergency requiring immediate protection of the airway due to the dependence of infants on nasal breathing (Figure 26.4). Unilateral disease may be detected in the neonatal period by failure to pass a flexible catheter into the nasopharynx on routine screening or later in life due to unilateral symptoms of nasal obstruction with thick mucous drainage (Figure 26.5).

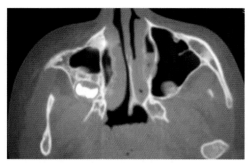

Figure 26.4 An axial CT scan at the level of the nasopharynx demonstrating left unilateral choanal atresia.

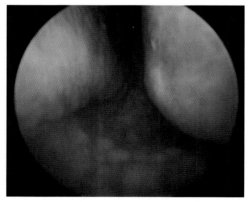

Figure 26.5 An endoscopic view of the left posterior nasal cavity shows the absence of the choanal opening into the nasopharynx.

DIFFERENTIAL DIAGNOSIS

Bilateral choanal atresia: pyriform aperture stenosis, bilateral vocal cord paralysis, and other congenital upper airway obstructions.

Unilateral choanal atresia: nasal foreign body, antrochoanal polyp, adenoid hypertrophy, and chronic sinusitis (Figure 26.6).

WORKUP

Choanal atresia is often suspected in newborns after failure to pass a small flexible catheter through the nose into the oropharynx. The airway in a neonate with bilateral choanal atresia may be secured using an oral airway taped in place or with endotracheal intubation. Once stable, a CT scan with 1 mm cuts through the nose and nasopharynx should be obtained to evaluate the site and degree of obstruction. A genetics consult should also be considered to help evaluate for concomitant findings characteristic of CHARGE syndrome including coloboma, heart defects, choanal atresia, retarded growth and development, genitourinary anomalies and ear abnormalities including hearing loss (Figure 26.7).

TREATMENT

Bilateral choanal atresia is generally treated with surgery early in the postnatal period with the goal of establishing nasal patency. For unilateral atresia, surgery may be delayed until early childhood. Transnasal endoscopic approaches are used most frequently and sometimes require drilling and removal of the posterior vomer depending on the amount of bony obstruction. Transpalatal approaches are also described, though used less frequently. Restenosis, usually over a period of 3–6 months, is common and may require additional surgery or dilation. Stents are commonly used postoperatively, though some authors have reported success without them (Figure 26.8).[6] The use of topical mitomycin C, an inhibitor of epithelial cell migration, has also been described in reducing renarrowing and stenosis, though recent studies have failed to demonstrate significant benefit.[7] Growth of the child will also help ultimately in maintaining choanal patency.

Congenital nasolacrimal duct cyst

DEFINITION AND CLINICAL FEATURES

Congenital nasolacrimal duct cyst is a very rare condition resulting from obstructed nasolacrimal ducts in the inferior meatus of the nose leading to nasal airway obstruction.

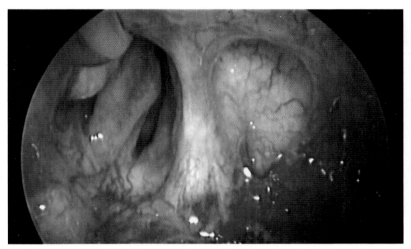

Figure 26.6 Obstruction of the left choana due to a bony atretic plate seen endoscopically from the nasopharyngeal side.

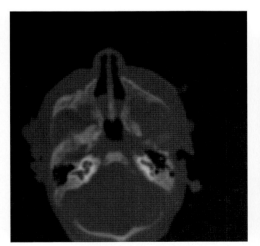

Figure 26.7 An axial CT scan demonstrating membranous choanal atresia, bilaterally.

Airway and feeding difficulties vary in severity (Figure 26.9).

DIFFERENTIAL DIAGNOSIS
Choanal atresia, congenital nasolacrimal duct cyst(s), and congenital nasal mass (glioma, meningocele, meningoencephalocele, vascular malformation).

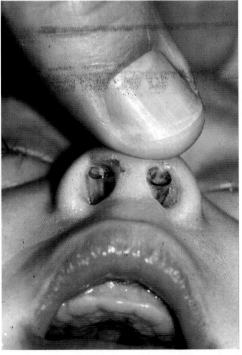

Figure 26.8 Stents created from endotracheal tubes secured with transseptal stitch.

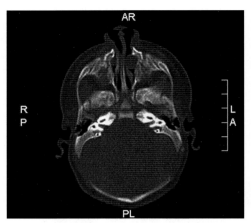

Figure 26.9 CT of congenital nasolacrimal duct cysts.

WORKUP

Diagnosis is suspected by physical examination. Anterior rhinoscopy may be normal in the neonate. The ability to pass catheters through the nose may be difficult but nasal endoscopy will reveal the problem. A complete airway evaluation is recommended immediately followed by surgical treatment. Imaging confirms the diagnosis and rules out other congenital nasal masses, which require more complicated management.

TREATMENT

Treatment is marsupialization of the cysts. Symptom resolution should be clinically confirmed and surveillance for recurrence should be assessed by nasal endoscopy (Figure 26.10).

Cystic fibrosis

DEFINITION AND CLINICAL FEATURES

Cystic fibrosis (CF) is an autosomal recessive genetic disease associated with numerous mutations of the CF transmembrane conductance regulator gene, which regulates the movement of sodium and chloride ions across epithelial membranes.[8] The results are dehydration and thickening of secretions affecting the respiratory tract, pancreas, liver, and intestines. In the paranasal sinuses and lungs, reduced and thickened secretions impair the normal function of cilia in mucociliary clearance, leading to recurrent cycles of infection and inflammation. Nasal polyps and chronic rhinosinusitis (CRS) are the hallmarks of ENT disease in children with CF. In addition to sinonasal symptoms, CRS may also contribute to pulmonary disease including recurrent bronchopneumonia and bronchiectasis (Figure 26.11).

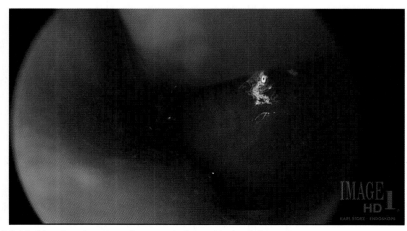

Figure 26.10 Nasal endoscopy of congenital nasolacrimal duct cysts.

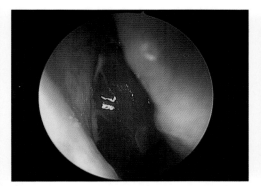

Figure 26.11 Endoscopic view of right nasal polyp at the middle meatus in a child with cystic fibrosis.

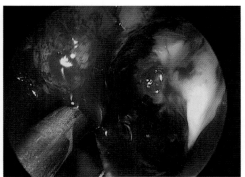

Figure 26.12 Intraoperative photograph of purulent fluid within the left maxillary sinus.

DIFFERENTIAL DIAGNOSIS

Primary ciliary dyskinesia, nasal polyposis, and chronic rhinosinusitis.

WORKUP

Children with nasal polyps or refractory CRS should be evaluated for CF with sweat chloride testing. Genetic testing for common genotypes is also available. A CT scan of the sinuses can be helpful for baseline evaluation as well as preoperative planning (Figure 26.12). Cultures obtained from the middle meatus or sinuses can be helpful in directing antibiotic therapy when needed.

TREATMENT

Sinonasal disease due to CF is treated with a medical regimen including nasal saline irrigations and topical nasal steroid spray. Surgery, such as adenoidectomy or functional endoscopic sinus surgery (FESS), is considered for nasal obstruction due to polyps, severe sinonasal symptoms, or the possible effects of sinus disease on the lungs, as might be demonstrated with decreased pulmonary function testing. The need for revision FESS is common in many CF patients (Figure 26.13).

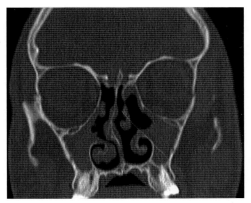

Figure 26.13 A coronal CT scan demonstrating the recurrence of disease within the maxillary sinuses despite prior endoscopic sinus surgery with adequate maxillary antrostomies.

Nasal dermoid sinus cyst

DEFINITION AND CLINICAL FEATURES

Nasal dermoid sinus cysts (NDSCs) are congenital nasal masses resulting from the inclusion of epithelial cells along the lines of embryonic closure (Figure 26.14). Containing both ectodermal and mesodermal elements, these cysts generally present along the midline nasal dorsum and are classically associated with a single

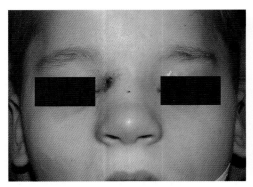

Figure 26.14 Infected nasal dermoid sinus cyst (NDSC) with skin breakdown and characteristic midline nasal pit and hair.

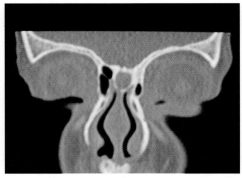

Figure 26.15 A coronal CT scan demonstrating a nasal dermoid sinus cyst (NDSC).

nasal pit and hair follicle. NDSC is present at birth in 40% of cases, while the remainder generally become clinically apparent by age 6.

Dermoid cysts can occur in other areas, including the brow, forehead, chin, and occiput, and may erode the skull.

DIFFERENTIAL DIAGNOSIS
Congenital teratoma, hemangioma, or other vascular lesions.

WORKUP
Both CT and MRI are helpful in further evaluating NDSC prior to excision. About 45% of cysts extend deep to the nasal bones, and up to 25% are associated with a tract connecting to the dura or more obvious intracranial extension (Figures 26.15 and 26.16).

TREATMENT
Because of the potential for infection, these cysts should be surgically excised along with any associated tracts or intracranial component. For cysts limited to the soft tissues of the nasal dorsum, local excision of the cyst and any associated pit or hair is generally sufficient. NDSC with deeper extension may require an external rhinoplasty incision or, rarely, a combined

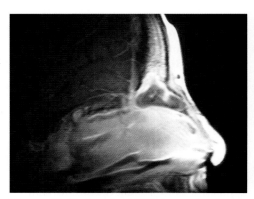

Figure 26.16 A sagittal MRI shows the close association of a nasal dermoid sinus cyst (NDSC) with both the dura and skin of the nasal dorsum.

craniofacial approach. Recent reports have also described the use of endoscopic techniques, either through the nose or via a small scalp incision, for the surgical treatment of NDSC (Figure 26.17).[9,10]

Nasal glioma and encephalocele

DEFINITION AND CLINICAL FEATURES
Nasal gliomas, or nasal glial heterotopia, are congenital malformations of displaced normal glial tissue with no residual intracranial

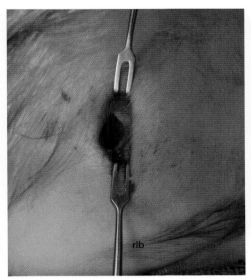

Figure 26.17 Erosion of the skull from a fore-head dermoid seen intraoperatively over the right lateral brow (rlb).

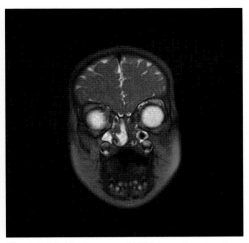

Figure 26.19 A coronal MRI reveals a nasal glioma with both intranasal and extranasal components, though no obvious intracranial connection.

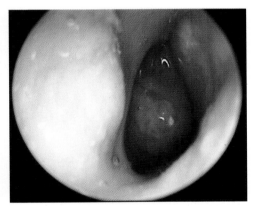

Figure 26.18 Anterior nasal exam demonstrating the intranasal component of a large congenital nasal glioma.

space and circulating cerebrospinal fluid (CSF). Encephaloceles may be present at birth like congenital nasal gliomas or develop later in life through traumatic or iatrogenic skull base defects. Unlike with NDSC, gliomas will often present lateral to the midline and are seen more commonly in males by 3 to 1. Thirty percent of gliomas are intranasal, while 60% are primarily external to the nasal bones. Ten percent demonstrate both intranasal and extranasal components (Figure 26.19). External gliomas can present anywhere along the glabella or length of the nose, while intranasal lesions typically present with unilateral nasal obstruction and can be seen on anterior rhinoscopy or with endoscopy. Enlargement with crying or straining, a positive Furstenberg sign, is characteristic of nasal encephaloceles and not seen with gliomas.

connections (Figure 26.18). In contrast, nasal encephaloceles are characterized by the herniation of neural tissue or leptomeninges through a defect in the skull base with a persistent connection to the subarachnoid

DIFFERENTIAL DIAGNOSIS

Nasal dermoid sinus cyst, teratoma, antrochoanal polyp, and nasopharyngeal hairy polyp.

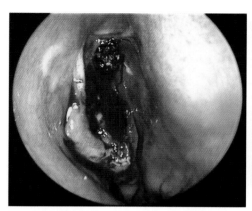

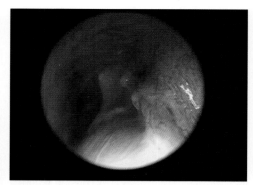

Figure 26.20 Intraoperative view following endonasal endoscopic excision of a right-sided nasal glioma.

Figure 26.21 Endoscopic photo demonstrating an intranasal encephalocele and its connection to the subarachnoid space superiorly.

Nasopharyngeal hairy polyp

WORKUP
CT scan is used to help narrow the differential diagnosis prior to any biopsy or surgery and can also be used later in the operating room for CT-image guidance. MRI is useful in demonstrating the extent of the lesion and can help to differentiate a nasal glioma from an encephalocele (Figure 26.20). Any associated clear rhinorrhea can be tested for beta-2 transferrin. This would confirm leakage of CSF, more commonly associated with an encephalocele.

TREATMENT
Both nasal gliomas and encephaloceles are treated with surgical excision. Endonasal endoscopic techniques are generally used, though external incisions may be necessary in some cases.[11] Fifteen to twenty percent of nasal gliomas have an associated fibrous tract that should also be removed to reduce any chances of recurrence. Following the excision of an encephalocele, the underlying defect in the skull base and dura must also be repaired to prevent further herniation of brain tissue and CSF leak. Topical fluorescein may be applied intraoperatively to help demonstrate the presence and source of any CSF leakage (Figure 26.21).[12]

DEFINITION AND CLINICAL FEATURES
Nasopharyngeal hairy polyp is a rare congenital benign hamartoma generally composed of skin and adnexal structures, though elements of the other germ cell layers may occasionally be found. This lesion is sometimes therefore described as teratomatous. This benign mass presents at birth with symptoms of intermittent respiratory and feeding difficulties. A mass can sometimes be appreciated behind the uvula on oral exam, though endoscopy may also be necessary to demonstrate the lesion.

DIFFERENTIAL DIAGNOSIS
Teratoma, vascular anomalies, nasal glioma or encephalocele, and rhabdomyosarcoma.

WORKUP
Evaluation with either CT or MRI can be helpful in narrowing the differential diagnosis prior to surgery. A careful fiberoptic endoscopy, demonstrating the characteristic hairs on the surface of the lesion, will help to confirm the diagnosis.

TREATMENT
Nasopharyngeal hairy polyps are usually attached only by a small fibrous stalk to the

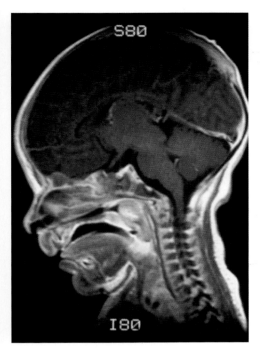

Figure 26.22 Transoral view of a large congenital nasopharyngeal hairy polyp extending behind the soft palate into the oropharynx.

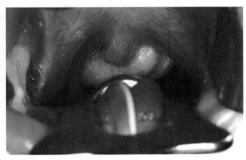

Figure 26.23 Sagittal MRI demonstrating a large soft tissue mass of the nasopharynx.

lateral nasopharynx, near the Eustachian tube orifice, or the posterior soft palate. Adequate exposure is achieved using a Dingman mouth retractor, along with red rubber catheters through the nose for elevation of the soft palate. Bipolar excision of the fibrous stalk close to its attachment with the

nasopharynx will free the mass completely and is curative. The endonasal or transoral use of endoscopes may aid in visualization (Figures 26.22 and 26.23).[13]

References

1. Muhlbauer W, Schmidt A, Fairley J. 1993. Simultaneous construction of an internal and external nose in an infant with arhinia. *Plastic and Reconstructive Surgery* 91(4):720.
2. Meyer R. 1997. Total external and internal construction in arhinia. *Plastic and Reconstructive Surgery* 99(2):534.
3. Cole RR, Meyer CM, Bratcher GO. 1989. Congenital absence of the nose: A case report. *International Journal of Pediatric Otorhinolaryngology* 17:171.
4. Palmer CR, Thomson HG. 1967. Congenital absence of the nose: A case report. *Canadian Journal of Surgery* 10:83.
5. Froehlich P and Ayari-Khalfallah S. 2007. Management of choanal atresia. In: Graham JM, Scadding GK, and Bull PD (eds) *Pediatric ENT*. Berlin, U.K.: Springer, Chapter 33, pp 291–294.
6. El-Ahl MA, El-Anwar MW. 2012. Stentless endoscopic transnasal repair of bilateral choanal atresia starting with resection of vomer. *International Journal of Pediatric Otorhinolaryngology* 76(7):1002–1006.
7. Newman JR, Harmon P, Shirley WP, Hill JS, Woolley AL, Wiatrak BJ. 2013. Operative management of choanal atresia: A 15-year experience. *JAMA Otolaryngology Head and Neck Surgery* 139(1):71–75.
8. Yankaskas JR, Marshall BC, Sufian B, Simon RH, Rodman D. 2004. Cystic fibrosis adult care consensus conference report. *Chest* 125(90010):1–39.
9. Re M, Tarchini P, Macri G, Pasquini E. 2012. Endonasal endoscopic approach for intracranial nasal dermoid sinus cyst in children. *International Journal of Pediatric Otorhinolaryngology* 76(8):1217–1222.
10. Manickavasagam J, Robin JM, Sinha S, Mirza S. 2013. Endoscopic removal of a dermoid cyst via scalp incision. *Laryngoscope* 10:1002.

11. Bonne NX, Zago S, Hosana G, Vinchon M, Van den Abbeele T, Fayoux P. 2012. Endonasal endoscopic approach for removal of intranasal nasal glial heterotopias. *Rhinology* 50(2):211–217.

12. Jones ME, Reino T, Gnoy A, Guillory S, Wackym P, Lawson W. 2000. Identification of intranasal cerebrospinal fluid leaks by topical application with fluorescein dye. *American Journal of Rhinology* 14(2):93–96.

13. Roh JL. 2004. Transoral endoscopic resection of a nasopharyngeal hairy polyp. *International Journal of Pediatric Otorhinolaryngology* 68(8):1087–1090.

CHAPTER 27

Pediatric Airway Disease

Carlton Zdanski

- **Congenital supraglottic airway obstruction**
- **Congenital glottic airway obstruction**
- **Acquired glottic airway obstruction**
- **Subglottic airway obstruction**
- **Tracheal obstruction**

Congenital supraglottic airway obstruction

Congenital supraglottic airway obstruction includes laryngomalacia, vallecular cysts, and saccular cysts. Symptoms include inspiratory stridor, airway obstruction, and feeding difficulties.

LARYNGOMALACIA
Definition and clinical features
Laryngomalacia is the most common cause of stridor in the newborn. It is characterized by a prolapse of the supraglottic structures (arytenoids, epiglottis) into the airway with inspiration. The exact cause in the neonate is not clearly defined at present and may be multifactorial. The airway obstruction is variable and may lead to significant feeding difficulties such as aspiration and failure to thrive. There may be an association with gastroesophageal reflux disease (GERD) as well.

Differential diagnosis
Pharyngomalacia, vallecular cyst, laryngocele, and saccular cyst.

Workup
The diagnosis is clinical: inspiratory stridor in the neonate. It can be easily confirmed with flexible laryngoscopy in the clinic or at the bedside (Figure 27.1). A feeding evaluation is recommended.

Treatment
Treatment is variable depending on the severity of the airway and feeding difficulties. Anti-GERD therapy should be considered.

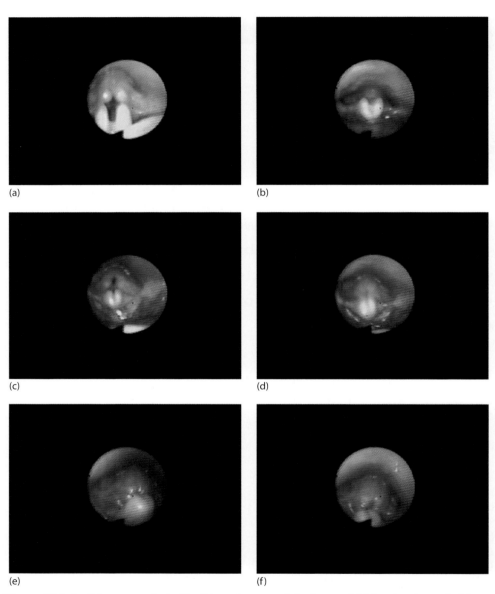

Figure 27.1 (a–f) Laryngomalacia. Flexible endoscopy of the larynx. (a) (showing the typical features of laryngomalacia with a curved or curvilinear-shaped epiglottis and shortened aryepiglottic folds) is at the beginning of inspiration and the sequence. (a–f) shows the progressive prolapse of the supraglottic structures into the airway with inspiration.

Most commonly, symptoms resolve with growth. However, if symptoms worsen or do not resolve, a complete operative airway evaluation is recommended as there is a high incidence of secondary airway lesions. Failure to thrive may result from feeding difficulties and work of breathing. In this event, or in the setting of significant airway obstruction, consideration should be given to surgical intervention (i.e., supraglottoplasty). Rarely, growth or surgery fails to improve symptoms and the placement of a tracheostomy or gastrostomy must be considered.

VALLECULAR CYST
Definition and clinical features
A vallecular cyst is thought to arise from a blocked mucous gland in the vallecula. The cyst may become quite large, causing upper airway obstruction with inspiratory stridor and concomitant feeding difficulties.

Differential diagnosis
Pharyngomalacia, laryngomalacia, thyroglossal duct cyst, lingual thyroid, laryngocele, and saccular cyst.

Workup
The diagnosis can be made with a lateral neck x-ray (Figure 27.2) or readily by flexible nasopharyngoscopy in the clinic or at the bedside.

Treatment
Treatment is surgical marsupialization of the cyst (Figure 27.3). Cysts can recur and surveillance with endoscopy in the clinic or operative setting is recommended.

CONGENITAL SACCULAR CYST
Definition and clinical features
A saccular cyst is thought to arise from a blocked mucous gland in the laryngeal ventricle. If a mass arising from the ventricle is air filled rather than mucous filled, then it is known as a laryngocele. These cysts may become quite large, causing airway obstruction with inspiratory stridor and

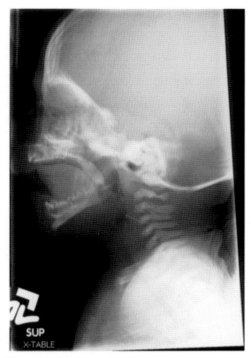

Figure 27.2 Lateral neck x-ray showing vallecular cyst.

concomitant feeding difficulties. In some cases, they may become infected causing fulminant life-threatening airway obstruction.

Differential diagnosis
Pharyngomalacia, laryngomalacia, and laryngocele.

Workup
The diagnosis can be made readily by flexible nasopharyngoscopy in the clinic or at the bedside. The extent of the lesion can be confirmed by CT scan (Figure 27.4).

Treatment
The marsupialization of the cyst results in a high rate of recurrence and so complete extirpation is recommended (Figure 27.5). This can usually be accomplished endoscopically. Cysts can recur and surveillance with endoscopy in the clinic or operative setting is recommended.

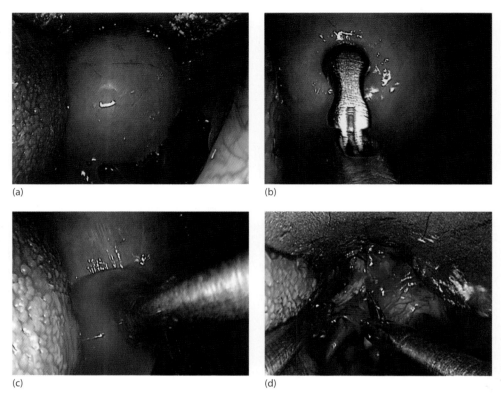

(a)   (b)

(c)   (d)

Figure 27.3 (a) Vallecular cyst. (b) Opening the cyst with cup forceps. (c) Thick fluid suctioned from cyst. (d) Marsupialization of the cyst.

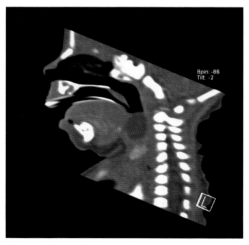

Figure 27.4 CT of saccular cyst.

Congenital glottic airway obstruction

Congenital glottic airway obstruction can arise from fixed lesions (webs) or impaired vocal fold mobility. Glottic airway obstruction typically results in biphasic stridor. Vocal fold immobility in particular may result in feeding difficulties, notably aspiration.

CONGENITAL GLOTTIC WEB
Definition and clinical features
A congenital glottic web is thought to occur from the incomplete canalization of the larynx during fetal development. If the glottis fails to recanalize at all, the condition is known as laryngeal atresia. Symptoms

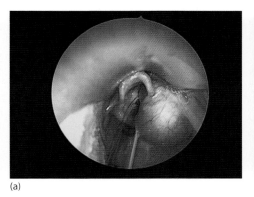

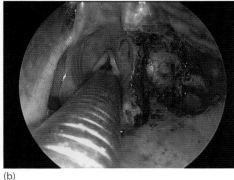

(a)   (b)

Figure 27.5 (a) Saccular cyst. (b) Saccular cyst status post resection.

vary depending on the extent of the web from simple dysphonia to airway obstruction. Feeding difficulties may also be present. Complete laryngeal atresia represents a life-threatening emergency and, if not diagnosed prenatally, has a high likelihood of neurologic injury and/or death. If diagnosed prenatally, then an EXIT (ex partum in utero) procedure can be performed to increase the likelihood of successfully securing an airway without injury or death.

Differential diagnosis
Subglottic stenosis and glottic neoplasm.

Workup
The diagnosis can frequently be made by flexible nasopharyngoscopy in the clinic or at the bedside, but smaller webs may easily be missed in this fashion. If symptoms are not explained by findings on flexible laryngoscopy, then operative direct laryngoscopy and bronchoscopy should be performed (Figure 27.6). If a web is found, then FISH assay for 22q11 deletion syndrome should be performed and genetics consult obtained. In the event of laryngeal atresia (Figure 27.7), a genetics consult is recommended as additional concomitant problems may be present.

Treatment
Treatment is surgical lysis of the web. It is critical to be aware that a high percentage of

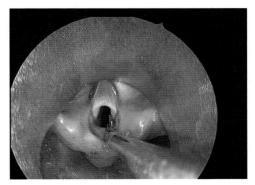

Figure 27.6 Laryngeal web. Intraoperative photo prior to lysis.

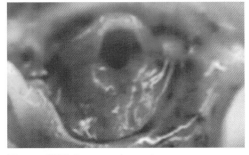

Figure 27.7 Laryngeal atresia, postmortem.

congenital glottic webs involve the subglottis, and therefore, simple endoscopic lysis of the "web" is not possible and will not result in airway or other symptom improvements (Figure 27.8). Webs can recur and

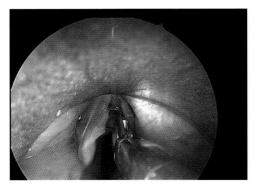

Figure 27.8 Laryngeal web status post attempted intraoperative lysis demonstrating subglottic involvement, which is common.

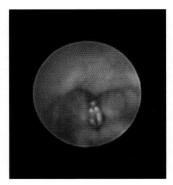

Figure 27.9 Vocal fold paresis with vocal folds in midline position resulting in airway obstruction.

surveillance with endoscopy in the clinic or operative setting is recommended. For laryngeal atresia, if the neonate survives, successful airway reconstruction may be attempted later in childhood.

VOCAL FOLD IMMOBILITY
Definition and clinical features
Vocal fold immobility can be unilateral or bilateral, partial or complete, and may result from neural problems or from physical impairment of mobility. Thus, immobility is the proper terminology until a diagnosis of the underlying cause is determined.

Differential diagnosis
Subglottic stenosis and glottic stenosis/web.

Workup
The diagnosis can be made with readily by flexible nasopharyngoscopy in the clinic or at the bedside (Figures 27.9 and 27.10). The larynx should be examined by operative direct laryngoscopy and bronchoscopy with palpation of the vocal folds to assess passive mobility and to rule out cricoarytenoid joint fixation and posterior glottic scar bands resulting in immobility. In the case of postoperative immobility (e.g., post-PDA ligation or neck surgery), consideration for diagnosis by flexible examination alone should be given. Anesthesia may

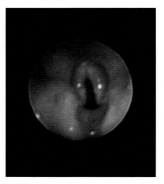

Figure 27.10 Vocal fold paresis with vocal folds in paramedian position resulting in dysphonia and aspiration.

impair vocal fold mobility and so care must be taken in making this diagnosis in the anesthetized child. Additional studies should include an MRI of the brain and brainstem to rule out Chiari malformation in neonates with bilateral immobility and in children with new-onset vocal fold immobility to rule out central nervous system lesions. A formal swallow evaluation is recommended to rule out and treat aspiration.

Treatment
Treatment is directed at symptoms. For life-threatening airway obstruction, a tracheotomy may be necessary. Dietary modification

or gastrostomy tube placement may be necessary to treat aspiration. Destructive or augmentative procedures of the larynx may be undertaken if function does not return, but judgment regarding the timing and extent of such procedures in the developing larynx is required. The utility of laryngeal EMG for prognostication is unclear.

Acquired glottic airway obstruction

Acquired glottic airway obstruction in children most commonly results from manipulation of the airway (i.e., intubation, surgery) or from infectious causes (recurrent respiratory papillomas [RRPs]). Symptoms are typical of glottic lesions: biphasic stridor, voice abnormalities, and possible aspiration.

ANTERIOR GLOTTIC WEB
Definition and clinical features
Acquired anterior glottic webs are most commonly the result of laryngeal surgery but may occur as a postintubation injury. Surgery that involves both sides of the glottis at the anterior commissure of the larynx causes demucosalized surfaces, which appose one another and have a propensity to scar together. It is characterized by symptoms as described earlier, which can be variable depending on the extent of the web and other associated airway problems. Voice is typically more affected than airway due to the location in the anterior or "phonatory" glottis.

Differential diagnosis
Vocal fold paralysis, RRP, vocal fold nodules, and vocal fold granuloma.

Workup
The diagnosis is suspected on clinical signs: voice abnormalities, stridor, and aspiration in a postoperative patient. It can sometimes be confirmed with flexible laryngoscopy in the clinic or at the bedside, but small webs can be easily missed. Operative direct

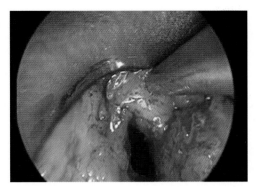

Figure 27.11 Acquired anterior glottic web in child with RRP.

laryngoscopy and bronchoscopy are recommended for patients with unexplained symptoms (Figure 27.11). A feeding evaluation may be indicated in some patients.

Treatment
Treatment is surgical: operative lysis of the web. Microflap techniques may be employed to reduce the risk of recurrence. Topical application of mitomycin C to reduce the risk of recurrence may be considered as well. Perioperative anti-GERD therapy should be considered.

POSTERIOR GLOTTIC WEB
Definition and clinical features
Acquired posterior glottic webs are most commonly the result of laryngeal surgery or postintubation injury. It is characterized by symptoms as described earlier, which can be variable depending on the extent of the web and other associated airway problems. Airway is typically more affected than voice due to the location in the posterior or "respiratory" glottis. Subglottic involvement may be present. Aspiration may also occur.

Differential diagnosis
Vocal fold paralysis, RRP, vocal fold granuloma, and subglottic stenosis.

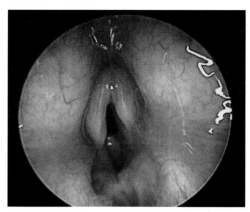

Figure 27.12 Posterior glottic scar secondary to intubation injury.

Workup

The diagnosis is suspected on clinical signs: stridor, aspiration, and voice abnormalities in a postoperative or previously intubated patient. It can sometimes be confirmed with flexible laryngoscopy in the clinic or at the bedside, but small webs can be easily missed. Operative direct laryngoscopy and bronchoscopy are recommended for patients with unexplained symptoms (Figure 27.12). A feeding evaluation may be indicated in some patients.

Treatment

Treatment is surgical: operative lysis of the web. Microflap techniques may be employed to reduce the risk of recurrence. Topical application of mitomycin C to reduce the risk of recurrence may be considered as well. A posterior cartilage graft (most typically costochondral) may be required particularly in the setting of failed endoscopic lysis of the web and can be placed endoscopically. A tracheotomy may be required intraoperatively or perioperatively. Perioperative anti-GERD therapy should be considered.

RECURRENT RESPIRATORY PAPILLOMATOSIS

Definition and clinical features

RRPs are an infection caused by the human papillomavirus. In small children, it is thought to occur from maternal to fetal transmission of the virus. In older children and adults, it may be transmitted as a sexually transmitted disease. It is characterized by symptoms as described earlier, predominantly voice change and stridor, which can be variable depending on the extent of the disease and other associated airway problems. Distal spread may occur to the tracheobronchial tree and lungs and pulmonary involvement is associated with a poor prognosis.

Differential diagnosis

Vocal fold paralysis, vocal fold nodules, vocal fold granuloma, and subglottic stenosis.

Workup

The diagnosis is suspected on clinical signs: progressive voice abnormalities and stridor. It can be confirmed with flexible laryngoscopy in the clinic or at the bedside but in uncooperative patients or in those with significant airway obstruction operative direct laryngoscopy and bronchoscopy may be necessary (Figure 27.13).

Treatment

Treatment is surgical but surgery is not curative. The goal of surgery is to maintain a patent airway until potential disease regression without causing iatrogenic airway

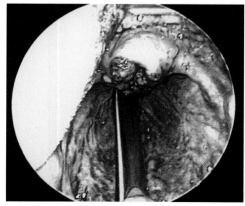

Figure 27.13 Total airway obstruction secondary to RRP.

obstruction secondary to intervention as the natural course of disease in juvenile RRP is eventual regression of disease in most cases. Multiple anesthetic techniques are utilized (native airway, jet ventilation, intubation) as well as surgical techniques (cold steel, microdebrider, laser) with good results. The effectiveness and utility of various medical treatments (interferon, indole-3-carbinol, cidofovir, mumps vaccine) are not well established and somewhat controversial. Tracheotomy may sometimes be necessary, but some feel it should be avoided as it may cause spread of disease to the distal tracheobronchial tree.

Subglottic airway obstruction

Subglottic airway obstruction may be either congenital or acquired. Clinical features include biphasic stridor and airway obstruction of varying severity depending upon the extent of the disease. Voice and/or cry may be normal if the glottis is not involved. Aspiration may be present depending upon the extent of the lesion. Treatment varies depending upon the extent of the disease and patient factors that make medical and surgical decisions complex and individualized.

Congenital subglottic airway obstruction includes subglottic stenosis and subglottic hemangioma.

Acquired glottic airway obstruction in children most commonly results from manipulation of the airway (i.e., intubation, surgery) or from infectious causes (RRPs). Symptoms are typical of glottic lesions: biphasic stridor, voice abnormalities, and possible aspiration.

CONGENITAL SUBGLOTTIC STENOSIS
Definition and clinical features
Congenital subglottic stenosis is caused by a congenitally malformed (elliptically shaped) cricoid cartilage. Symptoms, as described earlier, may be apparent shortly after birth or may not be present until later in infancy or childhood as recurrent croup. Not infrequently, the lesion will not be discovered until the child undergoes general anesthesia for an unrelated condition and there is difficulty with airway management. There is a definite association with trisomy 21.

Differential diagnosis
Vocal fold paralysis, subglottic hemangioma, croup, complete tracheal rings, and distal tracheal obstruction.

Workup
The diagnosis is suspected on clinical signs: biphasic stridor and recurrent croup. Flexible laryngoscopy in the clinic or at the bedside is an inadequate examination and operative direct laryngoscopy and bronchoscopy are necessary (Figure 27.14a and b). A chest or

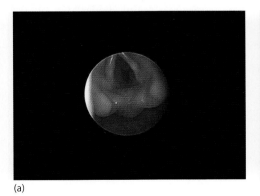
(a)

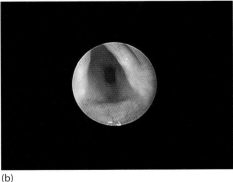
(b)

Figure 27.14 (a and b) Congenital subglottic stenosis ("elliptical cricoid").

cervical airway x-ray may reveal the problem. It is imperative to be completely prepared to manage fulminant life-threatening airway obstruction at the time of diagnostic airway evaluation.

Treatment

Treatment is individualized and can be heavily influenced by comorbid conditions. Simple observation with surveillance may be adequate until normal growth corrects the condition. Medical management with anti-GERD medications should be considered as well as caregiver possession of steroids for administration during acute "croup" episodes. Surgery may be necessary and typically takes the form of expansion laryngoplasty (laryngotracheal reconstruction with cartilage graft). Endoscopic procedures to "dilate" an abnormal cricoid cartilage with a small airway caliber seem ill advised.

SUBGLOTTIC HEMANGIOMA
Definition and clinical features

Subglottic hemangioma is caused by a congenital, infantile hemangioma located in the subglottis. As is typical with the natural history of infantile hemangiomas, the neonate is initially asymptomatic until the proliferative phase of the hemangioma is entered. This typically occurs at around 6–8 weeks of life with symptoms such as stridor and croupy cough with progressive airway obstruction causing respiratory distress. As with other causes of insidious airway obstruction, the child may be surprisingly tolerant of significant if not near total airway obstruction until presentation. The lesion may be associated with cutaneous hemangiomas and reportedly has an association with "beard distribution" infantile hemangiomas.

Differential diagnosis

Vocal fold paralysis, subglottic stenosis, croup, complete tracheal rings, and distal tracheal obstruction.

Workup

The diagnosis is suspected on clinical signs: new-onset biphasic stridor and croupy cough in a neonate. Cutaneous hemangiomas may or may not be present. Flexible laryngoscopy in the clinic or at the bedside may reveal the subglottic hemangioma, but this is an inadequate examination and operative direct laryngoscopy and bronchoscopy are necessary for unexplained symptoms (Figure 27.15). A chest or cervical airway x-ray may reveal the problem. It is imperative to be completely prepared to manage fulminant life-threatening airway obstruction at the time of diagnostic airway evaluation. MRI may be helpful postdiagnosis to evaluate the extent of the disease. Referral to hematology/oncology may be useful for evaluation of disseminated disease and for assistance with medical treatment.

Treatment

Treatment initially involves securing a safe airway. For small hemangiomas, observation may suffice while treatment is implemented. For larger hemangiomas, brief endotracheal intubation may be necessary until evaluation is complete and treatment is initiated. In the past, surgery with medical adjunct treatment was the primary modality

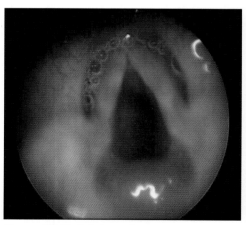

Figure 27.15 Subglottic hemangioma.

employed for treatment. Options included endoscopic laser or microdebrider resection of the mass, intralesional injection of steroids, open resection of the lesion with or without laryngotracheal reconstruction, and tracheotomy until eventual involution of the hemangioma. Endoscopic procedures in general needed to be repeated for control of symptoms. Medical adjuncts included the use of systemic steroids or chemotherapeutic agents such as vincristine. Recently, systemic use of propranolol has become the first-line option for the treatment of the disease with maintenance of therapy until the involution of the hemangioma. Medical management with anti-GERD medications should be considered as well as caregiver possession of steroids for administration during acute episodes of airway obstruction. Surgery may be necessary for lesions that do not respond to medical treatment.

ACQUIRED SUBGLOTTIC STENOSIS
Definition and clinical features
Acquired subglottic stenosis is caused by manipulation with subsequent scarring of the airway. The insult typically occurs during the course of normal and appropriate intervention, primarily endotracheal intubation. It may occur with surprisingly short exposure times (i.e., minutes), but risk increases with increasing length of intubation period and with increasing numbers of intubations or airway manipulations. A congenitally malformed cricoid cartilage (congenital subglottic stenosis) may be an unsuspected underlying predisposing element as inadvertent subglottic injury may occur when attempting to place an age- and size-appropriate endotracheal tube. Symptoms, as described earlier, may be apparent shortly after extubation or intervention but may not be present until later in infancy or childhood as recurrent croup or progressive stridor and airway obstruction with respiratory distress. Not infrequently, the lesion may not be discovered until the child undergoes a general anesthetic for an

unrelated condition and there is difficulty with airway management.

Differential diagnosis
Vocal fold paralysis, subglottic hemangioma, subglottic cyst, croup, complete tracheal rings, and distal tracheal obstruction.

Workup
The diagnosis is suspected on clinical signs: biphasic stridor and recurrent croup. Not infrequently, there is a history of asthma treated with bronchodilators without effect. Flexible laryngoscopy in the clinic or at the bedside is an inadequate examination and operative direct laryngoscopy and bronchoscopy are necessary. A chest or cervical airway x-ray may reveal the problem. The most common grading system utilized to characterize the degree of subglottic stenosis is the Cotton–Myer system: grade I is less than or equal to 50% airway luminal narrowing, grade II is between 51% and 70% airway luminal narrowing, grade III is between 71% and 99% airway luminal narrowing, and grade IV is complete subglottic stenosis (Figure 27.16a through d). It is imperative to be completely prepared to manage fulminant life-threatening airway obstruction at the time of diagnostic airway evaluation.

Treatment
Treatment is complex, multifactorial, and individualized. Factors involved in therapeutic decision making include the extent of the lesion, its underlying characteristics, its state of progression, the preferences and skills of the treating physicians, the resources of the treating institution and health-care system, the child's social situation, and the child's comorbid conditions. Simple observation with surveillance may be adequate until normal growth corrects the condition for mild lesions. More extensive lesions may require temporary or permanent tracheotomy. Endoscopic surgical options include laser or cold steel surgery and dilation with or

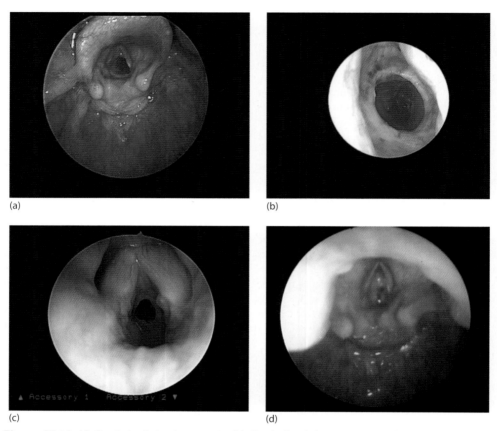

(a)

(b)

(c)

(d)

Figure 27.16 (a) Grade I subglottic stenosis. (b) Grade II subglottic stenosis. (c) Grade III subglottic stenosis. (d) Grade IV subglottic stenosis.

without application of mitomycin C and/or injection of steroid. A posterior cricoid split with graft placement can also be performed endoscopically. Open surgical options include one- or two-stage laryngotracheal reconstruction with anterior, posterior, or anterior and posterior grafts as well as cricotracheal resection. Cartilage grafts may be obtained from the auricle, septum, thyroid ala, and rib. Staged open procedures may be required for lesions with glottic involvement. Not infrequently, both endoscopic and open procedures are required for more extensive lesions. Medical management with anti-GERD medications is imperative and should be considered as well as surgical treatment for medically uncontrolled GERD. Eosinophilic esophagitis should be ruled out or treated.

SUBGLOTTIC CYST
Definition and clinical features
A subglottic cyst is caused by a blocked mucous-producing gland located in the subglottic region. They are typically associated with previous airway manipulation and may be singular or multiple. Symptoms, as described earlier, may be apparent shortly after airway manipulation or may not be present until later in infancy or childhood as progressive stridor or recurrent croup.

Subglottic stenosis may not infrequently be present as concurrent or perhaps contributing pathology.

Differential diagnosis
Vocal fold paralysis, subglottic hemangioma, subglottic stenosis, croup, complete tracheal rings, and distal tracheal obstruction.

Workup
The diagnosis is suspected on clinical signs: biphasic stridor and recurrent croup. Flexible laryngoscopy in the clinic or at the bedside may show the pathology, but this is an inadequate examination and operative direct laryngoscopy and bronchoscopy are necessary for unexplained symptoms (Figure 27.17). A chest or cervical airway x-ray may reveal the problem. It is imperative to be completely prepared to manage fulminant life-threatening airway obstruction at the time of diagnostic airway evaluation.

Treatment
Treatment is the marsupialization of the cyst. In small children, temporary intubation may be necessary to control airway edema. Associated subglottic stenosis may be present and may require significantly more complex airway management. Recurrence is common and operative surveillance should be strongly considered.

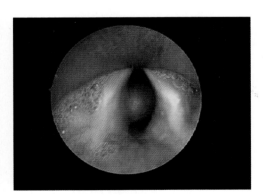

Figure 27.17 Subglottic cyst.

Medical management with anti-GERD medications should be considered.

Tracheal obstruction

Tracheal airway obstruction may be caused by intrinsic lesions or external compressive lesions. Symptoms are traditionally described as expiratory stridor, although biphasic stridor or wheezing may be present depending upon the clinical scenario.

TRACHEAL STENOSIS
Definition and clinical features
Tracheal stenosis is usually caused by manipulation with subsequent scarring of the airway. The insult typically occurs during the course of normal and appropriate intervention, primarily endotracheal intubation. Underlying tracheal pathology (such as tracheomalacia or external compression) may be associated or contribute to the development of the problem. Symptoms, as described earlier, may be apparent shortly after extubation or intervention but may not be present until later in infancy or childhood progressive stridor and airway obstruction with respiratory distress.

Differential diagnosis
Complete tracheal rings, tracheomalacia, tracheal tumor, and foreign body aspiration.

Workup
The diagnosis is suspected on clinical signs: expiratory or biphasic stridor. There may be a history of asthma treated with bronchodilators without effect. Flexible laryngoscopy in the clinic or at the bedside is an inadequate examination and operative direct laryngoscopy and bronchoscopy are necessary (Figure 27.18). A chest or cervical airway x-ray may reveal the problem. It is imperative to be completely prepared to manage fulminant life-threatening airway obstruction at the time of diagnostic airway evaluation.

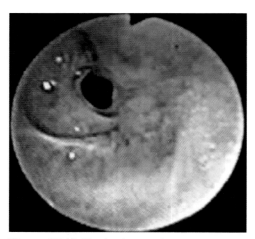

Figure 27.18 Tracheal stenosis.

Treatment

Simple observation with surveillance may be adequate until normal growth corrects the condition for mild lesions. More extensive lesions may require endoscopic or open surgery. It is important to realize that oroendotracheal intubation may not be possible nor placement of a tracheotomy to bypass the lesion. Endoscopic surgical options include laser or cold steel surgery and/or dilation with or without application of mitomycin C or injection of steroid. Open surgical options include tracheal resection or slide tracheoplasty. This might involve thoracotomy and possibly cardiopulmonary bypass. Medical management with anti-GERD medications is imperative and should be considered as well as surgical treatment for medically uncontrolled GERD.

TRACHEAL TUMOR
Definition and clinical features

Tracheal tumors may originate from the component structures of the trachea or invade from other mediastinal structures. Symptoms, as described earlier, may be present, but the relative rarity of the problem may make obtaining the diagnosis difficult.

Differential diagnosis

Complete tracheal rings, tracheomalacia, tracheal stenosis, and foreign body aspiration.

Workup

The diagnosis is suspected on clinical signs: expiratory or biphasic stridor. Apparent life-threatening events may precipitate the diagnostic evaluation. There may be a history of asthma treated with bronchodilators without effect. Direct laryngoscopy and bronchoscopy are necessary (Figure 27.19). A chest or cervical airway x-ray may suggest the problem; additional chest imaging may further define or delineate the pathology. It is imperative to be completely prepared to manage fulminant life-threatening airway obstruction at the time of diagnostic airway evaluation.

Treatment

Treatment is varied depending on the diagnosis. Securing a safe airway and obtaining tissue for diagnosis are the initial goals. Definitive management is pathology dependent and may require surgery, medicine, and/or radiation. It is important to realize that oroendotracheal intubation may not be possible nor placement of a tracheotomy to bypass the lesion. The involvement of an

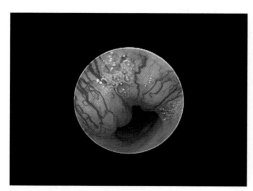

Figure 27.19 Tracheal tumor.

experienced anesthesia team and cardio-thoracic surgery is advised.

TRACHEOMALACIA
Definition and clinical features
Tracheomalacia is the result of a weakened or "floppy" tracheal wall that causes collapse of the trachea with obstruction on expiration. It may be the result of or associated with tracheoesophageal fistula, esophageal atresia, or external compression from the aortoinnominate artery. Symptoms, as described earlier, are variable in severity.

Differential diagnosis
Complete tracheal rings, tracheal tumor, and foreign body aspiration.

Workup
The diagnosis is suspected on clinical signs: expiratory stridor. Bronchodilators may exacerbate the condition by causing smooth muscle relaxation. Flexible laryngoscopy in the clinic or at the bedside is an inadequate examination and operative direct laryngoscopy and bronchoscopy are necessary (Figure 27.20).

Treatment
Simple observation with surveillance may be adequate until normal growth corrects the condition for mild lesions. More extensive lesions may require a tracheotomy and positive pressure ventilation. Medical management with anti-GERD and pulmonary medications should be considered as well as surgical treatment for medically uncontrolled GERD.

COMPLETE TRACHEAL RINGS
Definition and clinical features
Normally, the tracheal rings form about 3/5 to 4/5 of the tracheal circumference. Complete tracheal rings occur when these cartilaginous rings form the complete circumference of the trachea. A portion of or the entire trachea may be involved and the lesion may extend into the bronchial tree. In addition, the diameter of the trachea and subsequent growth of the trachea may vary as well. Concomitant cardiac lesions may exist as well as other congenital malformations. Symptoms, as described earlier, may be apparent shortly after birth or may not be present until later in infancy or childhood. Not infrequently, the lesion will not be discovered until the child undergoes general anesthesia for other conditions and there is significant difficulty with airway management.

Differential diagnosis
Vocal fold paralysis, subglottic stenosis, subglottic hemangioma, croup, tracheomalacia, and tracheal tumor.

Workup
The diagnosis is suspected on clinical signs: expiratory or biphasic stridor, croupy cough, respiratory distress, and failure to thrive. Operative laryngoscopy and bronchoscopy are necessary to make the diagnosis and evaluate its severity and extent (Figure 27.21).

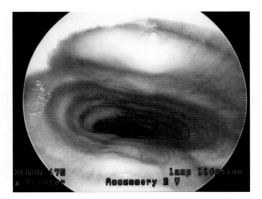

Figure 27.20 Tracheomalacia.

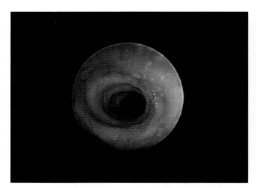

Figure 27.21 Complete tracheal rings.

It is imperative to be atraumatic in the evaluation and to be completely prepared to manage fulminant life-threatening airway obstruction at the time of diagnostic airway evaluation as endotracheal intubation and tracheotomy to bypass the obstruction may not be possible.

Treatment

Treatment is individualized and can be heavily influenced by comorbid conditions. Simple observation with surveillance may be adequate until normal growth corrects the condition. Medical management with anti-GERD and pulmonary medications should be considered. Surgery may be necessary and typically takes the form of slide tracheoplasty. This may require cardiopulmonary bypass and any coexisting cardiac lesions requiring surgery should be addressed concomitantly. Endoscopic procedures to address postoperative obstruction may be required to maintain airway patency.

FOREIGN BODY ASPIRATION
Definition and clinical features

Foreign body aspiration can cause hypoxic neurologic injury and death. It occurs more frequently in infants and toddlers due to their inexperience, exploratory nature, and tendency to experience objects orally. A witnessed aspiration event should lead to relatively expeditious diagnosis and treatment.

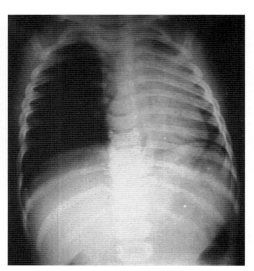

Figure 27.22 Chest x-ray showing left lung atelectasis from foreign body obstruction.

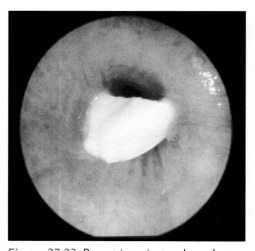

Figure 27.23 Peanut in mainstem bronchus.

Subtle signs of an unwitnessed aspiration event may cause delays and difficulties in diagnosis that can lead to significant complications.

Differential diagnosis

Reactive airway disease and tracheal tumor.

Workup

The diagnosis is suspected by history. Physical examination may reveal focal wheezing or decreased breath sounds. A chest x-ray may show the mass, atelectasis, or hyperinflation (Figure 27.22). Decubitus x-rays may demonstrate these findings more readily. A history of foreign body aspiration should lead to prompt endoscopic evaluation as physical findings and x-rays are often normal. Flexible bronchoscopy may lead to the diagnosis but rigid laryngoscopy and bronchoscopy are recommended for removal of the foreign body (Figure 27.23).

Treatment

Direct laryngoscopy and bronchoscopy with foreign body removal.

Oral and Oropharyngeal Disease

Lorien M. Paulson

- **Ankyloglossia**
- **Tonsillar hyperplasia**
- **Acute suppurative pharyngitis/tonsillitis**
- **Peritonsillar abscess**
- **Retropharyngeal abscess**
- **Base of tongue/vallecular cyst**
- **Ranula**
- **Suggested reading**

Ankyloglossia

DEFINITION AND CLINICAL FEATURES

Ankyloglossia, commonly referred to as "tongue tie," represents a restriction of tongue motion due to a tight or thick lingual frenulum. Symptoms vary from asymptomatic to impaired latching during breastfeeding and insufficient feeding. Although controversial, some feel that ankyloglossia may also contribute to speech difficulties later in life particularly if the tongue is unable to touch the upper incisors during articulation. There is also concern for oral hygiene if there is difficulty sweeping the tongue over the teeth and gingivobuccal sulci. Ankyloglossia is most often diagnosed at birth either on physical exam or after difficulties with breastfeeding. This may lead to prolonged, inefficient feeding sessions or painful chapped nipples. Affected infants will often have a tight frenulum and a "heart-shaped" tongue on attempted protrusion.

DIFFERENTIAL DIAGNOSIS

Anything causing restricted mobility of the tongue should be considered, including tongue weakness due to a variety of neurological disorders, primary tumors of the tongue, and cystic lesions of the floor of the mouth.

WORKUP

In the neonatal period, bedside oral motor exam by an occupational, speech, or lactation specialist may be very useful to determine or confirm latching difficulties. In older children, speech pathology or dental evaluation can assist in documenting difficulties in these arenas.

TREATMENT

Controversy exists over whether surgical intervention is necessary in many cases, although it is commonly performed due to the simplicity and low risk in the neonatal period. The procedure may be done at the bedside or in clinic with topical anesthesia alone. The baby may resume breastfeeding within minutes after this is complete and nipple pain is often immediately improved in appropriately chosen cases. Once the child becomes older than 5–6 months, clinic-based frenulotomy becomes more difficult due to both patient cooperation and growth/thickening of the frenulum. Simple excision with sutures or, in very thick or tight frenulums, a simple Z-plasty technique will provide appropriate release in selected patients (Figure 28.1).

Tonsillar hyperplasia

DEFINITION AND CLINICAL FEATURES

Hyperplasia refers to excessive growth of tonsillar tissue and in general is used in reference to the palatine tonsils. The palatine

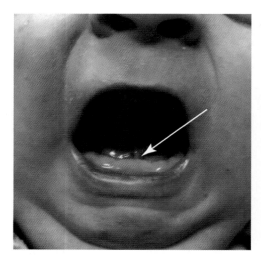

Figure 28.1 Ankyloglossia due to tight lingual frenulum.

tonsils, in conjunction with the adenoids and the lingual tonsils, form Waldeyer's ring, which is an organization of mucosa-associated lymphoid tissue (MALT) within the pharynx. MALT is part of the adaptive immune system and can be found in several areas of the body, including but not limited to the GI tract, the nasal cavity, the salivary glands, and the conjunctiva. The palatine tonsils typically grow throughout early childhood and decrease in size relative to overall craniofacial growth in late childhood.

Tonsillar hypertrophy in itself is not considered harmful. However, when tonsils become large enough, they may contribute to pharyngeal obstruction and sleep-disordered breathing. Obstructive symptoms include loud snoring, pauses in breathing, frequent awakening, mouth breathing, and drooling. Occasionally, large tonsils may cause "obstructive dysphagia," which may manifest as gagging or inability to swallow food, which is characteristically worse with solids.

Unilateral tonsillar hypertrophy is most commonly related to pseudohypertrophy as a result of differing anatomic boundaries, namely, the tonsillar pillars and the relative depth of the tonsillar fossae. Rapid unilateral growth of one tonsil over a course of weeks to months may be a warning sign for lymphoma, particularly if accompanied by ipsilateral lymphadenopathy.

DIFFERENTIAL DIAGNOSIS
Recurrent tonsillitis, sickle cell anemia–related tonsillar hypertrophy, posttransplant lymphoproliferative disorder, lymphoma.

WORKUP
A polysomnogram (sleep study) may assist in the diagnosis of obstructive sleep apnea, and examination of prior throat cultures is useful. Modified barium swallow exam may be considered to evaluate for obstructive dysphagia, if suspected. Unilateral hypertrophy that is progressive may require imaging and/or biopsy, particularly if other symptoms of malignancy such as lymphoma are of concern.

TREATMENT
Surgical treatment is typically reserved for cases of obstructive sleep apnea and recurrent/chronic tonsillitis. Tonsillectomy has been also shown to be effective for obstructive dysphagia when modified barium swallow demonstrates the tonsils to be the primary source of obstruction. Treatment involves removal of the tonsils and/or adenoids under general anesthesia (Figure 28.2).

Acute suppurative pharyngitis/tonsillitis

DEFINITION AND CLINICAL FEATURES
Suppurative pharyngitis may be defined as pharyngitis with visible exudate and is typically associated with reactive tonsillar hypertrophy. The vast majority of pharyngitis is caused by a host of viral entities, and although exudates can be present with viral infections, bacterial infections such as that seen with group A streptococcus tend to produce more exuberant exudates.

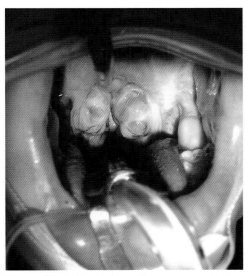

Figure 28.2 Marked tonsillar hypertrophy in a patient undergoing adenotonsillectomy for obstructive sleep apnea.

Viral pharyngitis is more likely to present as multifocal or diffuse respiratory or systemic symptoms, whereas bacterial infections alone tend to be localized. Fevers, malaise, odynophagia, and dehydration may be seen with either form of pharyngitis.

DIFFERENTIAL DIAGNOSIS
Viral pharyngitis, streptococcal pharyngitis, mononucleosis, influenza, peritonsillar abscess, chronic tonsillitis.

WORKUP
Throat swab with culture and rapid strep analysis. For negative cultures but prolonged symptomatology, monospot/EBV studies may be performed.

TREATMENT
Supportive care is essential, to include adequate hydration and antipyretics. With progressive symptoms or positive throat culture, directed antimicrobial therapy is recommended. Group A streptococcal infections may be treated with oral penicillin V

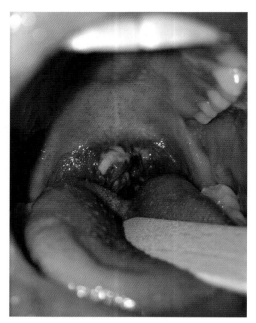

Figure 28.3 Acute suppurative tonsillitis.

or amoxicillin as first-line agents. Admission may be required if oral intake is insufficient, and intravenous fluids, intravenous antibiotics, and appropriate pain control should be delivered. For airway obstruction and/or persistently severe cases, intravenous corticosteroids may be very useful to decrease acute pharyngeal edema and increase comfort. Tonsillectomy is rarely done emergently and is typically reserved for recurrent or chronic cases of tonsillitis (Figure 28.3).

Peritonsillar abscess

DEFINITION AND CLINICAL FEATURES
A peritonsillar abscess is an abscess localized to the peritonsillar space. This is typically preceded by acute pharyngitis and presents with increasing pain, dysphagia, and progressive inability to take anything by mouth over course of several days time. Abscesses are unilateral in nature, with clinical exam revealing unilateral protrusion of the tonsil on the affected side, commonly in association with ipsilateral soft palate bulging and uvular deviation. Progression to the parapharyngeal and/or retropharyngeal space is possible, which may be suspected if symptoms progress to include trismus.

DIFFERENTIAL DIAGNOSIS
Acute tonsillitis, asymmetric tonsils, mononucleosis, parapharyngeal abscess, parapharyngeal or tonsillar tumors.

WORKUP
Workup should include workup of suppurative pharyngitis as well as ENT consultation. Imaging is not necessary in most classic cases of pediatric peritonsillar abscesses. Cases that may require imaging include suspected abscesses in adults or anyone with an atypical history, time course, risk factors, or symptoms, which may suggest tumors or spread outside the peritonsillar space. Depending on the suspicions, CT scan with or without contrast or MRI may be most helpful. ENT consultation prior to imaging is recommended to determine optimal imaging, if any.

TREATMENT
Incision and drainage under local or general anesthesia, depending on patient tolerance, is typically curative, and symptoms tend to resolve rapidly after drainage. Needle aspiration has been performed successfully in many studies as an alternative to incision and drainage although no comparison studies have been performed. Repeat peritonsillar abscesses may be managed with repeat incision and drainage with either concurrent or delayed tonsillectomy to prevent further occurrences (Figure 28.4).

Retropharyngeal abscess

DEFINITION AND CLINICAL FEATURES
Abscesses in the retropharyngeal space most commonly occur in toddlers and

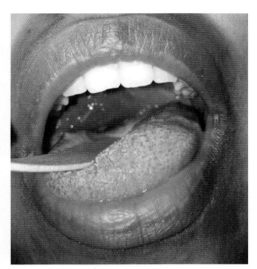

Figure 28.4 Right peritonsillar abscess: Note swelling and erythema of the ipsilateral soft palate; palpation reveals fluctuance in this region.

young children, as a result of suppuration of a retropharyngeal lymph node. In older children and adults, retropharyngeal abscesses may be more likely to result from direct spread from parapharyngeal space infections. Presentation is typically characterized by progressive odynophagia, dysphagia, and/or food aversion, in conjunction with fevers. Drooling, neck stiffness, and airway obstructive symptoms may evolve as the problem progresses. Clinical exam reveals a patient who appears ill, irritable, and lethargic and may be drooling. Trismus is often present if the infection involves the parapharyngeal space. Oropharyngeal exam may be difficult and may appear normal, although careful oropharyngeal exam with headlight and a trained eye may reveal asymmetry of the posterior pharyngeal wall.

DIFFERENTIAL DIAGNOSIS
Acute tonsillitis, parapharyngeal abscess, masticator space abscess, mononucleosis, foreign body ingestion ± pharyngeal trauma, tumor of the retropharyngeal or parapharyngeal space.

WORKUP
Lateral neck radiographs are quick and inexpensive and may reveal thickening of the retropharyngeal tissue. CT scan with contrast is useful if high level of suspicion. Throat and blood cultures may help direct antibiotic therapy.

TREATMENT
Small fluid collections may resolve on conservative therapy alone with aggressive IV hydration, antibiotics, and close monitoring. Expedited incision and drainage should be pursued for larger fluid collections, impending airway obstruction, progressively worsening symptoms, or failure to improve on conservative therapy. Most retropharyngeal abscesses may be approached from a transoral approach, although extensive or refractory cases may require formal external transcervical drainage with temporary drain placement (Figures 28.5 and 28.6).

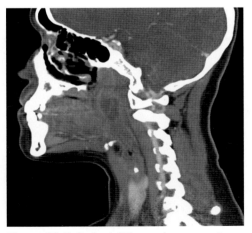

Figure 28.5 Sagittal CT scan demonstrating rim-enhancing fluid collection in retropharyngeal space.

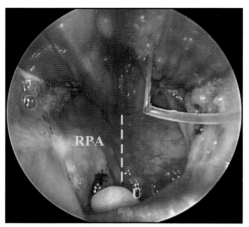

Figure 28.6 Intraoperative photo of posterior pharynx with left-sided retropharyngeal abscess. Dotted line = midline. RPA, retropharyngeal abscess; U, uvula.

Base of tongue/vallecular cyst

DEFINITION AND CLINICAL FEATURES

A vallecular cyst is a cystic lesion arising from the base of the tongue or vallecula. The presentation varies from asymptomatic and noticed on imaging or direct laryngoscopy to stridor, respiratory distress, dysphagia, and failure to thrive. Cysts may be simple or complex and most commonly arise from a blocked salivary gland.

DIFFERENTIAL DIAGNOSIS

Thyroglossal duct cyst, lingual thyroid, vascular or lymphatic malformation, teratoma, laryngocele, foregut duplication cyst.

WORKUP

Direct visualization in the operating room with or without biopsy is recommended. For midline cysts, an ultrasound of the thyroid is useful to ensure the presence of a normal thyroid gland and to evaluate the path of the thyroglossal duct. For unusual cases, CT or MRI may be chosen to evaluate involvement of surrounding structures or to rule out lymphatic malformation.

TREATMENT

Treatment is necessary only if symptomatic. Complete excision versus marsupialization via a transoral approach is typically sufficient with sharp techniques or CO_2 laser assistance. Due to location, endoscopic assistance with angled telescopes may be helpful for visualization (Figure 28.7).

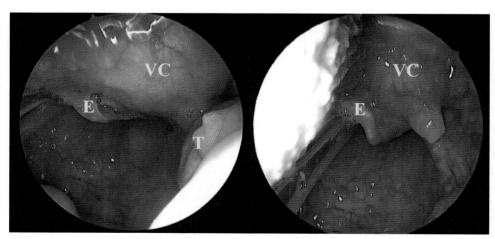

Figure 28.7 Vallecular cyst as seen on direct laryngoscopy. The endotracheal tube is visualized passing posterior to the epiglottis. VC, cyst; E, epiglottis; T, tonsil.

Ranula

DEFINITION AND CLINICAL FEATURES

A ranula is a term to describe a mucous retention cyst in the floor of the mouth. Typically, these are thought to occur from minor trauma to a duct associated with sublingual glands or, less commonly, minor salivary glands or the submandibular gland. Trapped mucoid secretions accumulate and form a cystic mass that can cause displacement of the floor of the mouth structures and tongue. Ranulas typically present as an asymptomatic floor of mouth swelling, which is lateral to midline and fluctuant and may take on a translucent or "blue" hue. Deeper ranulas may expand inferiorly around the myelohyoid muscle into the neck and present as a neck mass. These are often referred to as "plunging ranulas." Ranulas may become secondarily infected or burst and lead to recurrent swelling.

DIFFERENTIAL DIAGNOSIS

Vascular or lymphatic malformation, epidermal inclusion cyst, dermoid cyst.

WORKUP

Although physical exam may be sufficient for small or superficial ranulas, MRI is useful in defining soft tissue involvement in larger or complex ranulas. If the ranula appears to be associated with a concurrent mass, biopsy may be indicated. Fine needle aspiration of the fluid with analysis may aid in differentiation between ranula and lymphatic malformation.

TREATMENT

Surgical treatment of ranulas is indicated if symptomatic and typically involves removal of the sublingual gland on the affected side. In certain cases, marsupialization of the cyst may be sufficient although complete excision of the gland is the preferred method (Figure 28.8).

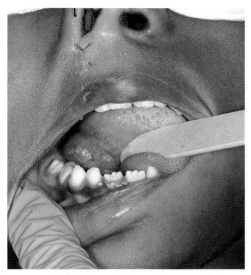

Figure 28.8 Right-sided ranula seen as bulging in the right floor of the mouth.

Suggested reading

Baugh RF, Archer SM, Mitchell RB et al. 2011. Clinical practice guideline: Tonsillectomy in children. *Otolaryngology—Head and Neck Surgery* 144(1 Suppl.):S1–S30.

Berkowitz RG, Mahadevan M. 1999. Unilateral tonsillar enlargement and tonsillar lymphoma in children. *Annals of Otology, Rhinology and Laryngology* 108:876–879.

Bouquot J, Brad WN, Douglas DD, Carl MA, Jerry E. 2002. *Oral & Maxillofacial Pathology*, 2nd ed. Philadelphia, PA: WB Saunders, pp. 391–392.

Clayburgh D, Milczuk H, Gorsek S, Sinden N, Bowman K, MacArthur C. 2011. Efficacy of tonsillectomy for pediatric patients with dysphagia and tonsillar hypertrophy. *Archives of Otolaryngology—Head and Neck Surgery* 137(12):1197–1202.

Clegg HW, Ryan AG, Dallas SD et al. 2006. Treatment of streptococcal pharyngitis with once-daily compared with twice-daily amoxicillin: A noninferiority trial. *Pediatric Infectious Disease Journal* 25(9):761–767.

Costales-Marcos M, López-Álvarez F, Núñez-Batalla F, Moreno-Galindo C, Alvarez Marcos C, Llorente-Pendás JL. 2012. Peritonsillar infections: Prospective study of 100 consecutive cases. *Acta Otorrinolaringologica Espanola* 63(3):212–217.

Dollberg S, Botzer E, Grunis E, Francis BM. 2006. Immediate nipple pain relief after frenotomy in breast-fed infants with ankyloglossia: A randomized, prospective study. *Journal of Pediatric Surgery* 41:1598–1600.

Herzon FS, Harris P. 1995. Mosher Award thesis. Peritonsillar abscess: Incidence, current management practices, and a proposal for treatment guidelines. *Laryngoscope* 105(8 Pt 3 Suppl. 74):1–17.

Hsieh WS, Yang PH, Wong KS, Li HY, Wang EC, Yeh TF. 2000. Vallecular cyst: An uncommon cause of stridor in newborn infants. *European Journal of Pediatric* 159(1–2):79–81.

Lalakea ML, Messner AH. 2003. Ankyloglossia: Does it matter? *Pediatric Clinics of North America* 50:381–397.

La'Porte SJ, Juttla JK, Lingam RK. 2011. Imaging the floor of the mouth and the sublingual space. *Radiographics* 31(5):1215–1230.

Messner AH, Lalakea ML. 2002. The effect of ankyloglossia on speech in children. *Otolaryngology—Head and Neck Surgery* 127(6):539–545.

O'Callahan C, Macary S, Clemente S. 2013. The effects of office-based frenotomy for anterior and posterior ankyloglossia on breastfeeding. *International Journal of Pediatric Otorhinolaryngology* 77(5):827–832.

O'Connor R, McGurk M. 2013. The plunging ranula: Diagnostic difficulties and a less invasive approach to treatment. *International Journal of Oral and Maxillofacial Surgery* 42(11):1469–1474.

Shulman ST, Bisno AL, Clegg HW et al. 2012. Clinical practice guideline for the diagnosis and management of group A streptococcal pharyngitis: 2012 update by the Infectious Diseases Society of America. *Clinical Infectious Diseases* 55(10):1279–1282.

Tuncer U, Aydoğan LB, Soylu L. 2002. Vallecular cyst: A cause of failure to thrive in an infant. *International Journal of Pediatric Otorhinolaryngology* 65(2):133–135.

Neck Disease

Lorien M. Paulson

Branchial cleft cyst

DEFINITION AND CLINICAL FEATURES

Branchial cleft cysts (BCCs) or sinuses represent remnants of ectodermal clefts, which serve to separate the pharyngeal arches during embryogenesis. When they fail to completely obliterate, a cyst or tract with epithelial lining may form at any point along the tract. When this is continuous with the skin, this is often visualized externally as a pit and is termed a sinus or, if continuous with the pharynx, is termed a fistula. If no external tract is identified, the cyst may present simply as a neck mass. Presentation varies and may present as asymptomatic pits, recurrent drainage, recurrent swelling, or progressive swelling. They may become infected and the patients often present with recurrent infections, which may have been initially treated with incision and drainage. BCCs typically present at any point throughout childhood but occasionally cysts do not become evident until adulthood.

Most branchial cleft anomalies arise from the second branchial cleft (90%–95%), which typically present as a submandibular mass, with external openings or pits, which may occur anywhere along the anterior border of the sternocleidomastoid muscle. Internally, the tract may open into the tonsillar fossa. First BCCs (5%–8%) may present either as postauricular swelling or abscess due to a duplication of the external auditory canal (type I) or as a preauricular, parotid, or submandibular mass (type II) with a tract passing through the parotid gland. Third and fourth BCCs are rare, predominantly left sided, and present most commonly as posterior triangle masses. Their courses lie posterior to the common carotid artery and enter the pharynx at the level of the pyriform sinus.

DIFFERENTIAL DIAGNOSIS
Suppurative lymphadenitis, thymic cyst, thyroglossal duct cyst (TDC), dermoid cyst, vascular malformation, laryngocele, sialocele, sialadenitis, cystic metastasis.

WORKUP
A CT scan is often useful in delineating the extent of the tract. Bilateral BCCs or sinuses may be associated with branchio-oto-renal syndrome, and therefore, otologic evaluation including an audiogram and renal evaluation including renal ultrasound, urinalysis, and serum electrolytes are recommended.

TREATMENT
Complete surgical excision of the tract with ligation at the level of the pharynx is curative, and the procedure varies based on location and extent of the tract. Direct laryngoscopy should be performed before or at the time of excision to confirm or deny an open tract into the pharynx. Cannulation with lacrimal probes or infiltration with methylene blue may help in aiding the identification of the tract intraoperatively. Occasionally, complete excision may be difficult due to location, scarring, inflammation, or persistent pharyngeal communication. Pharyngeal tracts seen on direct laryngoscopy may be cauterized circumferentially to induce scarring and prevent flow of saliva into the tract. In the case of second BCCs, a tonsillectomy may be required to access the pharyngeal opening (Figures 29.1 and 29.2).

Lymphangioma

DEFINITION AND CLINICAL FEATURES
Lymphangioma, otherwise referred to as lymphatic malformation or cystic hygroma, is a type of vascular malformation, which is formed from ectopic lymphatic channels that

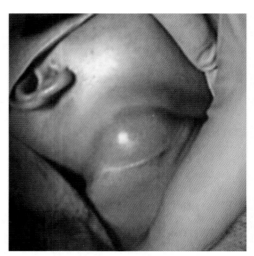

Figure 29.1 Second branchial cleft cyst.

become sequestered during lymphatic development in the embryo. Disordered growth leads to multiloculated cyst formation, which may be characterized as microcystic or macrocystic, or a combination of both. They present as a soft, nontender, irregular, fluctuant mass and most commonly occur in the soft tissues of the neck, throat, or lower face (75%–80%). They are typically diagnosed before the age of 2 and are the most common congenital lesion of the posterior cervical triangle. Lymphangiomas generally grow slowly with time but may fluctuate or swell rapidly in settings of increased lymph production such as during viral illnesses or with spontaneous or traumatic intralesional hemorrhage.

DIFFERENTIAL DIAGNOSIS
Venous malformation, hemangioma, arteriovenous malformation, BCC, TDC, thymic cyst, ranula

WORKUP
MRI with and without contrast will in most cases confirm the diagnosis and delineate the extent of involvement. Direct or indirect laryngoscopy may be useful to determine parapharyngeal involvement.

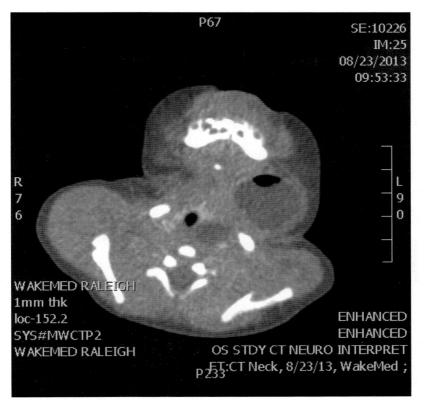

Figure 29.2 CT scan with contrast demonstrating fluid-filled cyst in the expected location of a third branchial cleft cyst. Axial CT scan with contrast demonstrating two sections of a fluid-filled cyst with a portion deep to the SCM and immediately adjacent to the airway, consistent with a third branchial cleft cyst.

TREATMENT

Treatment depends on symptoms and location. Patients with large lymphangiomas of the neck or pharynx, particularly in the suprahyoid region, have the potential to present with a difficult airway and may require tracheostomy for airway protection. Complete excision can be curative, although it is often extremely very difficult due to the infiltrative nature, irregular borders, and irreverence for soft tissue planes, making only partial excision possible in many cases. Sclerotherapy under ultrasound or x-ray guidance is useful for macrocystic lesions or macrocystic portions of the tumor but is generally unsuitable for microcystic tumors.

Patients who undergo sclerotherapy typically require multiple treatments over time, and although sclerotherapy may decrease the size of the tumor, it is not curative (Figures 29.3 and 29.4).

Thyroglossal duct cyst

DEFINITION AND CLINICAL FEATURES

TDCs occur when a portion of the primitive thyroglossal duct fails to involute completely. Although commonly located in the midline just anterior or inferior to the hyoid bone, cysts may be found anywhere along the embryologic descent of

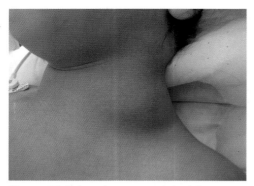

Figure 29.3 Lymphangioma of the left posterior triangle.

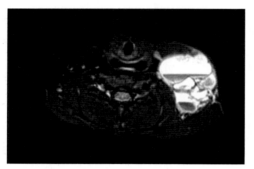

Figure 29.4 MRI scan T1-weighted image demonstrating multiloculated cyst in the left posterior triangle.

the thyroid, from the foramen cecum at the base of the tongue to its distal position at the pyramidal lobe of the thyroid gland. TDCs commonly present as painless midline enlarging masses, although they are reported as paramedian in approximately 25% of cases. They typically elevate with tongue protrusion. They may become infected and swell acutely or rupture. Rarely, TDCs are associated with malignancy, typically papillary thyroid carcinoma, which is found within an approximately 1% of excised specimens.

DIFFERENTIAL DIAGNOSIS

Dermoid cyst, teratoma, suppurative lymphadenitis, BCC, thymic cyst, vallecular cyst.

WORKUP

Serum TSH levels, as well as a thyroid and neck ultrasound, should be performed to evaluate the presence of a functionally and anatomically normal thyroid gland and to confirm the cyst anatomy. Occasionally, ectopic thyroid tissue may be present within the cyst, at the base of the tongue, or along the course of the duct, and occasionally, this tissue may represent the patient's only functional thyroid. If the ultrasound suggests abnormal thyroid anatomy, thyroid scintigraphy may be performed.

TREATMENT

Excision of the cyst alone has been found to lead to unacceptably high rates of recurrence, ranging from 38% to 70%. Surgical excision via a Sistrunk procedure is the recommended procedure, to minimize the chance of recurrence. In this procedure, the cyst is removed along with the central portion of the hyoid bone and the entire thyroglossal duct, which tracks from the pyramidal lobe of the thyroid gland to the foramen cecum at the base of the tongue. Recurrence using this technique in the literature ranges from

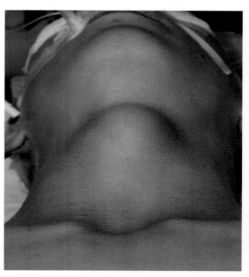

Figure 29.5 Thyroglossal duct cyst.

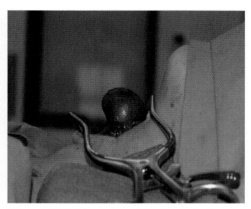

Figure 29.6 Thyroglossal duct cyst during excision.

2.6% to 5%. Aside from recurrence, risks include infection, pharyngocutaneous fistula, and injury to the hypoglossal nerve (Figures 29.5 and 29.6).

Neck abscess/suppurative lymphadenitis

DEFINITION AND CLINICAL FEATURES
Suppurative lymphadenitis is the most common cause of neck abscesses in children. This occurs from bacterial superinfection of a cervical lymph node, typically days to weeks after viral or bacterial URI, which subsequently results in central necrosis and pus accumulation within the node. Presentation typically involves progressive lateral neck swelling, with varying degrees of erythema. Fluctuance may be appreciated in superficial or large abscesses.

DIFFERENTIAL DIAGNOSIS
Lymphadenopathy with or without phlegmon, infected BCC, TDC, cat-scratch disease, scrofula (tuberculous lymphadenitis), lymphoma.

WORKUP
Simple suppurative lymphadenitis can be diagnosed by exam, CBC with differential,

and neck ultrasound. More complex or deeper abscesses may require CT scan with and without contrast, which reveals a rim-enhancing fluid collection and surrounding lymphadenopathy. If purulence is obtained, culture and sensitivities should be ordered.

TREATMENT
Admission to the hospital and intravenous antibiotics are necessary. Because the implicated pathogen in most acute cases is *Staphylococcus aureus* or *Streptococcus pyogenes* and the increasing incidence of methicillin-resistant and clindamycin-resistant *S. aureus* has been reported in this disorder, antibiotic coverage should be specifically tailored to culture results when possible. When culture results are not available, local antibiograms may be useful in determining antibiotic susceptibility. Small abscesses less than approximately 2.0–2.5 cm may improve with IV antibiotics alone, and many advocate an initial trail of medical management for these lesions. Larger abscesses or those that do not respond to conservative treatment should be managed with incision and drainage with temporary drain placement (Figures 29.7 and 29.8).

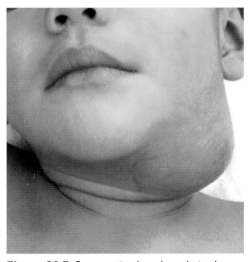

Figure 29.7 Suppurative lymph node in the anterior triangle.

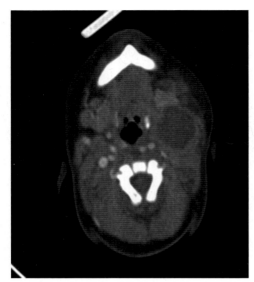

Figure 29.8 CT scan with contrast demonstrating rim-enhancing fluid collection and lymphadenopathy.

Acute bacterial sialadenitis/parotitis

DEFINITION AND CLINICAL FEATURES
Bacterial sialadenitis is an infection of the salivary glands, most commonly seen in the submandibular and parotid glands. Patients typically report several days of progressive unilateral pain and swelling of the affected gland, which worsens with eating and chewing. Fever and lymphadenopathy on the affected side are common. There may be a prior history of intermittent swelling of the gland, which raises suspicion for salivary duct stones or strictures.

DIFFERENTIAL DIAGNOSIS
Sialolithiasis, mucous retention cyst, mumps, HIV parotitis, Sjögren's syndrome, salivary tumor, suppurative lymphadenitis, first or second BCC.

WORKUP
A thorough exam should include examination of salivary flow through Wharton's and Stenson's ducts and palpation of the course of the duct to evaluate for masses or stones. Plain films may demonstrate radiopaque stones, although this cannot be ruled out with a negative study. CT or MRI should be reserved for complicated patients or where abscess or tumor is suspected. Sialography is a simple technique and may be considered to evaluate the ductal system in recurrent cases, although this may be poorly tolerated in young children.

TREATMENT
First-line treatment for simple sialadenitis is oral antibiotics, warm compresses, regular massage of the gland, and sialogogues (such as sugar-free lemon drops) to stimulate salivary production. Antibiotic choice should include coverage for *S. aureus* and oral flora, including anaerobes. Recurrent sialadenitis may indicate obstruction of the salivary duct by stones, strictures, or scar tissue. Small stones near the duct orifice may be removed in the office in compliant patients via incision of the duct to the location of the stone. In proximal obstruction, ductal dilation with or without sialoendoscopy may be performed. Stones and mucous plugs may be removed

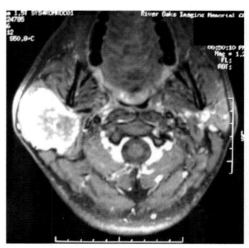

Figure 29.9 Asymmetric right parotid gland with diffuse post contrast enhancement on MRI consistent with acute sialoadenitis.

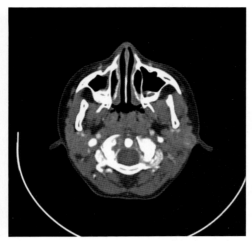

Figure 29.10 CT scan with contrast demonstrating a small mass in the superficial lobe of the left parotid gland.

with irrigation and endoscopic baskets or forceps via the sialoendoscope. Finally, complete excision of the affected gland is curative in refractory cases (Figures 29.9 and 29.10).

Suggested reading

Acierno SP, Waldhausen JH. 2007. Congenital cervical cysts, sinuses, and fistulae. *Otolaryngology of Clinical North America* 40:161–176.

Alexander AJ, Richardson SE, Sharma A, Campisi P. 2011. The increasing prevalence of clindamycin resistance in *Staphylococcus aureus* isolates in children with head and neck abscesses. *Canadian Journal of Infectious Disease Medical Microbiology* 22(2):49–51.

Cheng J, Elden L. 2013. Children with deep space neck infections: Our experience with 178 children. *Otolaryngology—Head and Neck Surgery* 148(6):1037–1042.

De Serres LM, Sie KC, Richardson MA. 1995. Lymphatic malformations of the head and neck: A proposal for staging. *Archives of Otolaryngology of Head and Neck Surgery* 121(5):577–582.

Enepekides DJ. 2001. Management of congenital anomalies of the neck. *Facial Plastic Surgery of Clinical North America* 9:131–145.

Fraser IP. 2009. Suppurative lymphadenitis. *Current Infectious Disease Report* 11:383–388.

Gillespie MB, Koch M, Iro H, Zenk J. 2011. Endoscopic-assisted gland-preserving therapy for chronic sialadenitis: A German and US comparison. *Archives of Otolaryngology of Head and Neck Surgery* 137(9):903–908.

Grasso DL, Pelizzo G, Zocconi E, Schleef J. 2008. Lymphangiomas of the head and neck in children. *Acta Otorhinolaryngolica Italica* 28(1):17–20.

Hawkins D, Jacobsen B, Klatt E. 1982. Cysts of the thyroglossal duct. *Laryngoscope* 92:1254–1258.

Iro H, Zenk J, Escudier MP et al. 2009. Outcome of minimally invasive management of salivary calculi in 4,691 patients. *Laryngoscope* 119(2):263–268.

Koeller K, Alamo L, Adair C, Smirniotopoulos J. 1999. Congenital cystic masses of the neck: Radiologic-pathologic correlation. *Radiographics* 9:121–145.

Mohan PS, Chokshi RA, Moser RL et al. 2005. Thyroglossal duct cysts: A consideration in adults. *American Surgery* 71(6):508–511.

Ossowski K, Chun RH, Suskind D, Baroody FM. 2006. Increased isolation of methicillin-resistant *Staphylococcus aureus* in pediatric head and neck abscesses. *Archives of Otolaryngology of Head and Neck Surgery* 132:1176–1181.

Papadaki ME, McCain JP, Kim K, Katz RL, Kaban LB, Troulis MJ. 2008. Interventional sialoendoscopy: Early clinical results. *Journal of Oral and Maxillofacial Surgery* 66(5):954–962.

Sistrunk WE. 1920. The surgical treatment of cyst of the thyroglossal tract. *Annals of Surgery* 71:121–122.

Telander R, Deane S. 1977. Thyroglossal and branchial cleft cysts and sinuses. *Surgery of Clinical North America* 57:779–791.

Telander R, Filson H. 1992. Review of head and neck lesions in infancy and childhood. *Surgery of Clinical North America* 72:1429–1447.

Wong DK, Brown C, Mills N, Spielmann P, Neeff M. 2012. To drain or not to drain—Management of pediatric deep neck abscesses: A case-control study. *International Journal of Pediatric Otorhinolaryngology* 76(12):1810–1813.

Craniofacial Disorders

Amelia F. Drake and Brent Golden

- **Down syndrome**
- **Pierre Robin sequence**
- **Cleft lip**
- **Cleft palate**
- **Craniofacial synostosis**
- **Mandibulofacial dysostosis**
- **CHARGE association**
- **Chromosome 22q deletion syndrome**
- **Congenital nasal pyriform aperture stenosis**
- **Oculo-auriculo-vertebral spectrum (craniofacial microsomia)**
- **Suggested reading**

Down syndrome

DEFINITIONS AND CLINICAL FEATURES

Down syndrome is the condition of duplication of the 21st chromosome or a translocation at this site and is also referred to as trisomy 21. The incidence of this condition is 1/700 live births making it the most common birth condition in the United States. In fact, some studies show that an increasing prevalence may be occurring in this country, especially in women over the age of 35.

Shott and others have delineated the common otolaryngologic findings in patients with Down syndrome, and these include small ear canals, small nasal passages and oropharynx, and relatively large-appearing tongue. The tongue is not as large as it appears but is located in the small oropharynx and oral cavity, giving the appearance of macroglossia.

DIFFERENTIAL DIAGNOSIS

The definitive diagnosis of Down syndrome is by karyotype of the chromosomes, indicating duplication of a part or all of chromosome 21 or translocation at this area. Several features, including the presence of epicanthal folds, a relatively large tongue, and single palmar creases, suggest the diagnosis.

WORKUP

Once a child is diagnosed with Down syndrome, certain concerns arise, including the high incidence of congenital heart disease, which can be evaluated with an echocardiogram and exam. Conductive hearing loss can also be an issue relating to Eustachian tube dysfunction or to ossicular abnormalities. Hearing assessment is important over time. Monitoring of growth and development should be done on separate growth charts existing for children with trisomy 21, as height and weight expectations are different. Next, polysomnogram can indicate if sleep disturbances exist.

TREATMENT

Treatment of the patient with Down syndrome should be directed at the clinical presentation, whether cardiac, respiratory, or developmental in nature. Otolaryngologic care includes determination of hearing and addressing breathing issues. Otologic care includes optimization of hearing, as conductive hearing loss can be corrected with tubes, when appropriate, hearing amplification, or surgery. The relative macroglossia and small oropharynx predispose to a higher incidence of obstructive sleep apnea. Weight issues, when present, can certainly exacerbate this.

Last, educational progress is an area where Down syndrome children may benefit

from an "individualized educational plan" to address areas of concern (Figure 30.1).

Pierre Robin sequence

DEFINITIONS AND CLINICAL FEATURES

Robin sequence (RS) is a phenotype comprised of the triad of micrognathia, glossoptosis, and airway obstruction (Figure 30.2). Highly associated with the condition is also a cleft of the palate that is characteristically U-shaped, although this is not universally viewed as a defining feature (Figures 30.3 and 30.4). Pierre Robin, a French stomatologist, was not the first to describe this association, since St. Hilaire reported a case over 100 years prior, but he is credited for bringing the condition to prominence and demonstrating the significant negative impact of its features.

The sequence is felt to originate with mandibular hypoplasia, which then leads to glossoptosis causing airway obstruction and cleft palate. Mandibular hypoplasia may result from external deformational causes or intrinsic malformation. Unfortunately, there is no set definition for what constitutes pathologic mandibular hypoplasia in the infant, and some degree of relative mandibular hypoplasia is considered normal. Taken together with the variability in features used to define RS, it is not surprising that the condition is subsequently heterogeneous with many different associations. Despite this, it is generally felt to be one of the more common birth anomalies occurring between 1/3,000 and 1/14,000.

DIFFERENTIAL DIAGNOSIS

RS is highly associated with syndromic diagnoses or features, and these cases account for about 50% of the total. The most frequently identified syndromes are the collagenopathies, of which Stickler syndrome is the most common occurring in 14% of infants with RS. Less commonly, the 22q11.2 deletion syndrome is concurrent. The remainder represents isolated RS with no known

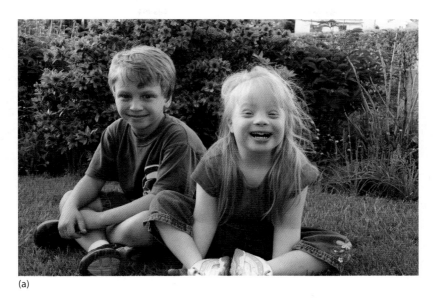

(a)

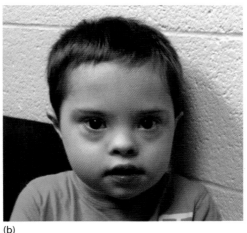

(b)

Figure 30.1 (a) Facial features of a girl with Down syndrome. (b) Facial features of a boy with Down syndrome.

associated anomalies. The condition must be differentiated from other craniofacial syndromes with known micrognathia.

WORKUP

The workup for RS requires a multidisciplinary approach involving the neonatologist, geneticist, pediatric otolaryngologist, pediatric pulmonologist, pediatric craniofacial surgeon, and speech therapist or occupational therapist specialized in infant feeding.

The initial concern in evaluating a child with RS is airway assessment and stabilization. Pulse oximetry, CO_2 monitoring, and inpatient monitoring are useful adjuncts in the newborn. Infants that appear to have a stable airway in the first days of life may exhibit a decline in status over the

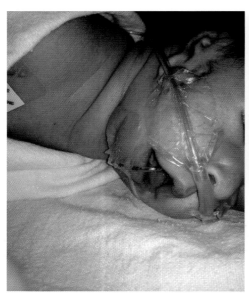

Figure 30.2 Small mandible with airway compromise in a patient with other craniofacial malformations.

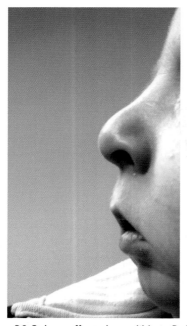

Figure 30.3 Less affected mandible in Robin.

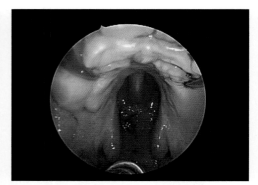

Figure 30.4 U-shaped cleft palate in Robin.

early weeks. Bedside clinical airway evaluation with or without laryngoscopy by the neonatologist and pediatric otolaryngologist may be sufficient for the mild to moderately affected cases early on. More severely affected cases or those with complicated courses may require intubation accompanied by direct laryngoscopy and bronchoscopy to direct therapy.

One-third to half of children with RS will exhibit problems with feeding significant enough to require gastric tube feeding. Assessment and cooperation with a speech therapist specializing in infant feeding are beneficial. Exacerbating feeding problems may be aspiration or reflux. Airway stabilization interventions are not primarily aimed at improving feeding, and some successfully treated for airway compromise will still need gavage support. Fortunately, the need for gastric tube nutrition rarely continues after the first year of life.

TREATMENT

Nonsurgical airway management is successful in the great majority of cases, perhaps as many as 70%. Prone or lateral positioning with airway monitoring may be sufficient without additional measures in half of affected children. In those who fail positioning with predominantly tongue base obstruction, a modified nasopharyngeal airway (NPA) can provide

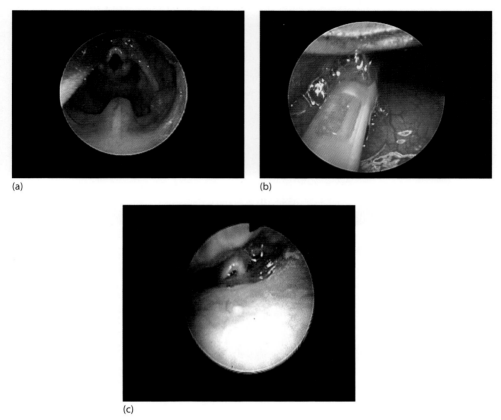

Figure 30.5 (a) Grade I laryngoscopy. (b) Grade IV laryngoscopy in neonate with PRS. (c) Flexible endoscopy in neonate with PRS and tongue-based airway.

adequate airway patency. With adequate education, parents can provide the care necessary to maintain a NPA at home for improved quality of life. Discontinuation of therapy is considered once the pediatric otolaryngologist determines the airway is sufficiently improved.

For infants with RS in whom neither positioning nor NPA therapy is sufficient, or in those who require intubation early on, surgical therapies may be the most predictable option. Prior to surgical therapy, direct laryngoscopy and bronchoscopy are required to evaluate for degrees of tongue base obstruction, laryngomalacia, tracheomalacia, or bronchial stenosis. The types

of surgeries that have been utilized include tongue–lip adhesion, infant mandibular distraction osteogenesis, and tracheostomy (Figure 30.5).

Tongue–lip adhesion is meant to prevent the retrodisplacement of the tongue base by anchoring the anterior ventral tongue to the lower lip. Its effectiveness is debated and wound breakdown can be troublesome. Mandibular distraction osteogenesis is a surgical means of increasing posterior airway space by elongating the mandible and thereby advancing the tongue. Over the course of one to three weeks, the mandible can be incrementally elongated with internal or external devices. After a consolidation phase,

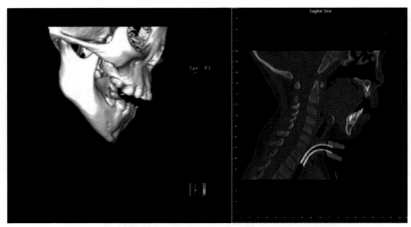

Figure 30.6 CT demonstrating micrognathia and tongue-based airway obstruction; a tracheostomy has been placed to secure the airway.

the distractors are removed. Depending on the technique, distraction procedures may place at risk developing tooth buds, the trigeminal nerve sensory innervation of the lower lip and chin, and the marginal mandibular motor innervation to the lower lip. Tracheostomy remains the gold standard for complete relief of airway obstruction, but morbidity and mortality remain real concerns. Palate repair typically is performed at the same time as isolated cleft palate, between 9 and 18 months based on speech development (Figure 30.6).

Cleft lip

DEFINITIONS AND CLINICAL FEATURES

An orofacial cleft represents the most common congenital craniofacial abnormality occurring approximately in 1 in every 550 live births. The incidence of a cleft of the lip with or without palate varies considerably based on geography and racial variability. The defect occurs as a result of a failure of the median nasal process to fuse with the maxillary process during the sixth week of development. The subsequent structural abnormalities have implications for both form and function that may negatively affect deglutition, respiration, speech, hearing, occlusion, facial appearance, and psychosocial development. To optimally address the complexity of effects, a multidisciplinary approach blending therapy and surgery is required. Since surgical interventions may have negative effects on growth, a staged surgical approach throughout childhood is required triggered by specific developmental goals.

The affected facial structures in the nasolabial cleft are displaced and variably hypoplastic, but largely present. Disruption of the nasolabial musculature is marked by abnormal orientation and insertion of the cleft side transverse muscles of the nose, levator muscles of the upper lip, and orbicularis oris muscle complex. In the unilateral cleft, the non–cleft side muscles have grossly normal insertions, but the resulting imbalance manifests in distortion of maxillary and nasal form bilaterally. Splaying of the alar base, inferior displacement of the alar rim, deviation of the nasal tip, and irregularity of the caudal nasal septum characterize the typical resulting nasal deformity. Abnormal fibrous insertions exist between the lateral crus of the lower lateral cartilage and the lateral piriform rim on the cleft side. In the bilateral cleft lip, the nasal tip is depressed, and the premaxillary segment can be variably displaced.

The upper jaw is deformed by the osseous discontinuity at the nasal base and dental alveolus, and dental anomalies are common. A missing lateral incisor is the most common finding occurring about 50% of the time, and missing second premolar teeth on the side of the cleft are increased in incidence as well. In a large minority of cases, supernumerary teeth complicate dental eruption.

DIFFERENTIAL DIAGNOSIS

In greater than 70% of cases, cleft lip with or without palate is an isolated birth defect that is not associated with any specific genetic diagnosis. The etiology of most isolated clefts of the lip is thought to be heterogeneous and multifactorial including genetic factors and environmental. The remainder may be related to one of more than 300 syndromic associations. Such syndromes that are most likely to be seen include trisomy chromosomal aberrations, the autosomal dominant Van der Woude with lip pit associations, and ectodermal dysplasia–clefting.

WORKUP

Initial evaluation for the child born with a cleft of the lip with or without palate should include a thorough family history and clinical exam. Any associated anomalies or positive history should trigger the involvement of a pediatric geneticist for more comprehensive assessment.

The full weight of evaluating the cleft patient is distributed throughout childhood and into adolescence with interdisciplinary contributions that are simultaneously applied, but variably emphasized. Early in childhood, hearing, speech development, and dental health assessments predominate. Middle childhood often represents a transition to maxillofacial and orthodontic management. Psychosocial and developmental assessments should be ongoing.

TREATMENT

The child with a cleft of the lip will require surgery to reorient and reconstruct the cutaneous structures of the upper lip and oral mucosa, the musculature of the oral sphincter and nasal base, and the nasal cartilaginous framework. The rotation advancement technique popularized by Millard remains the most common approach to primary surgical intervention for the unilateral cleft. In this approach, the medial cleft margin is rotated down and the repair incision inferiorly matched to the expected position of the philtral column. The lateral cleft lip is advanced to meet the medial lip and to fill any deficiency of tissue high in the philtrum below the columella. A preserved C-flap can be used to minimize the need for this advancement below the columella or to augment the nasal floor reconstruction. Bilateral cleft lip repair requires preservation of appropriate prolabial skin and mucosa, advancement of the lateral lip elements to fill the cleft defects, and recreation of a Cupid's bow by recruiting vermillion and white roll from the lateral lips. Aggressive nasal reconstruction in the infant is to be approached with caution. Closed treatment with release of the lower lateral cartilages from abnormal insertions from inside the lip incisions followed by resuspension using pexy sutures or bolsters is perhaps the most predictable approach, understanding that open technique secondary rhinoplastic intervention later in life is likely (Figure 30.7).

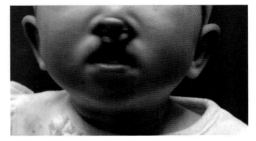

Figure 30.7 Infant with unrepaired bilateral cleft lip.

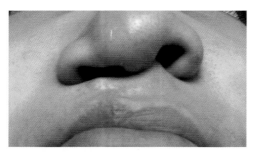

Figure 30.8 Cleft nose deformity.

When a palatal cleft is present, treatment proceeds as noted in the "Cleft Palate" section.

Since the development of the upper jaw is embryologically related to the upper lip, it is expected that bone graft construction of the cleft maxilla and palate will be beneficial in almost all patients with a cleft lip. In any case where there is insufficient bone to support erupting teeth, bone grafting is required. The primary objectives of bone grafting are to unify the maxilla, close any oronasal fistula, provide adequate bone to support eruption and orthodontic treatment of adult teeth, and provide appropriate nasal base support and symmetry. The ideal time for treatment is when the developing adult tooth adjacent to the cleft has a root that is half to two-thirds formed.

In addition to these primary reconstructions, some children will benefit from secondary interventions. Normalization of lip and nasal form may require a soft tissue revision of lip scars and proportions later in childhood. Secondary rhinoplasty in young adulthood is relatively common and is to be expected for bilateral cleft deformity (Figure 30.8).

Cleft palate

DEFINITIONS AND CLINICAL FEATURES

An orofacial cleft represents the most common congenital craniofacial abnormality occurring approximately in 1 in every 550 live births. The incidence of a cleft palate alone is closer to 1 in 2000, and interestingly, the occurrence is homogenous across racial populations. The defect occurs as a result of a failure of the palatal shelves to fuse or maintain fusion in the midline of the maxilla. The subsequent structural abnormalities have implications that may negatively affect deglutition, respiration, speech, hearing, occlusion, facial appearance, and psychosocial development. To optimally address the complexity of effects, a multidisciplinary approach blending therapy and surgery is required. Since surgical interventions may have negative effects on growth, the surgical approach is organized around specific developmental goals, specifically speech and language acquisition (Figure 30.9).

The affected oral structures in the palatal cleft are displaced and variably hypoplastic, but largely present. Disruption of the palatal musculature is dominated by abnormal orientation and insertion of the levator veli palatini, tensor veli palatini, and palatopharyngeus and palatoglossus muscles. Veau first recognized this in his cadaver studies where he described the "cleft muscle" and the understanding greatly enhanced in clinical practice by Kriens description of intravelar veloplasty.

The palate has been classified into two parts based on embryologic developmental

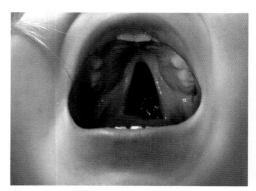

Figure 30.9 Unrepaired cleft palate.

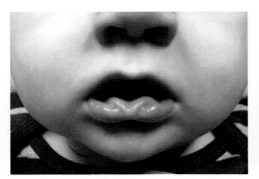

Figure 30.10 Lip pits associated with cleft palate.

patterns. The primary palate constitutes the maxilla and dental structures anterior to the incisive foramen and is formed by the same facial processes that form the lip and nose. The secondary palate includes the hard and soft palate tissues posterior to the incisive foramen and is distinct from the primary palate. An isolated cleft palate is complete if it extends into the hard palate approximating the incisive foramen; otherwise, it is considered incomplete. Vomerine fusion to the palatal shelves may be absent completely, present on one side only or present on both sides, depending on the degree of involvement (Figure 30.10).

A submucous cleft palate exists when the triad of bifid uvula, hard palate notching, and midline zona pellucida is present without an overt palatal cleft. The muscular disorientation continues to define the functional problems that may result, primarily velopharyngeal incompetency and Eustachian tube dysfunction (Figure 30.11).

DIFFERENTIAL DIAGNOSIS

It is important to remember the distinction between cleft lip and palate versus cleft palate alone. Cleft palate alone is notable for having a much greater association with syndromes, sequences, or additional malformations, occurring in approximately

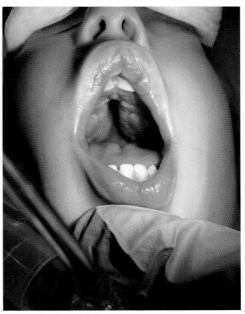

Figure 30.11 High-arched palate (at times mistaken for cleft palate).

50% of cases. The most notable because of frequency are Stickler syndrome, 22q11.2 deletion syndrome, and Van der Woude syndrome. Stickler syndrome is notable for ocular findings, hearing loss, midface deficiency, and arthritis. Because of this, early ophthalmologic exam in children with RS and cleft palate is advisable. The 22q11.2 deletion syndrome may also commonly be associated with cardiac anomalies, characteristic facies, developmental delays, and immune deficiencies.

WORKUP

Initial evaluation for the child born with a cleft of the palate should include a thorough family history and clinical exam. Any associated anomalies or positive history should trigger the involvement of a pediatric geneticist for more comprehensive assessment and possible genetic testing.

The full weight of evaluating the cleft patient is distributed throughout childhood and into adolescence with interdisciplinary contributions. Early in childhood, hearing, speech development, and dental health assessments are most critical. Middle childhood often represents a transition to maxillofacial and orthodontic management. Psychosocial and developmental assessments are perpetual.

TREATMENT

The child with an overt cleft of the palate will require surgery to reorient and reconstruct the musculature of the velopharyngeal mechanism, to resurface the cleft with healthy mucosa, and to eliminate middle ear drainage problems. The two most common techniques for closure of the palate with muscular reconstruction are the straight-line closure with intravelar veloplasty and the double-opposing Z-plasty technique of Furlow. In the straight-line closure, the hard palate may be closed with an early vomerine flap as advocated by Sommerlad, by lateral releasing incision in the style of von Langenbeck, or by two complete flaps pedicled off the descending palatine vessels as described by Bardach. The soft palate is closed in three layers with oral and nasal mucosa lining, a retrodisplaced levator veli palatini, and palatopharyngeus muscle sling. It is critical to separate this muscle unit from the posterior hard palate, from soft tissue attachment to the tensor aponeurosis, and from abnormal mucosal attachment to allow adequate reconstruction of the velopharyngeal muscle sling. Another means of accomplishing the same end is with double-opposing Z-plasty flaps. Furlow's description specifically managed the muscles by leaving maintaining their relationship to the mucosal flaps that are pedicled posteriorly allowing for retrodisplacement, closure under functional tension, and some added benefit of palatal lengthening, mild

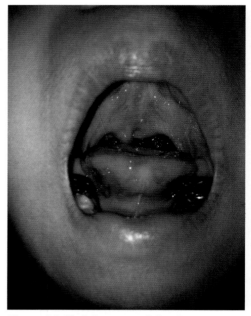

Figure 30.12 Submucous cleft palate.

sphincteroplasty, and disruption of any straight line scarring (Figure 30.12).

Myringotomy with placement of tubes is effective for treating Eustachian tube dysfunction, when present, and regular hearing checks, otoscopic exam, and tympanograms are necessary for longitudinal monitoring.

In addition to the primary reconstruction, all children benefit from regular developmental assessment by speech and language pathologists. Many will require speech therapy to maximize speech outcomes. A minority will have persistent velopharyngeal dysfunction that leads to secondary palatal surgery to lengthen the palate by secondary Z-plasty or to recruit extra tissue to the area via a pharyngeal flap, sphincter pharyngoplasty, or posterior pharyngeal wall augmentation.

Surgical repair of the submucous cleft palate should be pursued only when indicated for dysfunctional speech (Figure 30.13).

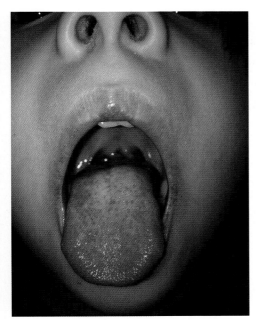

Figure 30.13 Bifid uvula associated with SMCP.

Craniofacial synostosis

DEFINITION AND CLINICAL FEATURES
Apert's, Crouzon's, and, less frequently, Pfeiffer's syndrome are some of the syndromes associated with craniofacial synostosis, or premature fusing of the sutures of the skull. Apert's syndrome was described in 1906, and Crouzon's syndrome was initially described in 1912 in a mother and son with exophthalmos, calvarial deformities, and facial anomalies. Not only do infants with these conditions have early closure of their sutures in their craniums, most often the coronal suture, but they also have fusion of sutures of the cranial base and midface, leaving them with shallow orbits and midfacial hypoplasia and the characteristic exophthalmos, which is a hallmark of these conditions.

DIFFERENTIAL DIAGNOSIS
The syndromic craniosynostosis have been found to be genetic in cause, with FGFR2 or FGFR3 mutations seen in most Crouzon's and Apert's patients. They are usually inherited in an autosomal dominant pattern with variable penetrance or represent a new occurrence. Involvement of the hands and feet, with severe symmetric syndactyly, occurs in Apert's syndrome. Patients with Crouzon can have a milder expression of their craniofacial condition and the facial features can be subtler.

WORKUP
Imaging, including CT scanning, is generally performed early to assess the degree of synostosis and the timing of intervention. Neurodevelopmental assessment is important to follow cognition. Routine ophthalmologic monitoring can evaluate vision as well as evidence of increased intracranial pressure over time. Hearing and speech evaluations help determine gains in those arenas.

TREATMENT
As any baby with potential nasal obstruction, an infant with midfacial hypoplasia should be monitored closely in the first few weeks of life for potential airway concerns and, with these, feeding challenges. Supportive care may be required early on in life.

Treatment of craniosynostosis is surgical, including neurosurgical, to prevent complications that can occur due to pressure on the brain by the limitation of growth of the cranium. Ideally, patients with a craniofacial condition would be followed by a craniofacial team and have the input of the surgeon, the psychologist, the speech pathologist, as well as the otolaryngologist. If a cleft palate presents, it would also be addressed. Recently, parameters of care have been outlined for craniofacial conditions with craniosynostosis (Figure 30.14).

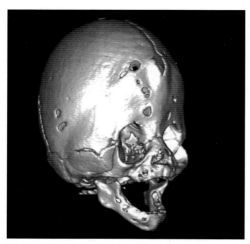

Figure 30.14 Craniofacial synostosis—3D reconstruction of CT scan.

Mandibulofacial dysostosis

DEFINITIONS AND CLINICAL FEATURES

A patient with mandibulofacial dysostosis was first described in 1889 by Berry, an ophthalmic surgeon focusing on colobomata of the lower eyelid. Treacher Collins, another ophthalmologist, presented two cases in 1900 with similar findings. The term mandibulofacial dysostosis appeared in the 1949 when Franceschetti and Klein began to more fully describe the condition and its facial characteristics.

Few have understood or characterized the deformity more fully than Tessier. In his review of over 60 cases, he describes the complete form to have typical features including the following: slant of the palpebral fissures, coloboma of the lower lateral eyelids, absence of the eyelashes medial to the coloboma, lateral canthal dystopia with shortening of the palpebral fissure, hypoplasia or absence of the malar bone, absence of the zygomatic arch, and numerous ear deformities. Extreme antegonial notching of the mandibular body is also characteristic. The incomplete form of the condition with expression of lower eyelid notching or coloboma combined with malar hypoplasia is still considered representative for diagnosis. The Nager form of mandibulofacial dysostosis (preaxial acrofacial dysostosis) is characterized by severe palatal hypoplasia and radial limb abnormalities in addition to the aforementioned.

The Treacher Collins type of mandibulofacial dysostosis has been characterized as most commonly arising from a mutation to the TCOF1 gene mapped to chromosome 5. The occurrence is felt to be between 1 in 25,000 and 1 in 50,000 live births. The condition is transmitted in an autosomal dominant fashion. Over half the cases are the results of a de novo mutation. Intelligence is often average or above average.

DIFFERENTIAL DIAGNOSIS

Mandibulofacial dysostosis must be differentiated from other conditions with lower facial hypoplasia such as RS and oculoauriculovertebral spectrum disorders. Of particular difficulty can be differentiating the bilateral form of oculoauriculovertebral spectrum disorders that may share in common mandibular hypoplasia, ear malformations, and macrostomia.

WORKUP

The workup for mandibulofacial dysostosis requires a multidisciplinary approach involving the neonatologist, geneticist, pediatric otolaryngologist, pediatric neuroophthalmologist, pediatric craniofacial surgeon, and speech therapist or occupational therapist specialized in infant feeding.

The initial concern in evaluating a child with mandibulofacial dysostosis is airway assessment and stabilization. Airway compromise may arise at multiple levels including tongue base obstruction from mandibular deficiency and increased nasal resistance from choanal atresia. Pulse oximetry and inpatient monitoring are useful adjuncts in the newborn. Bedside clinical airway evaluation with or without laryngoscopy by the neonatologist and pediatric otolaryngologist may be sufficient. More severely affected cases or those with complicated courses may require intubation accompanied by direct laryngoscopy and bronchoscopy to direct therapy. Mandibular distraction osteogenesis is used in selected cases to prevent tracheostomy or accelerate decannulation. Tracheostomy surgery remains the definitive means of airway protection.

Formal audiological testing should take place in the first days of life. Hearing aids should be fitted early on in the child's life. CT scanning to formally characterize the craniofacial skeleton and specifically the middle and inner ear anatomy should be obtained prior to attempts at surgically addressing the conductive loss.

Evaluation by a pediatric neuro-ophthalmologist is beneficial for comprehensive ocular evaluation and to protect the vision from unrecognized corneal exposure.

A formal evaluation by a pediatric geneticist is requisite given the heritable nature of the condition.

TREATMENT

Craniofacial reconstruction typically requires a staged approach based on the developmental progress of the facial skeleton. When necessary, cleft palate repair is performed around a year of life based on speech development. Specific to mandibulofacial dysostosis syndrome, Posnick's description of iterative surgery is most comprehensive. Orbitomalar reconstruction is optimally performed at or after ages 5–7 coincident with maturation of the orbits to near adult size. This is typically performed using fresh, autogenous nonvascularized grafts to reconstruct the lateral orbit and floor, while onlay bone grafts of the maxilla and malar region augment undercontoured areas. The maxillomandibular relationship is most predictably addressed through orthognathic surgery with coincident orthodontics during the adolescent years after the jaws have largely completed their growth potential. Rhinoplastic surgery, soft tissue

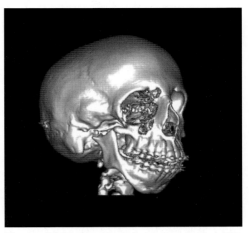

Figure 30.15 Mandibulofacial dysostosis—3D reconstruction of CT scan.

reconstruction of the eyelids, and otoplasty are reconstructive options. Treatment of conductive hearing loss, when present, should occur early by means of either amplification or surgery (Figure 30.15).

CHARGE association

DEFINITIONS AND CLINICAL FEATURES

CHARGE is an acronym whose letters stand for the constellation of features including coloboma, heart defect, atresia of the choanae (also known as choanal atresia), retarded growth and development, genital abnormality, and ear abnormality. The degree and involvement of malformations can vary among people with the disorder. The diagnosis of CHARGE syndrome is based on a combination of major and minor characteristics. The minor characteristics include heart defects, slow growth, developmental delay, and cleft lip with or without cleft palate. The condition is known as an "association" of clinical features, and hence, it can be variable in its presentation.

DIFFERENTIAL DIAGNOSIS

As an association of clinical characteristics, CHARGE presents in various degrees of

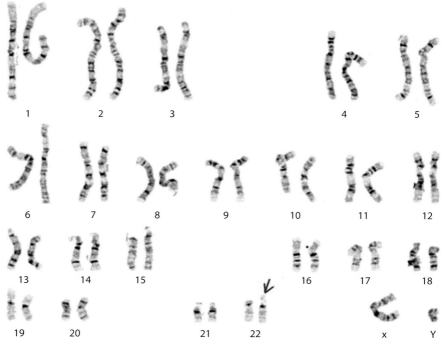

Figure 30.16 Karyotype from a patient with DiGeorge syndrome.

severity. Infants may present emergently if bilateral choanal atresia is present, as they are obligate nose breathers.

WORKUP

Most patients have a deletion or mutation at the CHD4 gene, though other genetic abnormalities can occur. If CHARGE is suspected, then attention to the heart, hearing, and renal and overall development is important.

TREATMENT

The first procedure necessary for patients may be the surgical repair of the choanal atresia, when this presents early on. As with any condition, the overall health of the infant should be assessed, with attention to feeding and growth. Hearing needs can be addressed with tubes or with amplification, when appropriate. More definitive

treatments can address the specific abnormalities that present (Figure 30.16).

Chromosome 22q deletion syndrome

DEFINITIONS AND CLINICAL FEATURES

Chromosome 22q deletion syndrome, also known as DiGeorge syndrome, velocardiofacial syndrome, or Shprintzen syndrome, is recognized as a spectrum condition with early names used for the various clinical presentations that may present. Today, support groups call for a better understanding of the spectrum in order to coordinate research and funding. For this microdeletion, the potential findings are diverse; these findings include psychological; immunologic, especially T-cell suppression; cardiac; and speech abnormalities specifically hypernasality and laryngeal webs (Figure 30.17).

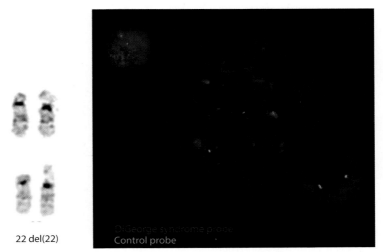

22 del(22)

DiGeorge syndrome probe
Control probe

Figure 30.17 Chromosome 22 and fluorescence in situ hybridization demonstrating DiGeorge syndrome deletion del(22)(q11.21q11.21).

DIFFERENTIAL DIAGNOSIS

The condition is to be considered when velopharyngeal insufficiency occurs without having a cleft of the palate necessarily appreciated. The abnormal function of the palate can more readily be seen on nasendoscopy; however, many patients present after extensive speech therapy or adenoidectomy.

WORKUP

The genetic finding of a deletion in the portion of the 22q chromosome can be found with fluorescence in situ hybridization, performed with karyotype. Rarely, duplication can occur.

As the deletion occurs in the region of the chromosome associated with thymic dysfunction, an affected patient can have abnormal immune function. The "facial" aspects of the velocardiofacial syndrome are variously described and include a broad nose and close-set eyes.

TREATMENT

Treatment of patients with 22q deletion syndrome is directed at the area of expression of the condition. If cardiac disease is present,

this is usually diagnosed and addressed in early childhood. Velopharyngeal dysfunction becomes evident as the child learns to talk and can be associated with a cleft palate, a submucous cleft palate, or a dysfunction of the velopharyngeal mechanism without visible clefting.

Congenital nasal pyriform aperture stenosis

DEFINITIONS AND CLINICAL FEATURES

First described by its current name in 1989, the condition of congenital nasal pyriform aperture stenosis represents the anterior nasal narrowing relating to its dental manifestation, the single central maxillary incisor (Figure 30.18). Usually the infant with bilateral nasal obstruction presents early and dramatically, with difficulty breathing when the mouth is closed. As the condition has become better understood, authors have suggested a more involved developmental midline defect in addition to the nasal obstruction, with other possibly affected organs including the pituitary.

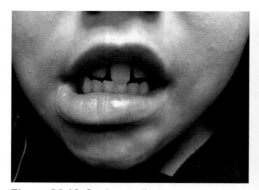

Figure 30.18 Single maxillary incisor.

DIFFERENTIAL DIAGNOSIS

Other congenital causes of nasal obstruction to be considered include choanal atresia, congenital nasolacrimal duct cysts, and congenital nasal masses (glioma, meningocele, meningoencephalocele, vascular malformations).

WORKUP

The diagnosis can be made clinically, as it is difficult to visualize into the nose or to place an endotracheal tube or nasal trumpet through the slit-like nasal openings. The diagnosis is also apparent in imaging studies obtained early on, as the associated single maxillary tooth is visualized even when unerupted, and its importance to this condition is understood. The nasal pyriform apertures are medially located and narrow, causing the nasal obstruction that is evident clinically (Figure 30.19). Authors have determined accurate nasal dimensions of young infants to help in the diagnosis of this condition. Generally, computed tomography will reveal a narrow pyriform aperture and measurement of less than 3 mm per pyriform aperture or less than 8 mm in aggregate confirms the diagnosis. As nasal pyriform aperture stenosis can be accompanied by pituitary dysfunction, it is important to be sure that the patient does not have disturbances of adrenal gland, growth hormone, or thyroid suppression. Monitoring growth and development is important in

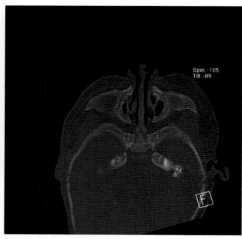

Figure 30.19 CT of a normal pyriform aperture.

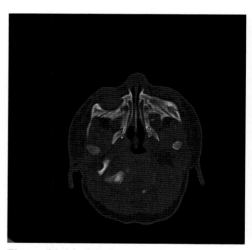

Figure 30.20 CT of a pyriform aperture stenosis.

this condition, as is treating any areas of deficiency. Genetics consult, endocrine evaluations, and MRI of the brain are recommended (Figure 30.20).

TREATMENT

Treatment to open the nose can include nasal decongestants, attempts at dilation, or tracheostomy tube placement to bypass the problem. Early efforts to surgically open the nasal airways were reported in the plastic surgery literature. More recently, sublabial repair of the nasal aperture stenosis is considered the standard approach to symptomatic nasal obstruction. Indeed, newer treatment options use advances that have been made in drill techniques and enhanced visualization that is present with endoscopic optics and light sources.

Oculo-auriculo-vertebral spectrum (craniofacial microsomia)

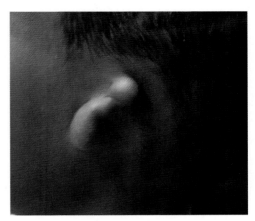

Figure 30.21 Microtia with ear canal atresia.

DEFINITIONS AND CLINICAL FEATURES
In 1963, Gorlin referred to oculo-auriculo-vertebral (OAV) dysplasia as a term to characterize patients with macrostomia, microtia, and hypoplasia of the mandibular ramus. Since then, other terms have been used to portray individuals with similar phenotypes, and the clinical spectrum has been expanded to include epibulbar dermoids and facial nerve palsies among others. Other terms used for this condition include hemifacial or craniofacial microsomia (CFM), Goldenhar syndrome, first and second branchial arch syndrome, and unilateral mandibulofacial dysplasia among others.

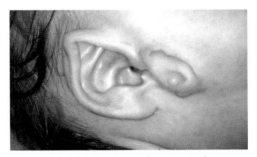

Figure 30.22 Microtia with preauricular tag.

CFM is phenotypical condition with a wide spectrum of soft and hard tissue hypoplasia affecting both hard and soft tissue components of the first and second branchial arch derivatives. More than half of affected persons have associated findings found outside the craniofacial region, most often cardiac, vertebral, or limb findings. Although universally accepted minimum diagnostic criteria do not exist, the condition is felt to be one of the more common craniofacial congenital anomalies, occurring in between 1:3000 and 1:5000 live births (Figure 30.21).

Characteristic craniofacial findings are ear anomalies (including microtia, preauricular or facial tags, aural atresia, and hearing loss), mandibular hypoplasia causing facial asymmetry and malocclusion, zygomatic and malar hypoplasia, eye and orbit anomalies, facial nerve weakness, asymmetric palatal function, and macrostomia/lateral facial clefts. Other craniofacial malformations including cleft lip and/or palate can be seen. Facial involvement is most often unilateral, but bilateral involvement is not rare. Even when bilateral, asymmetry is common (Figure 30.22).

DIFFERENTIAL DIAGNOSIS
Conditions that may commonly mimic CFM include the mandibulofacial dysostosis syndromes (Treacher Collins syndrome/Nager syndrome), Townes–Brocks syndrome, CHARGE syndrome, and branchio-oto-renal syndrome. Given the degree of overlap, a

number of these may represent a spectrum of developmental disturbance. Postnatal traumatic condylar injury may mimic the lower facial skeletal forms of more mildly expressed CFM.

WORKUP

The primary concern in the neonate with features of CFM is airway stability. For children with any signs of airway obstruction, a highly monitored environment such as a neonatal intensive care unit and early involvement of pediatric otolaryngologists is recommended. Formal evaluation of the airway, as well as noninvasive sleep studies, can be useful. Involvement of a pediatric geneticist is recommended. A renal ultrasound should be routinely obtained if CFM is suspected, and a low threshold should exist to obtain an echocardiogram with any concerning clinical findings.

Newborn hearing screening is ideally performed, and hearing will need to be closely monitored. For children with significant hearing loss or aural atresia, amplification can be pursued. In time, fine-cut CT evaluation of the temporal bone anatomy is useful to consider surgical planning. Also, baseline evaluation by a pediatric ophthalmologist is prudent given the high association of associated eye findings in the condition.

Feeding and nutrition may be significantly affected by a compromised airway, facial clefts, or jaw hypoplasia. Weight gain must be followed closely. Given the known association with cervical spine abnormalities, cervical spine imaging between ages 2 and 3 years should be completed.

Characterization of temporozygomatic and mandibular deformity can be screened with plain films (i.e., panoramic radiographs) and fully elucidated with CT imaging. Detailed analysis is undertaken based on the indication for treatment, not by a standard age. If surgery is indicated for ramus construction, then earlier assessment is needed than if the child has a functional condyle unit and needs only corrective jaw surgery.

TREATMENT

Children with OAV spectrum benefit from longitudinal interdisciplinary team care to address the hearing, communication, and potential developmental hurdles that they can have. There are numerous options for treatment. Craniofacial reconstruction typically requires a staged approach based on developmental progress of the facial skeleton and cognitive function. The earliest intervention that may be necessary is airway protection, and tracheostomy is sometimes required. Mandibular surgery in the infant using distraction osteogenesis has shown limited long-term value in the CFM patient. When necessary, surgical removal of facial tags and repair of any lateral facial clefting can be completed within the first 18 months of life. Surgery for palatal clefts typically occurs within the first year although this may be deferred for children with respiratory compromise (Figure 30.23).

Interventions to assess, protect, and maximize hearing are of critical importance in

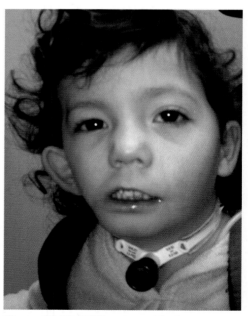

Figure 30.23 OAV patient with airway compromise.

the CFM child. With unilateral involvement, the uninvolved ear is critical for hearing and speech development. If one ear has normal function, amplification of the involved ear is not usually necessary. When conductive hearing loss is present bilaterally, bone-conduction amplification is initiated early. Throughout childhood and adolescence, developmental specialists should closely monitor children with CFM with a particular focus on speech and language development and any specialized needs related to hearing impairment. An oculoplastic surgeon may be needed to excise large epibulbar dermoids or those that interfere with vision (Figure 30.24).

The mandibular deformity exists on a spectrum from mild hypoplasia to complete atresia of the temporomandibular articulation and ascending ramus. Of particular importance is the function of the affected temporomandibular joint and airway patency relative to tongue base support. The spectrum of involvement of the lower jaw has been characterized by Pruzansky and modified by Kaban. For children who have a functioning articulation of the mandible to the cranial base, even if hypoplastic, reconstruction may proceed with conventional osteotomies or distraction osteogenesis to better position the tooth-bearing

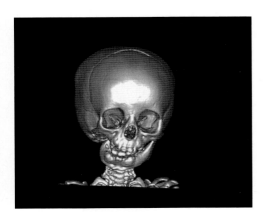

Figure 30.24 OVA spectrum—3D reconstruction of frontal CT scan.

segment and improve asymmetry and projection. This is most predictably done near the completion of growth during adolescence. If airway concerns are significant, earlier intervention can be undertaken with the understanding that revision is likely to be necessary by the mid to late teen years. For children without a functioning articulation, construction of a condyle/ramus and cranial base platform is needed. This is most predictable with costochondral autogenous grafting in conjunction with prolonged orthodontic splint-guided therapy. Rib grafts produce many challenges including resorption, infection, over or undergrowth, or ankylosis. Allowing for eruption of the adult first molars and incisor teeth provides significant utility for orthodontic assistance in protecting the graft. Surgery earlier than 6 or 7 years old remains quite unpredictable.

Otoplasty and ear reconstruction have become a relatively common component of treatment in the CFM patient. Even so, options exist ranging from no treatment to complex staged surgical reconstruction using autogenous costochondral cartilage. Camouflaging the area with hair is adequate for a number of patients. Implant-supported prosthetics are available. Surgical reconstruction provides a serviceable ear in many cases and can be considered as early as 6 years, when ear development nears adult size and position. Even so, it must be remembered that the burden of care with ear reconstruction is high for children who already must undergo many types of intervention.

Corrective jaw surgery in the mid to late teen years is beneficial in the majority of patients. Maxillary surgery is usually by conventional Lefort I osteotomy, and mandibular treatment is patient-specific but can often be accomplished with conventional ramus osteotomies. Soft tissue hypoplasia can be camouflaged with autogenous fat grafting by injection as described by Coleman, and this is most predictable when done following skeletal correction.

Suggested reading

Apert M. 1906. De l'acrocephalosyndactylie. *Bulletins et mémoires de la Société Médicale des Hôpitaux de Paris.* 23:1310–1313.

Arlis H, Ward RF. 1992. Congenital nasal pyriform aperture stenosis: Isolated abnormality vs developmental field defect. *Archives of Otolaryngology Head and Neck Surgery* 118:989–991.

Bardach J, Morris HL, Olin WH. 1984. Late results of primary veloplasty: The Marburg Project. *Plastic Reconstructive Surgery* 73(2):207–218.

Berry GA. 1889. Note on a congenital defect (coloboma) of the lower lid. *The Royal London Ophthalmology Hospital Report* 12:255.

Besser L, Shin M, Kucik J, Correa A. 2007. Prevalence of Down syndrome among children and adolescents in metropolitan Atlanta. *Birth Defects Research Part A* 79:765–774.

Birgfeld CB, Heike C. 2012. Craniofacial microsomia. *Seminars in Plastic Surgery* 26:91–104.

Birgfeld CB, Luquetti DV, Gougoutas AJ, Bartlett SP, Low DW, Sie KC, Evans KN, Heike CL. 2011. A phenotypic assessment tool for craniofacial microsomia. *Plastic Reconstructive Surgery* 127:313–320.

Brown OE, Myer CM, Manning SC. 1989. Congenital nasal pyriform aperture stenosis. *Laryngoscope* 99:86–91.

Calnan J. 1954. Submucous cleft palate. *British Journal Plastic Surgery* 6:264–282.

Caouette-Laberge L, Bayet B, Larocque Y. 1994. The Pierre Robin sequence: Review of 125 cases and evolution of treatment modalities. *Plastic Reconstructive Surgery* 93(5):934–942.

Chen H (ed). 2012. Crouzon syndrome. In: *Atlas of Genetic Diagnosis and Counseling*, Vol. 1. New York, Dordrecht, Heidelberg, London: Springer, pp. 529–535.

Cohen MM, Jr., Rollnick BR, Kaye CI. 1989. Oculoauriculovertebral spectrum: An updated critique. *Cleft Palate Journal* 26:276–286.

Coleman SR. 1997. Facial recontouring with lipostructure. *Clinical Plastic Surgery* 24:347–367.

Contencin P, Gumpert L, Sleiman J, Possel L, De Gaudemar I, Adamsbaum C. 1999. Nasal fossae dimensions in the neonate and young infant. *Archives of Otolaryngology Head and Neck Surgery* 125:777–781.

Costello BJ, Ruiz RL. 2004. Cleft lip and palate: Comprehensive treatment planning and primary repair. In: Miloro, M. (ed.), *Petersons Principles of Oral and Maxillofacial Surgery*. Toronto, Ontario, Canada: BC Decker Inc., pp. 839–858.

Devambez M, Alexis D, Pierre F. 2009. Congenital nasal pyriform aperture stenosis: Diagnosis and management. *The Cleft Palate-Craniofacial Journal* 46.3:262–267.

Douglas B. 1952. The relief of vestibular nasal obstruction by partial resection of the nasal process of the superior maxilla. *Plastic and Reconstructive Surgery* 9:42–51.

Esterberg ML, Ousley OY, Cubells JF, Walker EF. 2012. Prodromal and autistic symptoms in schizotypal personality disorder and 22q11.2 deletion syndrome. *Journal Abnormal Psychology* 122(1):238–249.

Evans KN, Sie KC, Hopper RA, Glass RP, Hing AV, Cunningham ML. 2011. Robin sequence: From diagnosis to development of an effective management plan. *Journal of Pediatrics* 127:936–948.

Franscechetti A, Klein D. 1949. The mandibulofacial dysostosis: A new hereditary syndrome. *Acta Ophthalmology* 27(2):143–224.

Friedman MA, Miletta N, Roe C, Wang D, Morrow BE, Kates WR, Higgins AM, Shprintzen RJ. 2011. Cleft Palate, retrognathia and congenital heart disease in velo-cardiofacial syndrome: A phenotype correlation study. *International Journal Pediatric Otorhinolaryngology* 75(9):1167–1172.

Furlow LT. 1986. Cleft palate repair by double opposing Z-plasty. *Plastic Reconstructive Surgery* 78:724–738.

Gennery AR. 2012. Immunological aspects of 22q11.2 deletion syndrome. *Cell Molecular Life Science* 69(1):17–27.

Gorlin RJ, Cohen MM, Jr., Hennekam RCM. 2001. *Syndromes of the Head and Neck*. Oxford, U.K.: Oxford University Press, 1344pp.

Grabb WC. 1965. The first and second branchial arch syndrome. *Plastic Reconstructive Surgery* 36(5):485–508.

Gray TL, Casey T, Selva D, Anderson PJ, David DJ. 2005. Ophthalmic sequelae of Crouzon syndrome. *Ophthalmology* 112(6):1129–1134.

Guimaraes CV, Donnelly LF, Shott SR, Amin RS, Kalra M. 2008. Relative rather than absolute macroglossia in patients with Down syndrome: Implications for treatment of obstructive sleep apnea. *Pediatric Radiology* 38(10):1062–1067.

Gundlach KK, Maus C. 2006. Epidemiological studies on the frequency of clefts in Europe and world-wide. *Journal Craniomaxillofacial Surgery* 34(Suppl. 2):1–2.

Heike CL, Hing AV. 2009. Craniofacial microsomia overview. In: Pagon, RA, Adam, MP, Bird, TD et al. (eds.), *GeneReviews*™ [*Internet*]. Seattle, WA: University of Washington, Seattle, 1993–2013.

Horgan JE, Padwa BL, LaBrie RA, Mulliken JB. 1995. OMENS-Plus: Analysis of craniofacial and extracraniofacial anomalies in hemifacial microsomia. *Cleft Palate Craniofacial Journal* 32(5):405–412.

Izumi K, Konczal LL, Mitchell AL, Jones MC. 2012. Underlying genetic diagnosis of Pierre Robin sequence: Retrospective chart review at two children's hospitals and a systematic literature review. *Journal of Pediatrics* 160:645–650.

Kaban LB, Padwa BL, Mulliken JB. 1998. Surgical correction of mandibular hypoplasia in hemifacial microsomia: The case for treatment in early childhood. *Journal Oral Maxillofacial Surgery* 56(5):628–638.

Katsanis SH, Jabs EW. 2004. Treacher Collins Syndrome. In: Pagon, RA, Adam, MP, Bird, TD, Dolan, CR, Fong, CT, and Stephens, K. (eds.), *GeneReviews*™ [*Internet*]. Seattle, WA: University of Washington, Seattle, 1993–2013.

Khong JJ, Anderson P, Gray TL, Hammerton M, Selva D, David D. 2006. Ophthalmic findings in apert syndrome prior to craniofacial surgery. *American Journal Ophthalmology* 142(2):328–330.

Khong JJ, Anderson PJ, Hammerton M, Roscioli T, Selva D, David DJ. 2007. Differential effects of FGFR2 mutation in ophthalmic findings in Apert syndrome. *Journal Craniofacial Surgery* 18(1):39–42.

Kriens O. 1970. Fundamental anatomic findings for an intravelar veloplasty. *Cleft Palate Journal* 7:27–36.

Leopold C, De Barros A, Cellier C, Drouin-Garraud V, Dehesdin D, Marie JP. 2011. Laryngeal abnormalities are frequent in the 22q11 deletion syndrome. *International Journal Pediatric Otorhinolaryngology* 76(1):36–40.

Markus AF, Delaire J, Smith WP. 1992. Facial balance in cleft lip and palate. I. Normal development and cleft palate. *British Journal Oral Maxillofacial Surgery* 30(5):287–295.

McCarthy JG, Warren SM, Bernstein J et al. 2011. Parameters of care for craniosynostosis. *Cleft Palate Craniofacial Journal* 49(Suppl):1S–24S.

Meazzini MC, Mazzoleni F, Gabriele C, Bozzetti A. 2005. Mandibular distraction osteogenesis in hemifacial microsomia: Long-term follow-up. *Journal of Craniomaxillofacial Surgery* 33(6):370–376.

Meyer AC, Lidsky ME, Sampson DE, Lander TA, Liu M, Sidman JD. 2008. Airway interventions in children with Pierre Robin sequence. *Otolaryngology Head Neck Surgery* 138(6):782–787.

Molina, F. 2009. Mandibular distraction osteogenesis: A clinical experience of the last 17 years. *Journal of Craniofacial Surgery* 20(Suppl. 2):1794–1800.

Parker SE, Mai CT, Canfield MA et al. 2010. Updated National Birth Prevalence Estimates for Selected Birth Defects in the United States, 2004–2006. *Birth Defects Research Part A* 88:1008–1016.

Posnick JC. 2000. *Hemifacial Microsomia: Evaluation and Treatment. Craniofacial and Maxillofacial Surgery in Children and Young Adults.* Philadelphia, PA: WB Saunders.

Posnick JC, Ruiz RL. 2000. Treacher collins syndrome: Current evaluation, treatment, and future directions. *The Cleft Palate-Craniofacial Journal* 37(5):434–434.

Randall P, Krogman WM, Jahina S. 1965. Pierre Robin and the syndrome that bears his name. *Cleft Palate Journal* 36:237–246.

Raulo Y, Tessier P. 1981. Mandibulo-facial dysostosis: Analysis; principles of surgery. *Scandinavian Journal of Plastic Reconstructive Surgery* 15:251–256.

Robin P. 1923. A drop of the base of the tongue considered as a new cause of nasopharyngeal respiratory impairment. *Academy National Medicine Paris* 89:37–41.

Robin P. 1994. A fall of the base of the tongue considered as a new cause of nasopharyngeal respiratory impairment: Pierre Robin sequence, a translation, 1923. *Plastic Reconstructive Surgery* 93(6):1301–1303.

Rollnick BR, Kaye CI. 1983. Hemifacial microsomia and variants: Pedigree data. *American Journal of Medical Genetics* 15(2):233–253.

Saal HM. 2002. Classification and description of nonsyndromic clefts. In: Wyszynski, DF (ed.), *Cleft Lip and Palate: From Origin to Treatment*, New York: Oxford University Press, pp. 47–52.

Sanlaville D, Verloes A. 2007. CHARGE syndrome: An update. *European Journal of Human Genetics* 15(4):389–399.

Shott SR. 2006. Down syndrome: Common otolaryngologic manifestations. *American Journal of Medical Genetics Part C* 142C(3):131–140.

Sommerlad BC. 2003. A technique for cleft palate repair. *Plastic Reconstructive Surgery* 112(6):1542–1548.

Spritz RA. 2001. The genetics and epigenetics of orofacial clefts. *Current Opinion in Pediatrics* 13:556–560.

Tolarova MM, Cervenka J. 1998. Classification and birth prevalence of orofacial clefts. *American Journal of Medical Genetics* 75:126–137.

Tortora C, Meazzini MC, Garattini G, Brusati R. 2008. Prevalence of abnormalities in dental structure, position, and eruption pattern in a population of unilateral and bilateral cleft lip and palate patients. *The Cleft Palate-Craniofacial Journal* 45(2):154–162.

Treacher-Collins E. 1900. Case with symmetrical congenital notches in the outer part of each lower lid and defective development of the malar bone. *Transactions of the Ophthalmology Surgery* (20):190.

Turvey TA, Ruiz RL, Tiwana PS. 2008. Bone graft construction of the cleft maxilla and palate. In: Losee, JE (ed.), *Comprehensive Cleft Care*, McGraw-Hill, pp. 837–865.

van den Elzen AP, Semmekrot BA, Bongers EM, Huygen PL, Marres HA. 2001. Diagnosis and treatment of the Pierre Robin sequence: Results of a retrospective clinical study and review of the literature. *European Journal of Pediatrics* 160(1):47–53.

Veau V, Borel S. 1937. *Division palatine: Anatomie—Chirurgie phonétique. By Victor Veau, Chirurgien de l'Hôpital des Enfants assistés*. Paris, France: Masson et Cie.

Verloes A. 2005. Updated diagnostic criteria for CHARGE syndrome: A proposal. *American Journal Medical Genetics Part A* 133A(3):306–308.

Vissers LE, van Ravenswaaij CM, Admiraal R et al. 2004. Mutations in a new member of the chromodomain gene family cause CHARGE syndrome. *National Genetics* 36(9):955–957.

Von Langenbeck B. 1861. Operation der angeborenen totalen spaltung des harten gaumens nach einer neuen methode. *Dtsch Klin* 8:231.

Zentner GE, Layman WS, Martin DM, Scacheri PC. 2010. Molecular and phenotypic aspects of CHD7 mutation in CHARGE syndrome. *American Journal Medical Genetics Part A* 152A(3):674–686.

Index